INTERVENTIONAL
RADIOLOGY

INTERVENTIONAL
RADIOLOGY
A SURVIVAL GUIDE

Fourth Edition

David Kessel MB BS MA MRCP FRCR EBIR
Formerly Honorary Clinical Associate Professor
University of Leeds
Leeds, UK

Iain Robertson MB ChB MRCP FRCR
Consultant Radiologist
Gartnavel General Hospital
Glasgow, UK

With a contribution by:
Des Alcorn, MBCHB, FRCS (Glasgow), FRCR
Consultant Radiologist
Department of Radiology
Gartnavel General Hospital
Glasgow, UK

ELSEVIER

ELSEVIER

ISBN: 978-0-7020-6730-3
E-ISBN: 978-0-7020-6888-1

Executive Content Strategist: Michael Houston
Content Development Specialist: Joanne Scott
Senior Project Manager: Beula Christopher
Senior Designer: Miles Hitchen
Illustration Manager: Karen Giacomucci
Illustrator: Marie Dean
Marketing Manager: Rachael Pignotti

your source for books, journals and multimedia in the health sciences

www.elsevierhealth.com

 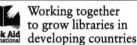

Working together to grow libraries in developing countries

www.elsevier.com • www.bookaid.org

Contents

Section 1: Core Interventional Skills

Section 2: Essential Equipment

Section 3: Principles of Intervention

Section 4: Intervention

Preface

Writing books is a lot like many of the practical tasks in Interventional Radiology. After the rush of excitement for the first few attempts you might be slightly less enthusiastic next time but you sure are a lot more experienced in what works and what doesn't! This is our fourth edition of *Interventional Radiology: A Survival Guide* and we are starting to get the hang of it (both writing books and Interventional Radiology).

Our aim remains for this to be the 'go to' book for the practical techniques of Interventional Radiology, written in a friendly, if sometimes slightly sardonic, style. (We each blame the other for that sardonic bit creeping in.) We share your pain. We have learned the lessons of successful procedures either by watching them unravel at our own hands or even worse, trying to retrieve a procedure which someone else has unravelled for you. The experience in this book cannot replace having a friendly experienced colleague standing nearby and cheering you on but we try to get as close as possible.

The way we interact with knowledge has changed. When we started the survival guide, all our attention spans were so much longer that readers actually started books from the front and, reasonably, often read all the way to the end. Can you imagine that? Now we all tend to dip in and out of knowledge sources – it's a miracle you've read this far in the preface alone!

To reflect these changes, the book has undergone a major rewrite, making it much more accessible and easier to dip in and out of. We have improved the format to include sections on essential equipment, and a principles section, which provide the foundations of Interventional Radiology. Many of the sections have been expanded to reflect the growth in Interventional Radiology. In particular, we have included much more on Interventional Oncology and we are hugely indebted to Dr Des Alcorn for his help and guidance with the sections on tumour ablation.

As always, we feel that having finished writing the fourth edition of the survival guide, we now understand much more about Interventional Radiology and hope that you will feel the same after reading it.

Abbreviations

AAA	abdominal aortic aneurysm	**MIP**	maximum intensity projection
AV	atrioventricular	**MPDSA**	multiposition DSA
CCA	common carotid artery	**MRA**	magnetic resonance angiography
CCF	congestive cardiac failure		
CECT	contrast-enhanced computed tomography	**MRI**	magnetic resonance imaging
		NSAID	non-steroidal anti-inflammatory drug
CE-MRA	contrast-enhanced MRA		
CFA	common femoral artery	**PA**	popliteal artery
CFV	common femoral vein	**PE**	pulmonary embolism
CIA	common iliac artery	**PFA**	profunda femoris artery
CTA	computed tomography angiography	**PIG**	peroral image-guided gastrostomy
CVA	cerebrovascular accident	**PTC**	percutaneous transhepatic cholangiography
DSA	digital subtraction angiography		
DVT	deep vein thrombosis	**PVA**	polyvinyl alcohol
EIA	external iliac artery	**RAO**	right anterior oblique
ERCP	endoscopic retrograde cholangiopancreatography	**RAS**	renal artery stenosis
		RHV	right hepatic vein
EVAR	endovascular aneurysm repair	**RIG**	radiologically inserted gastrostomy
FBC	full blood count		
FFP	fresh frozen plasma	**RIJV**	right internal jugular vein
FNA	fine-needle aspiration	**RPV**	right portal vein
FNAC	fine-needle aspiration cytology	**rt-PA**	recombinant tissue plasminogen activator
fps	frames per second		
GTN	glyceryl trinitrate	**RVEDP**	right ventricular end-diastolic pressure
IADSA	intra-arterial digital subtraction angiography		
		SFA	superficial femoral artery
IJV	internal jugular vein	**STD**	sodium tetradecyl sulphate
IM	intramuscular	**SVCO**	superior vena cava obstruction
IMA	inferior mesenteric artery	**SVT**	supraventricular tachycardia
IV	intravenous	**TIPS**	transjugular intrahepatic portosystemic shunt
IVC	inferior vena cava		
LAO	left anterior oblique	**TJB**	transjugular liver biopsy
LGA	left gastric artery	**TN**	tibial nerve
		TOS	thoracic outlet syndrome

Section One

Core interventional skills

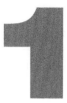

Planning safe procedures

Making the correct treatment plan

This chapter focuses on steps you should take to minimize risk and prepare yourself and the patient for successful and safe procedures. You may be tempted to skip past to get to the action and give this section little more than a perfunctory glance. Do so at your own peril, every patient has the right to expect that they will receive timely and correct treatment and that an appropriately skilled practitioner will perform their procedure. The adage 'Proper Planning Prevents Poor Performance' applies in interventional radiology and heeding it will help you maximize your chances of achieving a successful outcome for the patient. Before rushing off, needle in hand, stop and ask yourself the following questions:

- Does the patient really need/want an intervention?
- Have you and the patient considered and understood the pros and cons of the alternative treatment options?
- Is the proposed procedure the most appropriate in the clinical situation?
- Does the patient understand what is in store and the potential risks and benefits?
- Do you and the patient have similar and realistic expectations for the outcome?
- Are you and the team prepared for all eventualities?

If you are unsure or have answered no, then seek advice and make sure that you document your discussions with colleagues and the patient. It is always better and safer to delay or cancel a procedure than to rush headlong into the wrong option.

Preparing for successful and safe procedures

There are three distinct aspects to consider when preparing for procedures, these relate to:

- The patient
- The team who will perform the procedure
- The environment before, during and after the procedure, including recovery and destination ward.

These must be addressed in advance of every procedure in the outpatient department, at multidisciplinary team meetings, on the ward, in discussion with clinicians and members of the radiology team. The amount of planning will vary with the complexity of the procedure and the needs of the individual patient but clear documentation is mandatory at each stage.

Patient preparation

The key elements required to ensure that patients are properly prepared for a procedure are **evaluation** and **information**. Each assumes that you understand the procedure yourself.

Evaluation

The focus of evaluation is the identification of factors which may increase the risk of the procedure. Complex procedures should be discussed at multidisciplinary team meetings where all the different therapeutic options can be considered.

Screening tests Routine investigation (blood testing and electrocardiogram [ECG]) of all patients is unnecessary and merely increases the cost of patient care. In deciding whom to screen, consider the 'invasiveness' of the planned procedure and the likelihood of detecting an abnormality which would affect patient management. There is little evidence on which to base management, except in the case of prevention of contrast-induced nephropathy. The guidelines below are suggestions for screening and are not absolute; if in doubt, it is better to perform a non-invasive test.

Evaluation of renal function is indicated when the patient:

- Has a history of renal dysfunction
- Has a disease likely to impair renal function, e.g. hypertension, especially with peripheral vascular disease
- Is diabetic and has not had recent evaluation of renal function
- Has heart failure
- Is receiving nephrotoxic drugs.

Clotting studies are indicated when the patient:

- Has clinical evidence of a coagulopathy
- Has a disease likely to affect clotting, e.g. liver disease; therefore, it is unwise to perform a liver biopsy without knowing the coagulation status
- Is receiving medication that affects coagulation, e.g. heparin, warfarin or other anticoagulant or antiplatelet agents.

Platelet count is indicated in conditions that affect blood cell production or consumption, e.g. leukaemia, hypersplenism and cancer chemotherapy.

- Full blood count (FBC) is obtained in the context of bleeding but is less important than physiological status.

Alarm: Remember numbers may be misleading, e.g.:
- Haemoglobin can be normal for several hours after acute haemorrhage.
- Platelet number may be normal but function may be abnormal, particularly in patients on dual antiplatelet agents.

ECG is indicated when the patient:

- Has a history of cardiac disease
- Is to undergo a procedure likely to affect cardiac output or cause arrhythmia, e.g. cardiac catheterization.

Information

In order to decide whether to undergo treatment, patients need a basic understanding of their condition and how likely the proposed intervention is to alleviate symptoms or improve prognosis. They also need to understand the therapeutic alternatives and the relative risks and benefits of each approach to managing their condition. Expect patients to have researched their condition on the internet; your job is to help them to make sense of the bewildering mixture of fact and fiction they have found. For all but the most basic procedures it is best to see the patient in advance, either on the ward or in an outpatient clinic.

Be straightforward and honest about your ability and experience and do not be afraid to allow a patient the opportunity to seek a second opinion. Patients will respect this and it is the least you would expect from someone treating you.

Informed consent Patients have a right to be given sufficient information to make informed decisions about the 'investigation/treatment' (these terms will be used synonymously) options available to them. Your role is to provide relevant information in a way that they can comprehend. The laws regarding informed consent vary from country to country; these guidelines are based on the current situation in the UK but the ethos is broadly applicable.

Recent case law in the UK has changed the focus of consent to consider what the 'prudent patient' would be likely to want to know. This means that patients should be warned of 'material risks' associated with a procedure, even if they are uncommon. For instance, acute limb ischaemia is a recognized complication of peripheral arterial angioplasty; this may require surgery to restore flow and could conceivably lead to amputation or even result in death. Although uncommon, these risks must be mentioned and the likelihood of these events occurring must be put into perspective. In the UK at least, this has significant ramifications for consent.

Material risk In practical terms, a 'material risk' is anything that a 'reasonable person' in the patient's position would be likely to consider important. This includes the common and serious side-effects (and their management) of the proposed procedure. It also encompasses anything that the doctor would presume to be important to the individual patient. For instance, ischaemia of a fingertip would be expected to have particular relevance to a concert pianist, as it would potentially result in a loss of livelihood.

 Alarm: When considering 'material risk' ask yourself what you would want to know before agreeing to treatment. You should comment when the treatment is complex, unfamiliar or involves significant risk for the patient's health, employment, or social or personal life. Document the key elements of any explanation and record any other wishes that the patient has in relation to the proposed treatment.

Consent issues A qualified doctor who understands the risks and side-effects of the procedure should be responsible for obtaining consent for treatment. Usually the doctor performing the treatment is in the best position to provide this information. If this is not practicable, the doctor may delegate to an appropriately experienced colleague. You must provide a balanced explanation of the treatment and alternative management options along with the risks and benefits of each. Include things a prudent patient might want to know, such as:

- The general nature and purpose of the proposed treatment, including analgesia, sedation and aftercare
- Are there alternative therapeutic options? This might include doing nothing, optimizing medical therapy, surgery or other interventional approaches
- Information about those performing the procedure including:
  - The name of the doctor with overall responsibility for the patient
  - Names of the relevant members of the doctor's team, e.g. anaesthetist and surgeon
  - The experience of the operator/team with the procedure.
- What are the 'material risks' of the procedure and how common are they?

- Realistic expectations of the outcomes of the procedure, e.g.
  - What is the likelihood of the procedure being a technical success?
  - Will this have the clinically desired effect?
  - Is the treatment a cure?
  - What is the likelihood of recurrence?
- Will this treatment strategy impact on their future management?

The form of the explanation and the amount of information provided vary depending on the patient's wishes, their capacity to understand and the nature and complexity of the treatment. The patient should be allowed time to consider the information and must not be pressurized to make a decision. The patient must be told that they can change their mind or seek a second opinion at any time without prejudicing the care.

Review the patient's decision close to the time of treatment. This is mandatory when:

- Significant time has elapsed since consent was obtained. Many consent forms have a section to allow reaffirmation of consent.
- There have been changes that may affect the treatment strategy or outcomes.
- Someone else has obtained consent.

 Alarm: Compliance is not the same as consent! The patient's presence in the interventional suite does not indicate that the patient knows what the treatment entails. Documenting and checking the consent avoids misunderstanding and is the best defence in the event of litigation.

Special circumstances There are instances in which it is difficult or impossible to obtain informed consent. There are some general guidelines for what is acceptable procedure. If there is any doubt, legal advice should be obtained either from the hospital administration department or your medical indemnity provider.

Emergencies When consent cannot be obtained, you may only provide whatever medical treatment is necessary to save life or prevent significant deterioration in the patient's condition.

Capacity to make decisions This is the ability to understand and retain information for long enough to evaluate it and make a decision.

Inability to comprehend Seemingly irrational decisions and refusal of treatment are not evidence of a lack of capacity. Take time and review whether the patient has been provided with sufficient information or has not fully understood any of the explanation. Where doubt exists, seek advice; there is guidance for the formal assessment of capacity.

Fluctuating capacity When the patient's mental state varies and the decision can wait, consent should be obtained during periods of lucidity. This should be reviewed at intervals and recorded in the patient's notes.

In the UK, no one can give or withhold consent of treatment on behalf of a mentally incapacitated patient unless they have been legally authorized to do so. Try to establish whether the patient has previously indicated a preference, e.g. in an advance decision. If the patient complies, you may carry out any treatment that is judged to be in the patient's best interest. In these circumstances, it is prudent to seek a second opinion and for this to be documented in the patient record.

Children At the age of 16, the patient should be treated as an adult. Children below the age of 16 who are able to understand the nature, purpose and consequence of the procedure or its refusal have the capacity to make decisions regarding their treatment. In England, if a competent child refuses treatment, a person with parental authority or a court may give consent for any treatment in the child's best interest. Seek legal advice when doubt exists. A person with parental authority may authorize or refuse treatment for a child who is not competent to give consent. You are not bound by parental refusal; seek legal advice. In an emergency, proceed as above.

Managing high-risk patients

The role of interventional therapy is extending to some of the highest-risk patients, such as those with major bleeding from the gastrointestinal tract and secondary to trauma.

Risk management begins in advance of the procedure and starts by identifying which patients are at higher risk from the intervention (e.g. bleeding diathesis, allergy to contrast) and also whether they pose a risk to staff (e.g. infection control). It will also identify specific challenges such as the need for a hoist for a very heavy patient or a translator in case the patient speaks a different language.

In some cases, risk is evident from the nature of the procedure being undertaken. In other cases, it is necessary to seek out the relevant information from the patient, the referring clinicians or staff on the ward.

Most units will perform some form of screening for risk at the time of booking a procedure using a standard series of questions or proforma. This will identify the majority of the known conditions and risk factors. In addition to this, further checks should be performed once the patient is admitted to the hospital or day-case unit. This allows an additional opportunity to provide instructions for ward staff and the patient (e.g. the need for intravenous cannulation). If you use each of these opportunities and pay attention to detail few patients will cause surprises when they arrive for the procedure and your lists are more likely to go according to plan.

Having identified patients who are at increased risk, it is necessary to have strategies to manage them. Consider the risk in the context of the patient's condition. Clearly, there is a balance of risk; the risks of the procedure should be minimized, but the patient's wellbeing is paramount. You may be advised that 'the patient is too unstable to bring to radiology' but, for a patient with life-threatening haemorrhage, the time to stopping bleeding is key and there is seldom logic in delaying a potentially life-saving procedure! This section aims to help you keep the risk to the patient and to yourself as small as possible.

This list is not comprehensive, so pause to consider before every individual case and never hesitate to seek advice.

The patient's general condition

American Society of Anesthesiologists (ASA) status classification system

Anaesthetists will often quote ASA scores to you (see: http://www.asahq.org/resources/clinical-information/asa-physical-status-classification-system). The grading allows a common understanding of a patient's pre-procedure physical condition. The ASA score should not be used for prognostic indication, as actual risk will be affected by other factors such as age, body mass index, type of procedure, anaesthetic technique and operator experience.

In practice you need assistance with ASA IV patients (life-threatening condition), and ASA V (will not survive without intervention) patients require immediate attention!

The patient has a history of anaphylactic reaction to intravascular contrast This is fully discussed in Chapter 3. Consider alternative imaging strategies such as duplex ultrasound and magnetic resonance angiography (MRA), or another contrast agent such as gadolinium or carbon dioxide (CO_2).

The patient is anticoagulated or has a severe bleeding diathesis. The risk relates to the nature of the procedure; simple drainage and venous puncture are safer than arterial puncture or core biopsy. The risk of haematoma following angiography increases when the platelet count is 100×10^9/L. For surgery and invasive procedures, the platelet count should be $\geq 50 \times 10^9$/L.

Evaluate each case on its own clinical merit, consider postponing elective procedures to allow investigation and correction of the coagulopathy. Only intervene to correct the clotting if the procedure is urgent.

 Tip: Abnormal clotting is relevant mainly when the time comes to obtain haemostasis. Consider using a closure device (Ch. 37). Alternatively, leave a sheath in the artery until the clotting is corrected. An arterial line may be helpful for patients in the intensive therapy unit.

Diabetes Diabetic patients are at particular risk because of:

- The protean manifestations of diabetes, especially cardiovascular and renal disease
- Potential problems with diabetic control in the peri-procedural period.

Non-insulin-dependent diabetic patients The risks of lactic acidosis in patients taking metformin appear to have been exaggerated. The current UK recommendation from the Royal College of Radiologists (https://www.rcr.ac.uk/sites/default/files/Intravasc_contrast_web.pdf) has recently been revised. Guidance now states that renal function should be known; if the creatinine is normal or the estimated glomerular filtration rate (e-GFR) is >60 mL/min per 1.73 m² then metformin can be continued. If the creatinine is elevated or the e-GFR is <60 mL/min per 1.73 m² then the decision to continue or stop metformin for 48 h following contrast should be taken in conjunction with the referring team. Stopping metformin is not without risk and some patients will need to take insulin to control their diabetes over this period. In general, metformin should not be restarted until stable renal function has been confirmed 48 h after the procedure.

Insulin-dependent diabetic patients There are various regimens in practice and your hospital will have its preferred strategy. The following are simple principles that can be applied to most insulin-dependent diabetic patients:

- Avoid prolonged fasting
- If possible, schedule their procedure early in the morning. In this case they should take their long-acting insulin as usual but omit the short-acting insulin.
- If the procedure is later in the day, leave out the short-acting insulin and halve the dose of the long-acting insulin.
- A 5% dextrose solution should be infused to provide 5–10 g/h of glucose; this will usually maintain the blood glucose in the range 6–11 mmol/L.

 Tip: Ask the patient if they recognize when they are becoming hypoglycaemic. If they do, tell them to advise you if they develop symptoms. If not, then check the blood sugar periodically during the procedure.

 Alarm: Hypoglycaemia is more important than transient hyperglycaemia. Sweating, confusion and anxiety can all indicate significant hypoglycaemia. It is seldom unsafe to give the patient dextrose.

Renal impairment Chronic kidney disease (CKD) is common in very sick patients, the elderly and those with peripheral vascular disease. Roughly 50% of renal function has been lost by the time the creatinine rises above the normal limit. Estimated glomerular filtration rate (eGFR) is a better indicator of renal function. If the creatinine is elevated or the eGFR is <60 mL/min per 1.73 m^2 renal function is abnormal. Patients with CKD are at particular risk of developing contrast-induced acute kidney injury (CI-AKI). This is defined as a rise in an absolute rise creatinine of 0.3 mg/dL or 26 μmol/L or a 1.5 × increase within 48 h. In practice, if the patient is under 70 years old with no history of cardiovascular disease or renal dysfunction, the risk will be low, but ideally the e-GFR should be known for all patients undergoing elective procedures. Although few patients will require dialysis as a result of CI-AKI, prevention is better than cure. **The most important factor in protecting renal function is ensuring adequate hydration using normal saline.** If intravascular iodinated contrast is essential then non-ionic isosmolar agents probably minimize the risk. There is no evidence that any other pharmacological regimens reduce the incidence of contrast-induced acute kidney injury.

Alarm: eGFR is calculated using data including age, race and sex of the patient. If your laboratory does not provide eGFR reports, you can calculate it using online calculators (e.g. http://egfrcalc.renal.org).

1. **Is this the most appropriate investigation?** Consider using alternative tests (MRA, Doppler, CO_2). Remember that there is a risk of nephrogenic systemic sclerosis in patients given gadolinium-based contrast for magnetic resonance imaging (MRI) and non-contrast techniques should be considered, especially for angiography.
2. **Review medication. If possible consider stopping:**
   - Non-steroidal anti-inflammatory drugs (NSAIDs)
   - Angiotensin-converting enzyme inhibitors (ACE-Is) and angiotensin II receptor blockers unless there is severe heart failure
   - Metformin (stop for 48 h and restart if creatinine stable).
   Avoid loop diuretics if possible.
3. Act according to the severity of the CKD (based on e-GFR) and involve a nephrologist early:
   - **Stage 1 and 2 CKD, minimal risk e-GFR >60 (Cr <120)**
     Ensure hydration Oral fluids 1 L pre- and post-procedure
   - **Stage 3a and 3b, low risk e-GFR 30–59 (Cr 120–180)**
     Inpatient: Non-ionic contrast, IV normal saline 1 mL/kg per hour, 12 h pre- and post-procedure
     Outpatient: Iso-osmolar contrast (iodixanol). Encourage oral fluids 1 L pre- and post-procedure, if possible IV normal saline started on arrival 1 L over 4 h.
   - **Stage 4, intermediate risk e-GFR <30 (Cr >180 or renal transplant)**
     If possible admit for procedure: iso-osmolar contrast IV normal saline 1 mL/kg per h (caution if congestive cardiac failure [CCF]) 12 h pre- and post-procedure N-acetylcysteine 600 mg PO (two doses pre- and post-procedure).
   - **Stage 5, high risk, CrCl <15**
     Admit for procedure; as above. Repeat Cr at 7 days.
   - **Avoid further contrast exposure for 72 h if possible.**
4. Other risk factors, e.g. diabetes mellitus, multiple myeloma, CCF, cirrhosis: consider promoting to the next level of CKD.

Tip: Hydration – in the presence of CCF or cirrhosis with ascites, use 5% dextrose instead of saline.

Hypertension Hypertension is common and is exacerbated by anxiety and pain. Hypertension increases the risk of haematoma. Review the ward charts to check the normal baseline blood pressure (BP). The Society of Cardiovascular and Interventional Radiology (SCVIR) standards define uncontrolled hypertension as a diastolic pressure >100 mmHg. Systolic hypertension is present when the systolic pressure is >180 mmHg.

Controlling high blood pressure starts on the ward. The patient should take any antihypertensive medication (except loop diuretics) as normal. If they remain hypertensive in the angiography suite, they can be given 10 mg of nifedipine. Sedation and analgesia may also help blood pressure control. Aim to reduce the mean blood pressure by no more than 25%.

 Tip: If the blood pressure cannot be controlled by these simple measures, postpone elective cases until the patient is appropriately medicated on the ward.

Heart failure The patient's condition should be optimized before angiography. Diuretics should be avoided if possible to minimize the risk of nephrotoxicity. Limit the study to the essential details. If necessary, breathless patients can often sit up slightly; this can be compensated for by craniocaudal angulation of the C-arm. Give oxygen as necessary.

Gastric contents It is normal to fast patients before invasive procedures but the risk of aspiration of gastric contents is very small except in sedated patients. General guidelines are shown in Table 1.1. These are mandatory before conscious sedation or anaesthesia and advisable before other cases.

Table 1.1 General guidelines for fasting time before invasive procedures

Oral intake	Fasting time (h)
Solids and non-clear liquids	6–8
Clear liquids	2–3

In urgent cases, seek anaesthetic advice, avoid sedation and consider metoclopramide to promote gastric emptying, H_2 antagonists or proton pump inhibitors to increase gastric pH and antiemetics to minimize the risk of vomiting.

Patients with dementia, anxiety and agitation It is not safe to embark on an invasive procedure in a patient who cannot cooperate due to significant confusion or agitation. These patients may require sedation or general anaesthesia to allow the procedure to be performed successfully. Patients with anxiety will respond to sedation, those with dementia rarely do and in this case, general anaesthesia is usually the safest option for both the patient and staff. Consent issues are also relevant in this group of patients (see above).

Pre-procedure safety check

Formal and clearly documented safety checks and briefings are mandatory and essential if you want to reduce predictable and preventable errors during procedures. It has been clearly demonstrated that safety checks performed immediately before and after every surgical operation reduce patient morbidity regardless of the environment. The surgical safety checklist has been adopted worldwide and similar checks should be used in interventional radiology.

This chapter builds on the ethos of the surgical safety check and suggests reviewing complex elective cases in advance of the day of the procedure in addition to further formal reviews at the start and end of every day.

Advance planning

There are two separate aspects to advance planning: administrative and personal preparation.

Administrative preparation

This is usually the role of the radiographic or nursing staff. There should be a screening process aimed at identifying risk factors such as anticoagulation in advance of the procedure. The aim of this process is to avoid surprises on the day and thus prevent delays or cancellation. Screening is often carried out through a telephone checklist review with the patient or with their source ward. Once risk factors are identified, appropriate planning and mitigation should take place, e.g. converting a patient on warfarin to heparin or scheduling diabetic patients first on the list.

Personal preparation

It is always worth reviewing the imaging and mentally rehearsing the procedure. This is particularly true of more complex interventions and is mandatory for cases that require equipment which is not routinely stocked. This one habit prevents a lot of delay and disappointment and pre-rehearsal generates the opportunity to discuss cases where there is any uncertainty regarding the choice of treatment, how best to perform it and to consider potential problems and endpoints.

Advance review checklist

Always decide what you are aiming to achieve. Ask yourself the following questions, the answers will be useful when consenting the patient and carrying out the pre-procedure team briefing:

- Is this the correct procedure for this patient at this time? If there is any doubt, it is time to verify the clinical situation with the referring team; if there is still uncertainty, then discuss the case with your boss.
- What are the key steps and sequences in the procedure? Make sure you have a clear plan and know how to use the necessary equipment.
- What is the likelihood of the procedure having the desired technical and clinical outcome? Make sure that the patient and the referring team understand the limitations of the procedure, especially in cases where the clinical benefit is uncertain.
- What are the possible treatment strategies and which is most likely to succeed and least likely to cause harm?
- Does the case require specific equipment? If so, is it in stock or does it need to be ordered?
- What problems are likely to be encountered? Think about what you will do if there is a problem or you are not successful. You should always have a 'Plan B' and, if necessary, little plans C, D and E.
- Might you stop before your objective is reached? It is often better to 'live to fight another day' rather than ploughing on in a spiral of failure, especially if this might have an adverse clinical outcome for the patient – you did remember to warn them about this and document the discussion in the patient record didn't you?

Finally, ask yourself the ME question: would I be happy to have someone with my skill and experience undertake this procedure on me? If the answer is yes, then go ahead but if the answer is no, then either reschedule the patient on a more appropriate list or make sure that you have appropriate assistance from a colleague.

On the day: staff, equipment and room preparation

It is essential to review how the list will run and requirements for individual cases. There is no hard and fast way to do this as long as all of the key aspects are covered.

Daily safety check

Before the list begins Representatives from each of the teams who will be involved (radiologist, nursing, radiography, anaesthesia, surgery, etc.) should review all of the planned cases as a group. Some centres will choose to include a review of individual case management at this time.

It is the responsibility of these staff to disseminate important information to other members of their teams. The meeting should not take place in the absence of essential staff. One individual is responsible for recording the attendance and discussion and ensuring that the daily safety check is recorded in the radiology information system.

The purpose of this check is to:

- Review and agree the order of cases
- Consider complex or high-risk patients – this will include a review of your advance planning
- Consider risks to staff and other patients, such as infection control issues
- Verify that all required equipment is available.

The meeting should not take more than a few minutes assuming everyone has prepared.

Individual patient safety checks

The elements of the safety check are included in Table 2.1 and your institution will have its own version. What follows is intended to explain the ethos that lies behind the checks. If you understand this, you will be able to lead the team effectively through the process.

Table 2.1 Checklist for typical interventional cases

Task	Person responsible	Elements
Pre-procedure case review	Doctor	Review intended procedure: site, side, approach, etc.
	Nurse	Need for sedation, analgesia, anaesthesia
	Radiographer	Monitoring
		Anticipated equipment including patient-specific items, e.g. stent graft, chemoembolization
		Emergency equipment
		Potential difficulties
		Additional equipment, e.g. ultrasound machine
		Important elements of procedure
		Set of room: C-arm position, trolleys, etc.
Pre-procedure checklist	Nurse	Patient ID
		Patient notes
		Allergies/drug reactions
		Pre-procedure test results normal or inform doctor
		Intravenous access
		Hydration
		Premedication
		Antibiotic prophylaxis within previous 60 min
		Analgesia/sedation
		Check correct equipment available
		Bail out kit (covered stents, etc.)
	Doctor	Consent
		Medication required is prescribed
	Radiographer	Request available
		Imaging available
Post-procedure check	Doctor	Operative sheet completed showing procedure, outcomes, complications, aftercare
		Communication with patient, relatives and other carers
		Planned review stated
	Nurse	Sharps disposed safely
		Patient charts completed including prescribed drugs, monitoring
		Specimens labelled and handled correctly
		Handover to ward staff including instructions for aftercare/analgesia
		Patient given information sheets/instructions for care/contact numbers
	Radiographer	Images reviewed with doctor
		Images archived

Before starting

The team who will perform the case should convene and go through a safety checklist, this should be recorded on the radiology information system and a copy filed in the patient record. How you conduct the safety check is up to your team and it does not really matter so long as everyone takes it seriously and all the bases are covered.

If you use a white board to manage the list you can always call upon your artistic skills and draw a schematic overview of the case and list equipment and drugs. The key elements of the check are as follows.

Introductions Ensure that everyone knows each other. This is particularly important when working with another team from, e.g. intensive care staff coming to the interventional suite, or you are in an unfamiliar environment, e.g. when working in the operating theatre.

Patient identification and consent check Verify that the patient has been identified using appropriate two- or three-step checks (name, date of birth and address) and that there is a valid signed consent form.

Procedure plan Make sure that everyone knows the plan for the procedure, its steps and any anticipated difficult elements. Include patient positioning, the approach, site to be treated and the equipment you intend to use. Confirm that medications and blood products have been prescribed/administered/are available if required.

Equipment check Ensure the team has checked that all the anticipated and 'bale out' kit is available and in the room and that you are informed of anything missing or in short supply (e.g. balloons, stents, embolization coils).

Explanations If the case is complex, who will ensure that everyone knows their roles and responsibilities, e.g. patient monitoring, running nurse, scrub nurse? Pick your strongest team and ensure that the most appropriate individual is in each role.

Final confirmation Ask if anyone has any questions and check that everyone is happy to proceed.

Post-procedure check and aftercare

It is always tempting to think that once you have performed your technical wizardry your work is done. Unfortunately, this is not the case and now is the time for the less glamorous, but still important, aspects of the job.

As soon as the procedure is over, the post-procedure checklist (Table 2.1) should be completed, this can be completed by someone else while you obtain haemostasis, or even better, completed by you while someone you trained pushes on the groin. Following this is the time to sit down (in the UK with a cup of tea) and make an operative record. This should include technical details of the procedure and any implants. It is important to document complications, even if they have been resolved. It is good practice to keep a copy of the operative record on the radiology information system for future reference.

As well as the operative note, it is important to make sure that there is an adequate handover of care to the receiving ward and clinical team. Unlike the safety check, there is no particular ethos required and the individual elements to consider are set out below. It is essential that the person who actually hands over care to ward staff is aware of the key facts and also where you have your notes for handover.

- Will the patient require any special care or analgesia after the procedure?
- Have you handed over care to an appropriate colleague?
- Do the ward nurses require special orders for observations and patient monitoring?
- Do drains or lines need particular care or management?
- If there are potentially predictable problems what precautions are necessary and what actions should be taken if they occur?
- Who should be notified if there is a problem and how are they to be contacted?
- Will you be visiting to review the patient?
- When can the patient be discharged; has a discharge letter been provided and any medications prescribed?
- Is an outpatient appointment necessary, when and with whom?

A particular form of handover is communication with the patient/carer after an outpatient or day-case procedure. It is best to provide written instructions, especially if the patient has received sedation. Make sure that the patient/carer knows who to contact and how to contact them in the event of an emergency.

Table 2.1 indicates the typical elements that should be considered for almost every procedure.

 Tip: Fail to plan, plan to fail. Planning helps you and your staff to ensure procedures are performed safely and smoothly, with the minimum of stress for all concerned!

Contrast

Most vascular computed tomography (CT) and magnetic imaging resonance (MRI), the vast majority of angiographic procedures, and many nonvascular interventions rely on contrast media to reveal the anatomy. Contrast media can be broadly classified according to their use and also their chemical structure. X-ray contrast affects tissue X-ray attenuation, ultrasound contrast affects tissue and blood reflectivity and MRI contrast affects tissue relaxation times. The Royal College of Radiologists has issued pragmatic guidance on the use of intravascular contrast agents. Discussion in this chapter is confined to contrast media used for angiography and vascular diagnosis.

Intravascular X-ray contrast agents

The two principal categories of X-ray contrast both affect X-ray attenuation. Details of the chemical and physical properties of these agents are extensively discussed in many texts. It helps to be familiar with the different options and their indications, this will be most relevant in cases where there is kidney disease or a history of adverse reaction.

Positive contrast agents These are liquids containing iodine or gadolinium that have greater attenuation than the patient's soft tissues.

Negative contrast This has lower attenuation than the patient's tissues; at present, carbon dioxide gas is the only available option.

Basic principles for using intravascular contrast

Optimal demonstration of anatomy and pathology requires sufficient difference in attenuation between the target tissue and the surroundings, as well as X-ray equipment parameters, e.g. kV and mAs.

The aim is to adequately opacify the vessel but allow a level of grey-scale that allows branches/filling defects to be seen through the contrast. This requires the correct strength contrast in sufficient quantity (volume of contrast) delivered in the right place. If the contrast is too diluted, there will be insufficient change in attenuation, conversely too concentrated contrast can obscure lesions.

As a general principle, the contrast column should opacify the entire vessel segment. To achieve this, the total contrast dose and the duration of the bolus must be correct. Appropriate catheter positions, contrast volumes and flow rates are indicated throughout the diagnostic angiography sections. When the blood flow is slow, it may take several seconds for the opacified blood to pass through the vessel. Hence, a long contrast bolus is necessary. This is one of the reasons for increasing the volume of contrast to image the more distal vessels. Modern angiography equipment allows integration of multiple images, which has the same effect as increasing the length of the bolus, but it can reduce image quality due to minor degrees of patient movement between frames.

Iodinated contrast media

These are the most frequently used agents. Non-ionic contrast media are recommended in high-risk patients (see below).

Most diagnostic and therapeutic intervention is performed using '300 strength' contrast (300 mg/mL iodine). This density of contrast is fine for pump injections into large vessels where the contrast is diluted by rapid blood flow. For selective hand injections in the vascular system and for non-vascular examinations, 300 strength contrast is diluted with saline to 'two-thirds' or 'half strength'.

Contrast reactions with iodinated contrast media

There are two forms of contrast reaction: direct effects and idiosyncratic responses; these are more common in certain groups of patients and emphasis should be on identifying them, reducing risk and preventing reactions. Up to 2% of patients require treatment for adverse reactions to intravascular iodinated contrast agents. Fortunately, the majority of cases require only observation and minor supportive treatment. Less than 1% are severe but these require prompt recognition and immediate treatment.

 Alarm: Contrast reactions should be discussed during the consent procedure.

Direct effects Direct effects are secondary to the osmolality and direct chemotoxicity of the contrast, and they include heat, nausea and pain. More important are the effects on organ systems.

Renal Contrast-induced acute kidney injury (CI-AKI), defined as a rise in creatinine of 0.5–1 mg/dL or 44–88 μmol/L, is common and most likely in patients with chronic kidney disease. Strategies for preventing CI-AKI are discussed in Chapter 1.

Cardiac Cardiac problems are most likely to occur during coronary angiography and are usually manifest as arrhythmias or ischaemia. It is prudent to use non-ionic contrast in patients with ischaemic heart disease or heart failure.

Haematological Significant haematological interactions are uncommon. Non-ionic iodinated contrast can induce clotting if mixed with blood; hence, scrupulous attention to catheter flushing and avoidance of contaminating syringes with blood are essential.

Neurological Most neurological sequelae occur during carotid angiography and are related to angiographic technique. Genuine contrast-related problems are rare and are usually seen in patients with abnormalities in the blood–brain barrier.

Idiosyncratic reactions The mechanism of these reactions is uncertain; vasoactive agents such as histamine, serotonin, bradykinin and complement have been implicated but a causal role has not been established.

Idiosyncratic reactions are classified according to severity.

- **Minor:** Common, ~1:30, e.g. metallic taste, sensation of heat, mild nausea, sneezing; these do not require treatment.
- **Intermediate:** Common, ~1:100, e.g. urticaria; not life-threatening; these respond quickly to treatment.
- **Severe:** Rare, ~1:3000, e.g. circulatory collapse, arrhythmia, bronchospasm, dyspnoea; may be life-threatening; these require prompt therapy. Remember the A, B, C, D approach and do not hesitate to call for help.
- **Death:** Rare, ~1:40,000, mostly caused by cardiac arrhythmia, pulmonary oedema, respiratory arrest or convulsions.

Assessing the risk The risk of a contrast reaction varies depending on the circumstances of individual patients; however, the following are associated with an increased risk of a severe idiosyncratic reaction:

- Previous allergic reaction to iodine-containing contrast and shellfish allergy: 10×
- Cardiac disease: 5×
- Asthma: 5×
- General allergic responses: 3×
- Drugs: β-blockers, interleukin-2: 3×
- Age >50 years: 2× risk of death.

Remember that these factors increase the relative risk; the absolute risk remains very low.

Reducing the risk The vast majority of severe and fatal contrast reactions occur within 20 min of administration and therefore it is vital that patients are kept under constant supervision with a cannula in situ during this period. There have been a few isolated reports of delayed hypotensive reactions hours after contrast injection.

The ideal method of reducing risk is to avoid iodine-containing contrast examinations by using other imaging modalities, such as ultrasound or MRI. When this is not possible:

- **Prepare for reaction.** Ensure that resuscitation equipment and drugs are immediately available every time contrast is injected. Make sure that you are familiar with the management of the reaction; most catheter laboratories have charts on the wall to remind you in times of need (note: it is much less stressful to check it out in advance).
- **Use non-ionic contrast agents.** Non-ionic contrast agents certainly reduce the risk of minor reactions and may reduce the risk of more significant reactions.
- **Reassure the patient.** Explain that contrast reactions are unlikely and that the situation is under control. In severe anxiety, short-acting anxiolytic agents may be warranted.
- **Consider steroid pre-medication.** There is no conclusive evidence that oral steroid premedication reduces the risk of moderate–severe reactions but it pays to check whether your department has guidelines on steroid administration.

In the rare patient with a previously documented severe reaction:

1. Try to identify which agent was responsible (and make certain you do not use it again)!
2. Avoid iodinated contrast; use CO_2 or gadolinium or another imaging modality.
3. If this is impossible and the examination is essential:
   - If there is time, seek the opinion of an allergy specialist.
   - Ensure resuscitation personnel, equipment and drugs are immediately available. You may need expert assistance maintaining the airway, so consider enrolling anaesthetic assistance.
   - Monitor the patient carefully.
4. Use non-ionic contrast.

5. Consider steroid premedication in accordance with local guidelines.
6. Reassure the patient.

Treatment of contrast reactions

Warn patients that a sense of warmth, a metallic taste and transient nausea are all common after rapid IV injection of contrast and these effects wear off after a few minutes.

Minor reactions

- **Nausea and vomiting.** Active treatment rarely required. Reassure and monitor patient.
- **Urticaria.** One of the commonest contrast reactions. Localized patches of urticaria do not require treatment. Simply observe and monitor the patient (pulse, BP). Generalized urticaria or localized urticaria in sensitive areas, e.g. periorbital, should be treated by chlorphenamine 20 mg, given slowly by IV injection.
- **Vasovagal/syncope.** Monitor the patient's pulse, BP, oxygen saturation and ECG. Elevate the legs. Establish IV access. Give atropine 0.6–1.2 mg by IV injection for symptomatic bradycardia. Volume expansion with IV fluids for persistent hypotension. If hypotension persists, seek medical support.

Intermediate–severe reactions

Bronchospasm Monitor the patient's pulse, BP, oxygen saturation and ECG.

- Give 100% O_2.
- Treat initially with β-agonist inhaler, e.g. salbutamol.
- Give IV corticosteroids, e.g. 100 mg hydrocortisone. In acute reactions, steroids may work surprisingly quickly, although it can take a few hours for them to achieve full effect.

  If there is continuing bronchospasm seek assistance.

- Consider intramuscular epinephrine: 0.3–0.5 mL of 1:1000 solution.

Laryngeal oedema/angioneurotic oedema Seek anaesthetic assistance. Monitor the patient's pulse, BP, oxygen saturation and ECG. Give:

- 100% O_2 and watch the oxygen saturation closely.
- Chlorphenamine 20 mg by slow intravenous injection.

  Consider:

- Epinephrine intramuscularly (IM) 0.3–0.5 mL of 1:1000 solution.
- Get an anaesthetist to assess the airway. Tracheostomy may be required in severe cases.

Severe hypotension Call for support. Hypotension accompanied by tachycardia may indicate vasodilation and increased capillary permeability. Monitor the patient's pulse, BP, oxygen saturation and ECG.

 Alarm: Also consider other causes of hypotension related to the patient's underlying diagnosis or procedural complication e.g., bleeding or myocardial infarction.

- Rapid infusion of IV fluids is essential and several litres of fluid replacement may be necessary.
- Epinephrine IM 0.3–0.5 mL of 1:1000 solution. In the case of severe circulatory shut down IV epinephrine may be required. This is normally the preserve of expert anaesthetists/physicians but if the patient is severely shocked, consider epinephrine 1 mL (0.1 mg) 1:10000. This should be given with extreme caution by slow IV injection.

Cimetidine, the H$_2$ receptor antagonist, has been effective in severe reactions resistant to conventional therapy. The drug is given by slow IV infusion (cimetidine 300 mg in 20 mL saline). An H$_1$ receptor blocker, such as chlorphenamine, should be given first.

MRI contrast agents

Gadolinium

Gadolinium works well as an MRI contrast agent. Its use has been described in X-ray angiography but it is a poor X-ray contrast agent and is often difficult to see on fluoroscopy. Gadolinium is handled in the same way as conventional liquid contrast agents and can be injected by hand or with a dedicated injection pump.

There are many different gadolinium preparations and there is increasing interest in the use of 'blood pool agents' for magnetic resonance angiography (MRA). These have a longer dwell time in the circulation and this improves imaging in the venous phase.

Gadolinium-based agents are much more expensive than iodinated contrast, therefore their use is almost exclusively reserved for MRI and the occasional patient who needs a limited volume of contrast and has a genuine reason to avoid iodinated contrast, e.g. severe contrast reaction.

It is now recognized that gadolinium poses particular risks in patients with renal impairment. Gadolinium-based agents are nephrotoxic in their own right, especially when doses greater than 40 mL are used in MRA.

Nephrogenic systemic fibrosis (NSF)

NSF only occurs in the presence of impaired renal function. The following groups are most vulnerable:

- Patients with acute or chronic kidney disease. NSF has not been described in patients with GFR >60 mL/min per 1.7 m^2. This limits the utility of gadolinium-based agents for MRA and conventional angiography in patients with renal impairment
- Patients in the immediate postoperative period following liver transplant
- Neonates and infants
- Pregnant or breastfeeding women.

When a patient is deemed to be at high risk, there should be careful consideration whether an alternative test would be safer.

 Tip: If the patient requires angiography and you have a modern MR scanner, consider performing non-contrast MRA.

Those who require gadolinium contrast should be given the lowest diagnostic dose and a low-risk agent, e.g. a macrocyclic agent, such as gadoterate meglumine (Dotarem) should be used. Ideally, no further study should be performed within 7 days.

 Alarm: Informed consent should be obtained from high-risk patients requiring gadolinium-based contrast.

Negative contrast agents – carbon dioxide (CO$_2$)

Carbon dioxide angiography is exclusively performed as subtraction angiography (DSA) and additional software may be necessary to optimize the image. CO$_2$ dissolves rapidly in blood and is excreted through the lungs. Consider using CO_2 when there is a contraindication to conventional iodinated contrast and in a few circumstances where CO_2 is a superior contrast agent.

Carbon dioxide is most commonly used for the following reasons:

- History of severe reaction to iodinated contrast
- Renoprotection
- Where there is another advantage, such as the use of CO_2 for wedged hepatic venography.

 Alarm: There is a risk of cerebral toxicity with CO_2 and for this reason it should never be used intra-arterially above the diaphragm or intravenously in patients with right-to-left shunts.

Equipment

- Basic angiography set
- Medical-grade CO_2 from a disposable cylinder:
  - Reusable cylinders may be contaminated with water or rust particles; hence the need for a disposable system. The bacterial filter is a further safeguard. In an ideal world, one would use disposable stainless steel cylinders.
- Standard bacterial filter (from a blood-giving set)
- High-pressure connector
- Three-way tap
- Lockable stopcock for each syringe
- Sixty-mL Luer lock syringes.

The circuit is set up as shown in Figure 3.1.

 Alarm: The pressurized CO_2 must never be connected directly to the patient, as this risks inadvertent injection of a large volume of gas that may cause a 'vapour lock'.

Injecting CO₂

You can inject by hand or via a dedicated pump. CO_2 gas has very low viscosity and so is very readily injected even through small catheters. Injecting a colourless, odourless and invisible

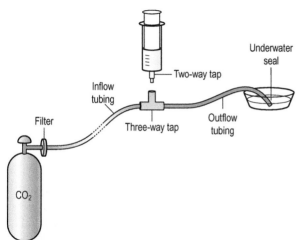

Fig. 3.1 Preparation of CO_2 for hand injection.

gas is disconcerting at first. It is essential to have a foolproof system for filling the syringes to prevent inadvertent air embolization.

Filling syringes with CO_2

Peripheral angiography typically requires a volume of around 50 mL CO_2 for each run, therefore use a 50-mL Luer lock syringe.

 Alarm: Never aspirate to fill the syringe, you might fill the syringe with air. Always allow the syringe to fill 'passively' under the pressure from the cylinder, this ensures that it can only fill with CO_2.

1. Allow a syringe to fill from the system.
2. Use the three-way tap to discard the contents three times to flush out any residual air in the system before finally filling.
3. Shut the lockable stopcock and disconnect the syringe from the three-way tap.
4. The syringe will now contain CO_2 at slightly above atmospheric pressure.

 Alarm: Avoid injecting air. Never aspirate to fill the syringe as air might be drawn into the system. The CO_2 in an open syringe will be replaced with air in about an hour! Always prepare CO_2 syringes just before use and keep the stopcock closed.

The catheter is flushed with saline as normal. As the filled syringe is connected to the catheter, the stopcock is opened; this has two functions:

- Air is flushed from the catheter hub
- The CO_2 in the syringe falls to atmospheric pressure and so the true volume of the gas is known.

The catheter is now gently flushed with CO_2; this expels the saline from the lumen. You will know when the catheter is flushed, as there is a marked fall in resistance. Close the tap and disconnect this syringe and discard its contents. Connect a fresh syringe of CO_2 and you are ready to inject. The volume and rate of injection are adjusted according to the size of the vessel, e.g. 50 mL for an aortic injection for peripheral angiography; 10–20 mL for an antegrade SFA injection. There is no dose limit as long as injections are restricted to 100 mL every 2 min.

If performing venography, always fluoroscope over the pulmonary artery to look for gas trapping.

Troubleshooting

Dependent vessels are not seen Intravascular CO_2 displaces blood rather than mixing with it like a liquid contrast. The CO_2 is buoyant and floats over the blood column; dependent branches tend not to fill and, in general, there is an underestimate of vessel size. If necessary, the patient can be turned to elevate the vessel of interest, e.g. side of interest up for renal angiography. C-arm angulation must be adjusted accordingly to compensate.

There is gas trapping The CO_2 collects above the blood and forms a 'vapour lock'. This reduces the surface area for the gas to dissolve. Potentially, this can lead to ischaemia or thrombosis. This is most likely to happen with large (>100 mL) injections of CO_2 or in capacious vessels with anterior branches, e.g. in an aortic aneurysm. If gas trapping occurs, simply turn or tilt the patient's head down so that the gas can disperse. If necessary, the gas can be aspirated via a catheter. Do not elevate the patient's head!

The gas column fragments This happens particularly in the distal vessels (Fig. 3.2). Use image summation techniques to integrate several frames onto the same image. Consider raising the leg, as this improves filling of the distal vessels.

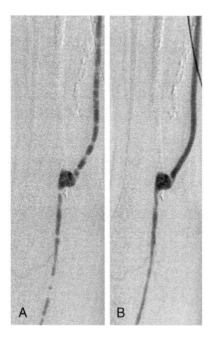

Fig. 3.2 ■ Gas fragmentation with CO$_2$ angiography. (A) Before multiple image summation. (B) After image summation.

The distal vessels cannot be seen CO$_2$ is a 'negative contrast' and not as good as conventional contrast media (otherwise we would use it all the time)! Sometimes bolus fragmentation and poor opacification require the use of a liquid contrast agent.

The patient experiences pain during injection. Try a slower injection rate.

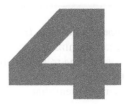

Sedation

Sedation is used to relax patients during procedures but does not relieve or prevent pain. Hence, sedation is often used in combination with analgesia. Sedation is useful in patients undergoing prolonged interventional procedures and can also be valuable in anxious or hypertensive patients.

Remember that sedation may result in respiratory depression and aspiration of gastric contents; in addition, there is a small but significant mortality. Children are at particular risk.

This chapter defines 'conscious sedation' and outlines patient selection and management within the radiology department. If you have any doubts about your ability to manage a particular patient, seek advice from an anaesthetist.

Conscious sedation

This refers to a controlled state of reduced consciousness throughout in which the patient retains the ability to make purposeful, verbal responses. Protective reflexes are preserved and the airway is maintained. Drugs used in conscious sedation should have a sufficient margin of safety to make unintended loss of consciousness unlikely.

 Alarm: If verbal responsiveness is lost, the patient requires a level of care identical to that needed for general anaesthesia and mandates anaesthetic assistance.

Deep sedation and anaesthesia These involve a further reduction in conscious level from which the patient is not readily roused and during which protective reflexes and the ability to maintain the airway may be lost, along with the ability to respond to physical and verbal stimulation. In terms of patient management, deep sedation should be regarded as a form of general anaesthesia.

 Alarm: Close clinical observation and monitoring are vital during conscious sedation; machines do not detect responsiveness. Someone must maintain verbal and tactile contact with the patient and assess the patient's mental state and alertness.

To sedate or not to sedate, that is the question

Practices differ widely between countries and cultures. Patient tolerance varies enormously; it is unnecessary to use sedation routinely. Try to establish whether sedation is likely to be required before starting the procedure. In this way, the patient can be properly assessed and risk minimized.

Take time to talk to the patient before, during and after the procedure and you will find that the majority of patients are not distressed if they are actively reassured and not in pain. Remind them that if they become anxious or distressed, sedation can be administered during the procedure. Consider sedation in the following circumstances:

- Prolonged procedures where the patient is likely to become uncomfortable
- Patients who remain very anxious despite explanation and reassurance
- Painful procedures. It is important not to equate sedation with analgesia, and if performing a painful procedure, give adequate analgesia. Remember that sedation and strong analgesia are synergistic, and take care
- Patients who are unlikely to cooperate, e.g. children. Now you have considered it, dismiss the idea – agitated or confused patients often become unmanageable following even light sedation. In these circumstances, you need anaesthetic support and general anaesthesia may be the safest option.

Sedation guidelines

- Assess the requirements and risks for each patient.
- Make sure the patient has IV access and pulse, BP and O_2 monitoring.
- Remember, benzodiazepines are more potent in patients >60 years: the dose should be reduced accordingly. Diazepam dosage is more predictable than midazolam in patients >70 years.
- Begin with a low dose and increase it as necessary. A large bolus is more likely to result in hypoxia (oxygen saturation <90%) and apnoea, e.g. use 1–2-mg aliquots of midazolam.
- Designated personnel should be responsible for monitoring the patient and maintaining records.
- Resuscitation equipment must be readily available and staff should be familiar with its use. It helps to have a designated staff member to respond in case of emergency.

 Alarm: Do not hesitate to seek anaesthetic assistance if you have any doubts about sedation; it is much better than having to deal with a problem during a case.

Patient selection

Most serious adverse events are not predictable and can occur in 'healthy' patients. Extremes of age and pre-existing cardiorespiratory disease and severe illness contribute to increased risk of sedation. Ask an anaesthetist to assess high-risk patients; a general anaesthetic may be safer for them than sedation. Do not forget that aspiration of gastric contents is associated with significant morbidity in patients who are not fasted.

Care and monitoring of sedated patients

Care It is essential that there are adequate numbers of trained staff and appropriate facilities to allow constant monitoring of the patient's condition. Radiologists often take responsibility for sedation; this is unsatisfactory during interventional procedures when your attention is focused elsewhere.

Monitoring A named member of staff is responsible for ensuring responsiveness and monitoring each patient. They must be capable of recognizing and managing important changes in the sedated patient's condition. Many of the complications caused by sedation can be avoided if the patient is closely and responsively observed during the procedure and in the recovery period. The following parameters should be monitored:

Pulse oximetry and respiratory rate Allows prompt recognition of hypoxia long before it is clinically obvious. Prompt action should be taken when the oxygen saturation falls below 95%. The patient should be encouraged to take some deep breaths and oxygen should be administered by mask or nasal cannulae. If this fails, try to establish an airway using the jaw thrust manoeuvre or a plastic airway. Seek assistance sooner rather than later.

 Tip: Give oxygen routinely to sedated patients; this saves an unseemly scuffle when the pulse oximeter alarm starts to ring.

Cardiac monitoring The ECG demonstrates heart rate and cardiac rhythms and detects signs of myocardial ischaemia. It is invaluable in the management of cardiac arrest and arrhythmia. It is not uncommon for you to hear a change in rate and rhythm before anyone else notices.

Pulse and blood pressure These are best monitored by an automatic device. Warn the patient that this is:

- Uncomfortable
- Normal practice and not a sign of impending problems.

   Most machines have alarms that can be set to respond to significant increases or falls in blood pressure. Record the pressure every 5 min and make additional recordings during procedures likely to affect the blood pressure. **NB Tachycardia and hypertension are usually the response to pain but may also reflect hypercapnea.**

 Alarm: Make sure that your staff notify you of any upward or downward trends in the record and warn them if you are going to do something likely to affect the values, e.g. give hyoscine butylbromide (Buscopan) or a vasodilator.

Aftercare

Remember that sedated patients require close observation until they are alert and oriented and able to drink. Inpatients may return to the ward as soon as they are stable enough to be cared for on the ward, but this varies considerably with the type of ward. Baseline observations should be stable for at least 1 h before discharge. Outpatients should not drive or operate machinery for 24 h and must be accompanied by a responsible adult. Clear instructions should be provided for the carer, detailing what to expect in the post-procedural period. State clearly who should be contacted (and how to contact them) in case of problems.

5

Pain control and analgesia

Pain control – forward planning

Many interventional radiology procedures do not require any analgesia; some procedures are intrinsically painful, especially if they are prolonged, and others are unpredictably uncomfortable. The procedure will be simpler and the patient less distressed if pain can be kept to a minimum; they will be even happier if pain can be avoided altogether. Preventing severe pain is likely to increase everyone's confidence in you! Remember pain and anxiety affect the patient pre-, peri- and post-procedure to a varying degree, so there is no 'one size fits all' solution. As always, forward planning is the key to success; recognize which procedures and which particular stages are likely to require analgesia.

If a procedure is predicted to be painful, e.g. uterine artery embolization:
- Explain this to the patient in advance and reassure them that this is normal and that effective pain control will be provided.
- Prophylactic analgesia should be given to minimize/prevent it. Combinations of non-steroidal and opiate analgesics are often used.
- Prescribe appropriate medication before starting (e.g. analgesic, antiemetic, sedative).
- Have someone check regularly whether the pain control is effective. Give additional analgesia and pain control as necessary. Patient-controlled analgesia (PCA) is useful here.
- Suitable analgesia should be prescribed for the post-procedural period.

 Tip: If you anticipate giving intravenous drugs on several occasions during a procedure, attach a low-pressure connector to the venous access and locate it in an easily accessible position. This means you will not have to interrupt the procedure while someone rummages around under the drapes trying to find a cannula each time a drug is given. Remember that a saline flush is needed or the drug will just sit in the tubing!

If a patient experiences unexpected pain during or after a procedure
- Establish what is causing the pain and what can be done to resolve it, e.g. stress-related angina may respond to the usual glyceryl trinitrate spray.
- Treat pain swiftly and effectively. This is not the time for oral paracetamol (acetaminophen); **intravenous opiate analgesics** are the order of the day, so remember to ensure that venous access is obtained in advance.

If a procedure is likely to have painful consequences
- Plan for this in advance by prescribing a suitable analgesic regimen. This is particularly important following embolization.
- Review the patient to ensure that clinical evolution is satisfactory.

You should become familiar with the regimens and preparations in use at your institution. Remember that the actions of sedatives and analgesics are often synergistic (antidotes to reverse the effects of both are available). Anaesthetists are expert at managing pain and should be consulted if there is any doubt regarding appropriate medication or the need for adjunctive procedures such as epidural or spinal anaesthesia.

Some typical regimens

Pre-procedure medication for painful procedures, especially those likely to induce inflammation, e.g. embolization of solid organs.

Non-steroidal anti-inflammatory drugs (NSAIDs), e.g.:
- Intravenous (IV) paracetamol 1 g
- Per rectum (PR) diclofenac 25–50 mg.

Opiate analgesics, e.g.:
- Morphine 1–5 mg is estimated according to patient size (e.g. little old lady, 1 mg).
- Fentanyl (Sublimaze) usually given in 20–40 µg aliquots. Fentanyl has faster onset and shorter duration of action and is almost 100× more potent than morphine.
- **Caution:** Start with a low dose and increase as necessary. Elderly patients are often very sensitive to the sedating properties of these drugs. Opiates and sedatives have a synergistic effect.
- **Consider concomitant antiemetic therapy.** Cyclizine (50 mg), ondansetron (4 mg), metoclopramide (10 mg), are all effective.
- **Monitor.** Pulse, BP and oxygen saturation.
- **Reversal.** Naloxone 100–200 mg (1.5–3 mg/kg) by IV injection. If the response is inadequate, give increments of 100 mg every 2 min. Repeat as necessary.

Patient-controlled analgesia

PCA is an important weapon in your armamentarium; in essence, following an initial loading dose, the patient self-medicates whenever they feel pain. To prevent overdose, there is typically a 'lockout period' of 5–10 min, during which the patient cannot administer further drug.

PCA can be set up simply to give dosage on demand or to give a background infusion dose, which can be supplemented on demand (Table 5.1). Many hospitals will have a standard prescription chart for PCA.

During a procedure a suitably trained member of staff should regularly assess the patient to gauge the effectiveness of pain control and to administer further analgesia in accordance with your local protocol.

Table 5.1 Patient-controlled analgesia (PCA) dosage table

Drug	Loading dose	Background infusion dose/h	Patient-administered dose	Lockout time (min)
Fentanyl (µg)	10–50	0–10	5–20	3–10
Morphine (mg)	1.0–2.5	0.2–0.4	0.2–0.4	5–15

After a procedure there is a tendency for interventional radiologists to forget this component of patient care or to devolve it to others who may not be familiar with the needs of patients post-intervention. Post-procedure pain control is essential. Make sure that the patient will be cared for on a ward that is appropriately staffed and equipped to monitor and manage the patient.

Drugs on discharge

If a patient has required opiate analgesia during a procedure, then PCA may be continued overnight. When patients have been treated on an outpatient, day-case or overnight stay basis, then an oral opiate analgesic such as oxycodone hydrochloride is prescribed to take, on discharge. This is normally taken in conjunction with an NSAID agent such as diclofenac (25–50 mg, 8–12-hourly). Oxycodone is very useful when there is moderately severe pain, for example following uterine artery embolization. A suitable dose is 25–50 mg every 6 h. When prescribing opiate analgesia to take home, a maximum of 3 days' supply is provided, the patient should be advised who to contact if pain is not controlled or if significant pain persists longer than this.

 Tip: It is prudent to review any patient in whom pain does not settle in the expected timeframe, in case of complications.

Recognition and management of complications

Oh dear, we are still in the introductory section and already complications are rearing their ugly heads. One thing is certain, during a career in interventional radiology, there will be cases which do not follow the script. There are of course many things that can and do go wrong. Your job is to:

- Minimize predictable/preventable errors
- Recognize problems as early as possible
- Limit damage to the minimum
- Call for assistance in a timely fashion
- Learn from the experience.

An earlier section dealt with patient preparation and pre-procedure checklists; these are key to avoiding preventable errors. The remainder of this section deals with complications that arise in the course of a procedure. As the manifestations of complications are protean, it is helpful to have some form of classification to help recognize them.

Complications

Specific to a procedure

You need to be familiar with the predictable complications of a procedure, how they are likely to manifest and how they are managed; reviewing these should be part of your advance planning. Specific complications will be considered in the relevant sections.

Predictable complications range from the minor, such as a small bruise, to serious, life-threatening emergencies, which are difficult to manage. Many of these complications will feature as 'material risks' during discussions about the procedure and should be documented as part of the consent process.

What is clear is that it would be negligent not to rapidly diagnose and begin to manage a recognized complication. A good example is iliac rupture during angioplasty. There are typically clear symptoms and signs and there is a straightforward management algorithm to be followed to minimize the impact. When treated promptly, iliac rupture can usually be managed with relatively little clinical impact. Conversely, failure to recognize the problem and initiate treatment can lead to death.

 Alarm: It is your responsibility to be familiar with the recognized complications of a procedure and to be able to initiate an appropriate immediate response while seeking assistance.

Related to drugs used during a procedure

The majority of these complications are predictable from the pharmacology of the agent, sometimes in conjunction with patient comorbidities. Among the commonest are those related to sedation, analgesia and anticoagulation. It is essential to know how to reverse these agents. Contrast reactions are also a form of 'drug reaction' and it is important to be able to treat these promptly.

 Tip: Patients with renal failure will accumulate opiates and peak toxicity may occur after a delay of several hours. Consider alternatives for pain relief.

Related to the patient's underlying condition

These complications can often be anticipated with a knowledge of the underlying disease. We will commonly work with patients who have generalized vascular disease – it is important to remember that the same process affecting the leg vessels may well be evident in the coronary or cerebral circulation, e.g. a patient with peripheral arterial disease having a myocardial infarction during an intervention. Probably the most important complications to consider are those related to diabetes mellitus, in particular hypoglycaemia, as this can be fatal if not rapidly recognized and treated.

Sometimes the procedure is the direct cause of the complication, e.g. precipitation of a carcinoid crisis during therapeutic embolization of carcinoid liver metastases. These 'predictable' complications are particularly relevant, as they can sometimes be prevented, for instance by pre-treating the carcinoid patient with octreotide.

Unpredictable complications

These complications are the most difficult and require you to be able to think on your feet. It is important to stay calm and make a clinical assessment and then to consider appropriate first aid measures as well as more definitive treatment.

Seeking assistance

The key to management of complications is to recognize them as early as possible. Common sense, knowledge of pathology, pharmacology and the risks of the procedure will point you in the direction of the correct diagnosis in the majority of cases. You should not spend a long time trying to work out what has gone wrong, as this can lose valuable time managing the situation before it escalates. When you know something is wrong but cannot figure out exactly what, is the right time to call for help.

Equally, if you recognize that you have a major complication, such as rupture of an iliac artery during angioplasty, it is much better to call the vascular surgical team to the interventional suite early. The worst that can happen is that you tell them they are not required because you were able to place a stent graft and have used a closure device to seal the arterial puncture. Conversely, if you delay calling them until the patient is in shock and the anaesthetist shakes their head and announces American Society of Anesthesiologists (ASA) grade 4, you will not win any friends.

 Alarm: Call for help when you are uncertain what is happening or unsure how best to respond or if you have a major potentially life-threatening complication. It is never wrong to call for assistance or a second opinion.

Post-procedure debrief

Members of the team may be upset when a complication has occurred. Complications should be discussed at the end of the procedure. Remember to do this with sensitivity, a public forum is not the time or place to attribute individual blame. However, if there are significant performance issues, then these must be addressed through the correct channels. You may need to seek advice on how to do this. If there is a malfunction of consumable equipment, keep hold of the packaging and any components that remain and store these safely. If there is a problem with the imaging equipment, ensure this is documented and rectified before recommencing.

Discussion with patients

In the UK, doctors have a 'duty of candour' to patients. This simply means providing an honest and straightforward account of any complication that has occurred. At this stage, stick to the material facts, i.e. a complication has occurred and the immediate implications and any change in management this entails. Indicate that you will discuss this and any longer-term implications at a later time and in a more suitable environment, e.g. on the ward.

This discussion is not an admission of liability. However, the discussion should take place even if you are aware, or suspect, that you may be at fault for a complication. In these circumstances, you should seek advice from senior colleagues and may need to inform your employer and indemnity provider before discussing this with the patient.

Documentation of complications

Important complications must be documented in the operative record and in the patient's case records. You must include explanations to the patient, relatives and clinical colleagues.

Learning from complications

Remember an old aphorism, *'those who don't learn from their mistakes are destined to repeat them'*. So, whenever you have a complication, make sure that you reflect on the causes and the management. Work out what went well and why it was successful and remember to do that again. Equally, think about aspects that could have been managed better and think what you would do differently on a future occasion. It often helps to review the case with a supportive senior colleague. This type of informal debrief should focus on learning from the event and providing support. Some incidents will be categorized as serious adverse events and undergo local investigation; try to approach such investigations as openly as possible.

It is always better to learn from the mistakes of others rather than your own. Every Interventional Radiology unit should have a structured Morbidity and Mortality (M&M) meeting. Errors are rarely due to one factor and a systematic analysis in the M&M meeting is invaluable in developing shared learning and improving outcomes.

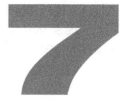

The interventional radiology clinic

Outpatient clinics are an essential component of contemporary practice. Some interventional radiologists have held outpatient clinics for many years but for others, this will be a new experience. The functions of the clinic should simply be extensions of various aspects of daily practice. The challenge of the clinic is to deliver this in time-limited encounters. Broadly speaking, the roles of the clinic can be understood as shown below.

The roles of the clinic

Establish what the patient expects

You should ask the patient what they understand about why they have been referred to you and perform a quick reality check that this corresponds with why you think you are seeing them. If there is a mismatch, then the first priority should be to try to rectify this.

Confirm the diagnosis

This requires you to have reviewed all of the information provided, including the referral document, patient records and also the imaging. Try to look at the imaging yourself rather than just relying on the reports.

In many instances, the diagnosis will be certain and it will be evident how this relates to the patient's symptoms. However, this is not always true, sometimes information from the referring team will be unclear or perhaps even incorrect. If there is doubt then obtain further history and perform clinical or perhaps even ultrasound examination as part of the clinic assessment. When there is uncertainty you will need to communicate this to the patient.

 Tip: A useful strategy is to spend a few minutes reviewing the clinical request, the patient record and relevant imaging before bringing the patient into the clinic. This way, there will be fewer surprises during the consultation.

Confirm symptomatology

Remember that symptoms may have changed in the interval between referral and the patient seeing you, e.g. claudication may have resolved following successful exercise therapy. Always make sure you verify the current symptomatology and any impact on the patient's life and work.

Discuss with the patient their concerns, wishes and expectations

Doctors have a tendency to assume that they understand a patient's concerns and that they will be similar to their own. This is often incorrect, so ask the patient what they are worried about. Many patients with peripheral vascular disease are very concerned that it will lead to amputation and relatively untroubled by their claudication or their walking distance. In this case, they should be reassured and placed on best medical therapy rather than reaching for angioplasty balloons and stents.

Find out what the patient wishes to know about their condition and what they hope to achieve from treatment. Do not be surprised to find that some patients are incredibly well-informed and you may even learn from them. Expect to be asked to explain the prognosis of the condition in the context of a variety of treatments.

Patient expectations vary widely from the very modest to highly demanding. It is essential to deal with any 'expectation gap' by providing clear and realistic explanations regarding what can be achieved and the limitations of treatment.

Provide realistic information

Interventional procedures

This will often be the principal focus of the clinic and builds on the discussions above. As a minimum you should be able to discuss the following questions:

- Whether the treatment is feasible for this patient?
- Whether it will be inpatient or outpatient?
- Will it be painful during or afterwards? (e.g. uterine artery embolization)
- The likelihood of technical success?
- The likelihood of symptom relief?
- Whether the treatment is curative or palliative?
- Whether the treatment is a 'one off' or whether a series of treatments may be necessary?
- How quickly symptoms will resolve and the likelihood of recurrence of symptoms/the disease?
- Whether the treatment can be repeated?
- The 'material risks' of the procedure (see consent), i.e. anything that any prudent patient would want to know and anything that this particular patient would be expected to want to know.
- How long it takes to recover after the treatment?
- The place of this treatment compared with alternative treatments?
- Whether this treatment will impact on other therapies?

Alternative therapeutic strategies

In many cases, there will be a number of therapeutic options, ranging from doing nothing at all through to major surgery. There will be pros and cons to each approach. Remember that you are there to help the patient work out which is best for them and not to promote interventional radiological treatments above other strategies. In fact, once you start considering the individual patient, you may find that interventional radiology is not the answer.

The consultation presents a lot of information and it is impossible for the patient to remember everything. Your clinic may come with a supply of printed information sheets; if not, you can either arrange to send them out later with a summary of the discussion or direct them towards websites with the relevant information.

Obtain consent

It is best practice to obtain consent in advance of the procedure. This is especially important for complex procedures where there is a lot of information for the patient to consider. Consent can be obtained in the outpatient clinic or alternatively in a dedicated 'consent clinic'. Just remember that the person obtaining consent must be trained to do this.

Book appointments for treatment

The commonest question after a long discussion of the pros and cons of treatment is often 'How long will I have to wait?' Some clinics may allow direct booking of appointments. Alternatively, give the patient an indication of the likely waiting time. Enquire whether the patient is able to attend at short notice if there is a cancellation. Find out if there are any times the patient will not be available, e.g. booked holidays.

Patient follow-up after intervention

One of the joys of being a doctor is seeing patients after successful treatments and reviewing their progress. The news is not always good, so be prepared to hear that the symptoms did not improve or recurred rapidly, this is particularly common following angioplasty for claudication. It is also good to review patients in whom there were complications to see how these are resolving.

Clinic records

Make accurate records and make sure that you send letters to the patient's referring team and general practitioner (GP). Consider either copying the correspondence to the patient or sending them a separate summary of the key points discussed and additional information. This is particularly useful if the patient was going to consider whether they wished to proceed with a particular treatment.

Further review

Sometimes you will find that it is impossible to cover everything in the allotted clinic time. Quite often the patient will indicate that they would like a family member, friend or carer to attend, to consider the information. In either case, consider offering the patient a longer appointment at a later date. Patients will usually appreciate this option and it beats running impossibly late.

Clinics running behind schedule

Everyone is familiar with this; either the administrators book patients ludicrously short appointments or you will find several patients arrive at once. If you are running late, you risk being left with a waiting room full of increasingly irritated patients. You know exactly how this feels from personal experience in a clinic or when your flight is delayed. If you are running behind, it pays to let any patients who are waiting know what is happening and when they can expect to be seen. Sometimes a patient will not be able to stay, in which case apologize and offer an early repeat appointment at the start of the list. On occasion a patient will be implacable and in this case you should continue apologizing and explain how they can make a complaint.

Discharge from the clinic

There comes a time when there is little value in repeat appointments. Usually it is fairly obvious that you have fulfilled all of the above roles. When a patient is discharged you should always indicate that you will be happy to review them again if the circumstances change, e.g. if symptoms recur or if they decide that they desire treatment in the future. Do not forget to inform the referring team and GP what is happening.

Section Two

Essential equipment

Essential equipment: Puncture needles

Purpose

Puncture needles are vital for getting from the skin to the target as a prelude to access with a guidewire, aspiration of fluid or placement of a drain. Not all needles are equal and you need to know what to request.

Description

One-part, two-part, sheathed

One-part needles have a cutting bevel (think needles used for taking blood or injecting local anaesthetic). These are commonly used as a prelude to passage of a guidewire into a vessel. **Two-part** needles have an outer shaft and inner stylet, which extends up to or beyond the tip of the outer shaft. **Sheathed** needles feature a plastic outer sheath; this usually stays in place after the needle is removed (think intravenous cannula), the needle component may be one- or two-part.

Usually, one-part needles are used for simple access procedures, such as arterial puncture during angiography. Two-part systems are commonly used for deeper punctures, especially when using smaller-calibre needles.

Most needles have Luer lock hubs to allow attachment to a connecting tube. Some needles' hubs have wings to aid manoeuvrability.

 Tip: One-part needles have a sharp cutting bevel – do not swivel it side-to-side when looking for the vessel – you can tear the vessel wall.

Measurements

Puncture needles are usually described by their outer diameter, e.g. 21G (gauge)/18G. Sizing is counterintuitive, the larger the number, the smaller the needle. The 21G is the smallest in most IR departments. The inner diameter of a needle depends on the gauge and wall thickness but, in general, the higher the gauge the smaller the lumen and a 21G will only take a 0.018-inch wire.

Needles also vary in length. Generally, they have been getting longer as the population gets wider. It is certainly worth thinking about needle length, especially for deeper procedures, such as nephrostomy.

 Tip: If in doubt, perform an ultrasound to assess depth of the target and choose a long enough needle.

Know what to ask for

Angiography Vascular procedures nearly always start with a 19G single-part needle; this allows passage of a standard 0.035-inch guidewire. Standard needles are generally about 7 cm long but you may require a longer needle, particularly for antegrade puncture in the larger patient.

Many non-vascular procedures will use a sheathed needle system; these are usually a bit bigger, e.g. 16G.

If faced with a difficult puncture, then a smaller initial needle is often the best option. These are the least traumatic way to hit a target (or the innocent bystanders) and cause less deflection of the target wall. They are most often chosen when the target is small, the risk of bleeding is high or the structure is under low pressure, e.g. venous puncture. The most obvious advantage is that these create a smaller hole in case repeat puncture is required.

The downsides of using a smaller-gauge needle are:

- They are much less rigid and more difficult to steer after a significant part of the needle is in the track.
- You will have to start with a 0.018-inch guidewire. These are harder to manipulate and more prone to kinking during passage of dilators.

Access kits, such as the vascular mini access set or Neff/AccuStick, are designed to simplify conversion from a 0.018-inch wire to take a 0.035-inch wire (see Ch. 10).

Know how to use it

Location, location, location Plan your approach to the target and take time to get the patient and the guidance in the best position. Large needles tend to follow the planned trajectory, while smaller-calibre needles are flexible and it is less easy to change direction once you have started down the tract.

If at first you don't succeed, pull the needle back along the tract stopping short of the skin and then re-direct. Try not to aspirate until the target is reached, as it risks drawing soft tissue/ blood into the needle and blocking it.

Essential equipment: Biopsy needles

Purpose

The ideal biopsy needle provides a diagnostic tissue sample at the lowest possible risk.

Description

Needles are usually characterised by their mechanism of action into aspiration and core biopsy needles.

Aspiration needles

Purpose

To safely provide a sample of a few cells for cytological, biochemical and microbiological analysis. Cytology can be enough to confirm malignancy but doesn't give any "architectural" information.

Description

Most aspiration samples are taken with standard 21 G needles or spinal/ Chiba needles.

Measurements

Length (cm)

Gauge: from 20-25G Most aspiration samples are taken with standard 21 G needles or spinal/ Chiba needles. Simply choose a suitable size and length to reach your target. There are more specialised cutting needles available for aspiration that probably appear more often in textbooks than departmental shelves but are certainly worth considering if an initial aspiration gives scant cellular tissue (Fig. 9.1).

A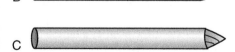

B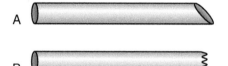

C

Fig. 9.1 Biopsy needles. (A) Conventional Chiba needle. (B) 'Crown'-type needle with serrated edge. (C) Stylet-type needle with serrated tip.

Know how to use it

The needle is placed into the lesion under imaging guidance and then attached to a 20-mL syringe. Draw a full vacuum on the syringe while the needle is passed back and forward through the lesion (Fig. 9.2). If you have an assistant, use a connecting tube or a 21G butterfly needle and get the assistant to aspirate the syringe while you manipulate the needle under guidance.

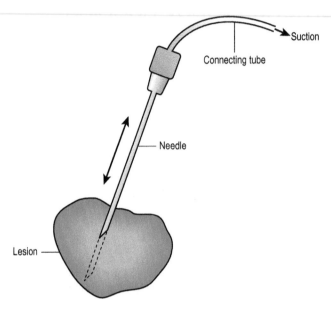

Fig. 9.2 Aspiration technique. The needle is passed into the lesion under ultrasound control. A connecting tube and 20-mL syringe are attached to the needle. Draw a full vacuum on the syringe and then pass the needle back and forward through the lesion. Slowly release the vacuum as the needle is withdrawn or the tiny sample will disappear into the syringe.

Tip: Maintain gentle suction whilst withdrawing the needle, then remove the syringe. Vigorous suction results in the tiny sample being lost in the syringe; without suction, the sample stays in the patient.

Place the sampling needle onto a slide and gently eject the needle contents onto the slide with an air-filled syringe. Also put any fluid in the sampling syringe onto a slide. Specimens may be simply air-dried but specimen preparation varies from centre to centre; check the preference of your cytologist. Specimens only contain a few cells and therefore it is best to make at least two passes.

Cutting biopsy needles

Purpose

Obtains a larger specimen for histological analysis.

Description

The cutting needle consists of two parts: an outer cutting shaft and an inner stylet (Fig. 9.3). There are a variety of devices but most centres use automated devices, which rely on a spring loaded mechanism to automatically fire the outer cutting needle at the push of a button. Manual biopsy needles operate in the same way but are less reliable and slower. Remember

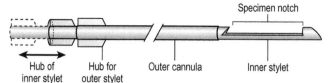

Fig. 9.3 ■ Construction of a cutting biopsy needle. Tissue prolapses into the specimen notch and is cut by advancement of the outer cutting needle shaft.

for some of the designs, the needle advances when fired to take the specimen from 1-2cm beyond the firing position. The needles are always single use but the mechanism may be disposable or reusable. It is very important to understand if you have a static or forward throw device in your hand.

Measurements

Needle length (cm): make sure your needle is long enough to reach the target.

Tip: Choose the shortest length of biopsy needle that will reach the target. Particularly in computed tomography (CT), needles that are too long flop about during repeat scanning and are more likely to get accidentally pushed in too far.

Specimen length: this is typically 10-20mm and is governed by how far the inner stylet advances. Longer needle throws tend to result in more reliable specimens. Consider a shorter needle throw when performing a biopsy close to important structures.

Gauge: Core biopsy needles vary from 14G- 20G in size, 18G are the most commonly used and yields a core of approximately 1mm diameter.

Know what to ask for

It's all about the individual patient situation and using the safest device possible. If you are confirming metastatic disease from a known primary or sampling in tricky areas eg through bowel then aspiration will probably do the trick. Start with the shortest standard needle. If that fails then it might be worth hunting through the department for one of those fancier cutting needles. If you are trying to confirm the cell type for a new primary lesion, diagnose lymphoma or preserve architecture eg for a diagnosis of cirrhosis then a core biopsy will be likely to be more successful. Histologists do vary in the size of sample that keeps them happy but in principle always use the smallest core needle possible.

Know how to use it

Individual biopsy needles vary and we can't list them all. Get familiar with the devices in the department before starting the procedure- it's not good for a patient to see you read the instructions for use. It's even less good, if you fail to get the biopsy because you didn't use the device properly. Advice on hitting the target is given in the section in hitting the target (Ch25 imaging guidance).

The following general principles apply:

The needle is advanced under imaging guidance to the edge of the target (Fig. 9.4a). Once in position the central stylet is advanced into the lesion (Fig. 9.4b) followed by the outer sleeve (Fig. 9.4c). There are two principal mechanisms of action which differ in how the central stylet is advanced:

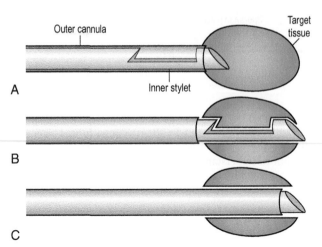

Fig. 9.4 ▇ Mechanism of action of a cutting needle. (A) Needle is advanced to the edge of the target tissue. (B) Inner stylet is advanced into the target tissue. (C) Outer cutting shaft is advanced to re-sheath inner stylet and cut the specimen core.

Semi-automatic: This is typified by the Temno needle. In this device, the inner stylet is manually advanced into the target. At this stage, resistance is felt and further pressure on the trigger mechanism fires the outer sleeve to cut the core. Manual needles also work in this way but the outer sleeve is advanced manually whilst holding the stylet in position. Important points to note are:

- the precise position of the core is ascertained before the biopsy is taken; this is particularly important in proximity to hazardous areas
- it is an integral system. There is no handle to attach and detach, but it remains relatively small and light. This is an important consideration for CT biopsy, where the patient must be rescanned to confirm needle position.

Fully automatic: This is most commonly used type of system. The needle tip is advanced to lie at the proximal edge of the area to be biopsied. At the push of the button both the inner stylet and then, almost instantaneously, the outer cutting shaft rapidly advance, taking the biopsy. Some automated systems now allow the operator to select between these two different modes on the same disposable device. Other systems allow the operator to determine the length of the specimen, i.e. the forward throw of the needle – very useful if the biopsy is close to a vital structure.

- The core is obtained 10-20mm ahead of the needle tip when it is fired.

Some automated systems now allow the operator to select between these two different modes on the same disposable device. Other systems allow the operator to determine the length of the specimen, i.e. the forward throw of the needle – very useful if the biopsy is close to a vital structure. Make sure you familiarize yourself with the systems in your hospital and get the best out of the devices.

Alarm: Remember that with a fully automatic system, the biopsy is taken from the tissue 10–20 mm in front of the needle tip, depending on the size of the specimen notch.

10

Essential equipment: Access kits

Purpose

An access kit allows the least traumatic (i.e. smallest) initial needle puncture of the target and provides a method to convert the 22G puncture to standard 0.035-inch guidewire access.

Description

A typical set comprises:

- A one- or two-part 22G needle for the initial puncture
- A short 0.018-inch guidewire with flexible tip and supportive shaft
- An interlocked dilator system. This varies from kit to kit. Those for hepatic and renal work often come with a metal stiffening cannula in addition to a coaxial inner dilator with a tapering tip inserted through a larger outer dilator, which will accept a 0.035/0.038-inch guidewire.

 Tip: Remember to remove the inner dilator to allow insertion of the 0.035-inch wire.

Know what to ask for

Vascular access sets

Mini-access set This set is usually used for vascular access and has an inner 3F dilator and an outer 4F dilator. This permits introduction of the 0.035-inch wire.

Pedal access kit This is very similar but has been specifically designed to help access the smallest of vessels. The needle is only 4 cm long and this makes back bleeding more obvious when the lumen has been accessed. The pedal access kit comes with a 0.021-inch wire, the coaxial dilator has an outer diameter of 4F and also a removable haemostatic valve, which allows this to be converted to a 2.9–3F 'mini-sheath'.

Non-vascular access sets

Coaxial access set (neff/accustick) This is the one to ask for if you are performing non-vascular intervention. Not only do you get a longer puncture needle but the sheath system has an inner metal stiffener to help prevent kinking of the guidewire and support the catheters as they pass through tissues/organs into deeper structures. In most of the kits, the final sheathed dilator will be at least 6F and often have a radio-opaque end-marker.

Alarm: The tip of the 0.018–0.021-inch guidewire is very easily kinked, and once kinked, it can be difficult to withdraw through the needle again. Be careful – it is possible to shear off the tip of the wire!

Know how to use it

Techniques vary slightly between individual kits but essentially the same principles apply. Puncture and ensure that the wire is inserted far enough that the entire floppy section (usually the most radio-opaque) and ideally a few centimetres of the stiff section, are in the target.

Once the guidewire position is secure, remove the needle leaving the wire in place. Then insert the interlocked dilator system over the wire.

Alarm: The coaxial catheter will only advance into the target over the stiff part of the wire so the entire floppy portion of the wire must be in the target.

Separate the inner dilator and remove it along with the guidewire making sure to keep the outer catheter in position in the target. You can now insert the standard guidewire through the outer sheath.

If you are using a version with an inner metal stiffener, the procedure is essentially the same. Use the stiffener in the straight portion of the tract – it is not designed to go round corners and is more likely to kink the guidewire if you attempt this. The coaxial catheters can be separated from the stiffener and then advanced over it, exactly like placing a venous cannula.

11

Essential equipment: Guidewires

Purpose

Guidewires are used in conjunction with catheters to navigate to a target, in addition they provide support and in the majority of cases, catheters, balloons and other devices are advanced into position over a previously positioned wire. Nearly all guidewires are constructed with a relatively flexible tip section of variable length and a less flexible shaft of variable stiffness. The performance of a guidewire depends on the relative properties of its tip and shaft.

Description

Guidewires broadly divide into functional groups:

- **Non-steerable guidewires:** these generally have a J-shaped or straight tip. They provide a supportive rail that allows the catheter to be advanced into position but are not designed to negotiate stenoses or select branch vessels.
- **Steerable guidewires:** these have shaped tips, the wire is constructed with good torque control so that when the shaft is rotated the tip turns a corresponding amount allowing responsive 'steering'.
- **Hydrophilic guidewires:** these are mostly steerable wires, which have a slippery 'hydrophilic' coating. This allows the wire to cross even the tightest stenosis if used properly.
- **Stiff guidewires:** these are heavy-duty wires with particularly supportive shafts. A stiff wire may be required to support catheters/devices as they pass through occlusions/scar/fibrotic tissue or around challenging anatomy. The length of the flexible tip varies considerably and there is a transition between this and the stiff and more supportive wire shaft. In some wires, the transition point is visible on fluoroscopy as the flexible tip is usually more radio-opaque. Stiff wires are not normally used for primary selective catheterization but are introduced once a stable catheter position has been achieved.
- **Hybrid guidewires:** these are a more recent development combining a steerable floppy tip with a supportive shaft. As with all devices designed to do two things, they often are not quite as good as the original separate wires but they are pretty close and save both money and wire exchanges.

Wire tip

Standard non-selective guidewires have a J-shape or straight tip. The J-tip is intended to be atraumatic as it is advanced but cannot be steered.

Steerable wires usually have a tip pre-shaped to a specified angle. Some wires are made of a material that will let you (with care) custom-shape the wire tip. A correctly chosen steerable hydrophilic angled guidewire can make even the least coordinated operator look as though they have been given a gift by the gods.

Stiffness

For non-steerable wires, this is the biggest factor in choice and there is huge variation between the wires. The correct choice is made by matching the stiffness with your task, e.g. a 4–5Fr catheter can normally be advanced over a Bentson or standard hydrophilic wire; passing a 6F stent over the aortic bifurcation may require something more robust and advancing a 21Fr stent graft needs a heavy duty wire at the other end of the spectrum, e.g. Lunderquist wire (Fig. 11.1).

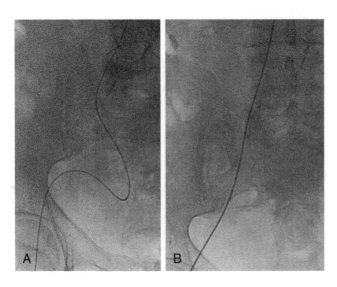

Fig. 11.1 ▓ (A) An extremely tortuous iliac artery with an Amplatz super-stiff guidewire in situ. (B) Following exchange for a Lunderquist guidewire, the artery has straightened markedly.

 Tip: You can readily get an idea of the relative stiffness of a guidewire by looking at the diameter of its delivery holder. Unsurprisingly, stiffer wires coil around a greater diameter.

 Alarm: Stiff guidewires should always be introduced through a catheter that has been placed over a conventional guidewire. Do not attempt to steer a very stiff wire through even mild curves.

Hydrophilic guidewires

The key to success with a hydrophilic wire is to keep it wet. A wet hydrophilic wire is incredibly slippery – so be careful that success does not literally slip through your fingers. The wire is usually lubricated by flushing with heparinized saline while it is still in its delivery holder (keeping it in this and flushing periodically when not in use helps). Wipe the wire with a wet sponge as you remove it and wet it again each time it is used. Dry hydrophilic wires are very sticky, making it hard to advance catheters over them; worse still they will adhere to your gloves and can easily be pulled out from a hard-won position.

Tip: If a catheter sticks on a hydrophilic wire as it is being introduced, try wetting the wire ahead of the tip. If this does not do the trick, have an assistant gently inject flush through the catheter hub until the catheter comes free.

Measurements

There are two factors to consider: diameter and length.

Guidewires come in a range of diameters, from 0.014 inches to 0.038 inches. Small-calibre wires of 0.014–0.018 inches are used with microcatheters and rapid exchange (monorail) systems; they do not have the same strength as larger wires. The 0.035-inch guidewires are used for the majority of cases and will fit through a 4Fr or larger catheter. The 0.038-inch wires were used frequently in the past but are falling out of favour – remember 0.038 wires will not always fit through a 4/5Fr catheter.

Length is important The length of the wire becomes critical when trying to exchange catheters, especially if in a hard-fought-for selective position. A standard 180 cm length wire is fine for most uses; however, longer wires, e.g. 260 cm, may be needed when:

- Working in the upper limb from the groin
- Working in the visceral/renal/hepatic circulation and needing to exchange catheters
- Working with 90 cm+ guide-catheters or angioplasty balloons
- Using through-and-through wires (body flossing).

Tip: The minimum length of guidewire necessary to allow catheter exchange = the length of the catheter + the length of the guidewire in the patient plus a few centimetres for comfort and control.

Know what to ask for

The easy bit is deciding the diameter and length of the wire. The next decision is on a support wire or a steerable wire, i.e. do you need to deliver a catheter/device/drain or select a target vessel?

Support non-steerable guidewires – in increasing stiffness

- **Platinum plus** The 0.018-inch equivalent of the Amplatz wire. Excellent and very supportive low-profile wire for monorail procedures, e.g. renal/mesenteric stents. The tip can be shaped but there is little to no torque control.
- **Bentson wire (0.035)** This wire has a very floppy, atraumatic 5-cm distal tip. If the end of the wire engages a branch vessel, often gently continuing to advance the wire under fluoroscopy forms an atraumatic loop within the main vessel, which pushes the wire tip out of the branch. It is sometimes used in combination with steerable catheters to negotiate stenoses and occlusions, as it does not readily dissect.
- **J-guidewire (0.035)** The 3-mm J-tip wire is one of the most frequently used wires and often the first choice to pass through a puncture needle. The J-tip does not dig up plaques and misses small branch vessels. The 3 mm refers to the radius of the curve of the 'J'. Larger (5-, 10- and 15-mm) J-curves are sometimes used to avoid branch vessels, e.g. a 15-mm J will avoid the profunda femoris artery during antegrade puncture (Fig. 11.2).

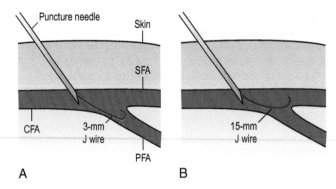

Fig. 11.2 ■ (A) During antegrade puncture of the common femoral artery (CFA) the 3-mm J wire will often enter the profunda femoris artery (PFA). (B) The increased radius of curve of the 15-mm J wire usually will pass directly down the superficial femoral artery (SFA).

- **Straight wire (0.035)** The length of the flexible tip varies from 1 cm to 6 cm, depending on the particular wire type. Take care when passing plaques and branch vessels. Straight wires are not steerable on their own but can be directed using a shaped catheter.
- **Other 'heavy-duty' guidewires, e.g. Rosen wire, Coons wire (0.035)** These come as straight or J and provide extra support for advancing a catheter. 'Heavy duty' is a relative term, moderately stiff wires are useful for inserting a guide-catheter or drainage catheter but are not strong enough for an aortic stent graft.
- **Amplatz super-stiff wire (0.035)** A very useful wire for stents, peripheral stent-grafts and other devices. Amplatz wires are available with a 1-cm or 6-cm floppy tip; choose the correct length depending on the length of target vessel available as an anchor.
- **Meier wire/Lunderquist wire (0.035)** Serious stuff, essential for large-calibre stiff devices, such as aortic stent grafts, but need to be handled with great care.

Steerable guidewires

- **SV5 (0.014/0.018)** This has a shapeable floppy tip and can be steered. It is not as supportive as the Platinum plus but is not as stiff either, so will follow more tortuous vessels.
- **Terumo angled hydrophilic wire (0.035)** The archetypal 0.035-inch steerable wire and benchmark against which others must be judged.
- **Terumo advantage (0.018/0.035)** Hydrophilic and steerable hybrid wire; the first 25 cm are hydrophilic but the main shaft is nitinol, which offers better support and torque.

Know how to use it

This is covered in more detail in Chapter 30.

Steerable wires have a shaped 'angled' tip, which is intended to be rotated to face a target vessel. Unless you can defy the laws of physics, this is best achieved using a pin vice attached to the wire shaft a few centimetres behind the catheter hub. Give the wire some space to work. If only a few millimetres of wire extend beyond the catheter, then the wire will not turn correctly and will be too stiff to flex through a stenosis; back the catheter off until you achieve the desired effect. Shaping the wire is useful and gives you a general air of both mastery and mystery – how did the master know that shape would work? Only some guidewire tips can be shaped and this is done by placing the wire tip over some forceps and pulling it back between the forceps and your thumb. Do this gently or the result will be a spiral wire that is destined for the bin.

Non-steerable wires need to be matched to the task and the anatomy. Support wires are not designed to lead through the vessel; judgement is needed here but, generally, any wire stiffer than a Rosen or Coons wire should be put in place through a catheter. There is a balance between the stiffness to deliver the device and the flexibility needed to get through the curves of the anatomy. Therefore, in a tortuous anatomy, a stiff wire may simply not advance through the catheter, usually when trying to go over a curve like the bifurcation. Do not just push harder, this will just mean losing position. Employ the grey cells and think about using a slightly less stiff wire, as this will flex enough to go around the curves. In this situation, a stiff hydrophilic wire can be very helpful, as this reduces the friction between the catheter and the wire.

Stiff wires only work if the transition between the floppy and stiff portion is within the target vessel. Remember to think about the floppy tip length when choosing the wire – if this is too long it will extend out of the target vessel, too short and it will be harder to introduce and more likely to cause dissection.

 Alarm: Stiff guidewires should always be introduced through a catheter that has been placed over a conventional guidewire. Do not attempt to steer a very stiff wire through even mild curves.

12

Essential equipment: Catheters

Purpose

Non-selective catheters with multiple sideholes are used for rapid injection of contrast into large–medium-sized arteries. Selective catheters may have sideholes or just a single endhole; they are shaped to allow the catheter to enter branch vessels or direct guidewires into them.

Description

Catheters come in a wide range of shapes, sizes and constructions. Simple rules govern catheter choice. Most interventional radiologists rely on a relatively small selection of catheters to perform almost all cases.

Catheter construction influences handling. You will need to experiment with different equipment until you find what works for you. Small-calibre catheters may be less traumatic in terms of the size of the puncture site but the cost is reduced ability to control rotation of the catheter tip in response to turning the catheter hub. This 'catheter torque' is also affected by many other factors, including catheter material, catheter length and the number of curves it has to negotiate.

Most non-selective angiograms can be performed with 3Fr catheters but selective catheterization, particularly if tortuous vessels are involved, usually requires 4Fr catheters or larger.

Construction considerations

Many of the common catheter shapes are available with different constructions. These change the handling characteristics markedly. In the absence of a known favourite, consider the following.

Braiding Braided catheters have a wire reinforcement, which gives increased torque and some kink resistance. The downside is that they tend to be rather rigid and more prone to 'ping in and out of vessels'.

Coating Hydrophilic catheters (and wires) have a slippery coating when they are wet; this tends to be most useful at the extremes of scale, e.g. for inserting very large devices, such as stent grafts and when using coaxial microcatheter systems. Hydrophilic-coated catheters, when used in combination with a hydrophilic wire, can be advanced into small vessels of the distal arterial bed.

Visibility It can be very difficult to see a small catheter in a large patient – opacity vs scatter. Some catheters have a barium coating or a platinum band to show the tip position.

Non-selective catheters

- **Pigtail catheter:** The workhorse of diagnostic angiography. The catheter has an endhole and multiple, much smaller sideholes extending down onto the distal 1–2 cm of the shaft. The distribution of sideholes produces a homogeneous contrast bolus (Fig. 12.1). The pigtail straightens out when the catheter is advanced over the guidewire and forms when the guidewire is withdrawn in a large enough vessel. If the pigtail does not form, simply push the catheter forward while twisting. Pigtails come in a variety of diameters, those used for diagnostic angiography measure approximately 15 mm across; this catheter should not be used in vessels smaller than this diameter. In practice, the endhole has greater flow than the sideholes and hence power injection of contrast should only be performed when the pigtail is properly formed. The pigtail shape minimizes inadvertent catheterization of small branch vessels and allows the catheter to be manoeuvred in a suitably sized vessel without a guidewire.
- **Pigtail variants:** Some pigtail catheters, such as the Grollman catheter, have a shaped shaft a few centimetres from the pigtail; this allows a degree of steering and also stability in the pulmonary arteries. In another variant of the pigtail, the distal end of the pigtail is turned back to face out of the loop – these catheters are intended to help place a guidewire across the bifurcation and can be useful if there is not a shaped catheter to hand.
- **Straight catheter:** Endhole only or with multiple sideholes on a straight shaft (Fig. 12.1). This catheter is used in vessels too small to form a pigtail but with reasonably rapid flow, e.g. the iliac arteries.

 Tip: A test injection of contrast is made to verify that the endhole is not in a small branch before the rapid injection of a contrast bolus.

Flow rates for non-selective catheters Maximum flow rates vary between catheters, depending on the internal diameter and length and number of sideholes. The maximum flow rate and injection pressure (psi) relate to the use of pump injectors – even the strongest will not exceed them with a hand injection! The measurements are usually on the catheter packaging ± catheter hub – check them before giving everyone a contrast shower. Typical maximum flow rates for pigtail catheters are: 3Fr 6–8 mL/s, 4Fr 16–18 mL/s, 5Fr 20–25 mL/s.

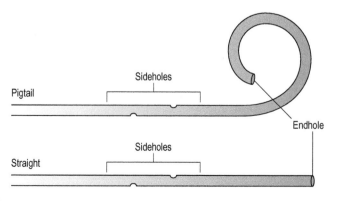

Pigtail

Sideholes

Endhole

Straight

Sideholes

Fig. 12.1 Pigtail and straight multi-sidehole catheters. Unless the catheter is flushed briskly, the flush exits via the proximal sideholes and will not flush the catheter tip, with resultant clot formation.

Selective catheters

Endhole vs sideholes

Selective catheters come in two main designs: endhole only and end- and sidehole. Unlike the multi-sidehole catheters above there are typically only two sideholes located close to the tip of the catheter. Endhole catheters are used for hand-injected, diagnostic angiograms and embolization procedures. Pump injections are potentially hazardous with endhole-only catheters, as the high-flow jet coming out of the single endhole is likely to displace the catheter and may dislodge plaque or cause dissection.

End- and sidehole catheters deliver a rapid, safe bolus of contrast and are used for pump-injected runs (e.g. superior mesenteric artery angiograms); however, sidehole catheters should not be used for embolotherapy: coils may become trapped in the sideholes and particulate matter may escape to non-target territory via the sideholes.

 Tip: Endhole catheters will not aspirate if the catheter tip rests against the vessel wall. Gently pull back/rotate the catheter and try again.

Top five selective catheters

These catheters have different shapes in order to point the tip in a specific direction. Once you understand how to choose these and to use them, you will seldom require anything else. Remember that catheters only adopt that shape when unconstrained. Passing a wire through a catheter or the catheter through a guide sheath or catheter will alter the direction in which the tip points by straightening out any curves. This phenomenon can be used to your advantage to increase the range of directions in which you can aim.

 Tip: A vascular simulator is a good place to learn the concept of selecting an appropriate catheter shape and using it to catheterize branch vessels. Use this to get the general idea but do not be fooled into thinking that success on the simulation equates to expertise on patients!

Cobra An invaluable catheter for visceral and peripheral selective arteriography (Fig. 12.2). The cobra is simple to use, does not need to be formed and can be used for selective

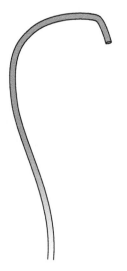

Fig. 12.2 Cobra catheter.

catheterization. The tip points slightly backwards and the Cobra shape forms as soon as the catheter is unconstrained in a large enough vessel. Cobra catheters can also be used in small vessels but the tip will only have a slight forward-facing curve.

The catheter is pulled down to engage a vessel but is pushed forward over a guidewire to allow deeper catheterization. Cobra catheters come in three flavours: C1–C3, each with a progressively widening curve; in practice, most people simply use a C2. Consider the use of a wider loop if you find the catheter backing out of your selective position when trying to advance a wire; the wider loop can sometimes get support from the contralateral aortic wall.

Simmons 'Sidewinder' This is a very useful tool for visceral angiography. The Sidewinder reverse curve comes in three sizes: S1–S3, with progressively larger curves and longer limbs (Fig. 12.3). There are two other catheters that are very similar in shape and function to the Sidewinder: the SOS Omni catheter and the Uni Select (USL). Re-forming the reverse curve can be difficult for the uninitiated. The smaller catheters, Sidewinder 1, SOS Omni and USL 1, can be formed in the thoracic aorta, within an abdominal aortic aneurysm (AAA) or sometimes even the abdominal aorta. For the larger catheters, there are a variety of techniques and these are outlined below.

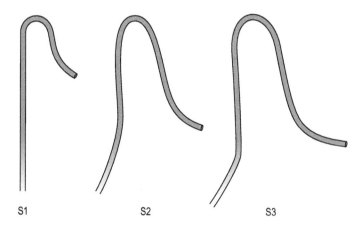

S1   S2   S3

Fig. 12.3 ▨ Sidewinder catheter.

Vertebral Endhole only; the tip is angled and therefore at its best when catheterizing forward-facing vessels, such as the aortic arch vessels (Fig. 12.4). This is one of the simplest catheters to use – just point and shoot; it is remarkably versatile for super-selective catheterization. The Berenstein catheter is similar but has a tip angle closer to 90 degrees but otherwise functions almost identically.

Renal double curve (RDC) As the name suggests, this is designed for selective renal work (Fig. 12.5). The tip points more steeply downwards than the cobra and therefore it is very useful for getting across the aortic bifurcation. At least one of the authors thinks this is a useful catheter for inferior mesenteric artery catheterization. The RDC is used much like a cobra catheter.

Headhunter This catheter has a forward-facing primary curve and is available with and without sideholes (Fig. 12.6). It is primarily used to catheterize the head and neck vessels. The catheter is usually advanced beyond the target vessel, then slowly withdrawn while applying torque; the catheter tends to spring into vessels, which can be alarming for the unsuspecting.

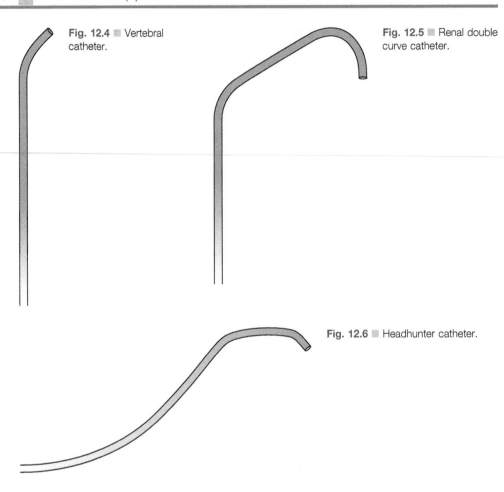

Fig. 12.4 ■ Vertebral catheter.

Fig. 12.5 ■ Renal double curve catheter.

Fig. 12.6 ■ Headhunter catheter.

Measurements

There are three important factors concerning catheter size and one relating to catheter construction; fortunately, the catheter packaging should help you find all these values, although you may have to look hard to find it. In addition, size and length and psi are often printed on the catheter hub.

- **Length:** the length of the catheter in centimetres refers to the length from the hub to the tip (obvious really). Beware, some devices, stents in particular, quote both the usable length (X cm) and total length (X + Y cm) of the delivery system. Make a mental note of these and you will be able to select an appropriate length of guidewire = length of wire in the body + total length of delivery system + 5–10 cm to manipulate.
- **Outer diameter:** the size of the hole or sheath required. This is usually given as the French (Fr) size, which is the outer circumference of the catheter shaft in millimetres.
- **Inner diameter:** relates to the lumen, hence the maximum diameter of catheter or guidewire that will pass through the catheter. To make things confusing, lumen and wire are usually given in inches, e.g. a 0.035 catheter will accommodate a guidewire of 0.035 inches or less.
- **PSI:** psi (pounds per square inch) is the maximum injection pressure the catheter construction has been designed to tolerate. In practice, this is the maximum pressure to set on the pump injector.

Tip: Translating from French For easy reference, the diameter in mm is approximately the French size divided by 3, e.g. 6Fr is ~2 mm. The majority of diagnostic catheters in current use are 5Fr or smaller.

Know what to ask for

Two simple questions:

Do I need a non-selective injection to opacify multiple branch vessels? Use a pigtail unless in a vessel that is less than the size of the loop (12–15 mm depending on the catheter), in which case ask for a straight multi-sidehole.

Not that easy? OK, you need a selective catheter; do not pick at random. Think about the angle of the vessel (see Fig. 30.1) and make your choice from there.

Know how to use it

This is sufficiently fundamental and important that you should really turn to Principles of using catheters and wires (Ch. 30).

13

Essential equipment: Microcatheters

Purpose

Microcatheters allow catheterization and delivery of embolic material to the smallest and most tortuous of vessels (Fig. 13.1). Microcatheters are ideal for super-selective hepatic, visceral and peripheral catheterization.

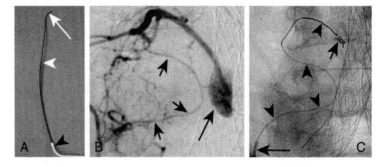

Fig. 13.1 ▓ (A) Microcatheters will negotiate the most tortuous vessels; 4Fr guide-catheter (black arrowhead), microcatheter (white arrowhead) and wire (white arrow). (B) Tiny iliolumbar collaterals (short black arrows) causing type II endoleak (long black arrow) following endovascular aortic aneurysm repair. (C) Microcatheters will negotiate the most tortuous vessels. Microcatheter (arrowheads) delivering embolization coils (short black arrow) into the lumbar artery. 4Fr guide-catheter in the iliolumbar branch of the internal iliac artery (long black arrow).

Description

Microcatheters are essentially an elongated highly flexible catheter. They most often come with a straight tip and are steered into vessels using 0.014–0.018 guidewires. Angled-tip microcatheters are now more widely available but there is a limit to the amount of torque possible from a microcatheter and even these need a steerable wire.

Measurements

They are sized in similar units to conventional catheters; length in cm and outer diameter in Fr. Microcatheters always need to be longer than conventional catheters and usually have a minimum length of 130 cm. Outer diameters vary a little between gradations of 2–3Fr but there are important variations in the inner lumen diameters (measured in thousands of an inch) that can make a difference to embolic or device delivery – as always, it is all on the packet.

Know what to ask for

Most units and operators will need only a small selection of microcatheters. For everyday work, the most popular microcatheter is probably the Progreat (Terumo), which is a hydrophilic catheter with an integrated nitinol guidewire. This is a good catheter and will get you most places but be aware, for special occasions and those really hard to reach spots, there are even better microcatheters available. They are beyond the scope of a survival guide but have a chat with your local interventional neuroradiologists and they will reveal the stunning kit available (at a cost).

 Tip: Avoid being 'so near but yet so far'! Passing a 130-cm-long microcatheter through a 100-cm-long conventional catheter leaves only about 25 cm free; this may not be sufficient to deeply catheterize the target vessels. Make sure that you choose a catheter combination able to reach the target site.

Know how to use it

A conventional catheter is initially used to selectively catheterize a branch of the proximal circulation; it then serves as a guide-catheter (sometimes referred to as the mother catheter) through which the microcatheter is advanced. It is important to achieve a stable catheter position; meaning the mother catheter should not back out when the microcatheter hits the first (or second or third) bend! A Tuohy–Borst adaptor can be used to maintain haemostasis; it is good practice to infuse saline down the side-arm as it will reduce the friction between the mother catheter and the microcatheter. To be honest, for non-neuro intervention, side-arm infusion is less frequently used than it should be. Always advance the microcatheter over the wire and use a steerable wire to access the target vessels.

14

Essential equipment: Sheaths and guide catheters

Sheaths and guide-catheters are designed to allow the coaxial passage of other devices. There is overlap between the structure and function and recently, introducer guides have developed as a crossover group. There are differences in sizing and usage, so the devices will be discussed separately.

Sheaths

Purpose

Sheaths act as atraumatic access conduits for other equipment. There are two main designs: the vascular access sheath and the peel away sheath.

Vascular sheaths

Vascular sheaths are often the primary vascular access; they are invaluable for any case that is likely to use more than one catheter, as they greatly simplify catheter exchange, maintain guidewire position and prevent bleeding at the puncture site.

Description

The sheath comprises two parts, they are often packaged with a short guidewire, which is only used for insertion.

- A hollow plastic tube connected to a haemostatic valve with a side-arm for flushing (Fig. 14.1). Some sheaths have marker bands at the end of the sheath, which can help if you will potentially have to perform an intervention close to the tip of the sheath. Some sheaths have thicker, kink resistant walls and greater column strength than simple access sheaths.

Dilator hub
Sheath hub   Sheath   Dilator

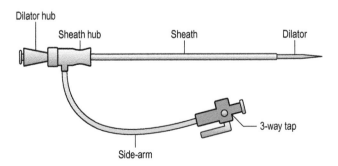

3-way tap

Side-arm

Fig. 14.1 ▪ Vascular sheath with side-arm for flushing.

- A central dilator. This usually 'clicks' into place in the sheath hub. The dilator has a tapered tip to facilitate passage over a guidewire into the access vessel and minimize transition to the sheath tubing.

Tip: Familiarize yourself with how to assemble the sheath and remove the dilator.

Measurements

Diameter (French size): this varies from tiny 2.7Fr microaccess sheaths to behemoths of over 20Fr.

Remember that the sheath size describes the calibre of catheter it will accept, e.g. a 5Fr sheath takes a 5Fr catheter but clearly will have a larger external diameter. A typical thin walled 5f sheath has an approximately 6Fr outer diameter, a braided reinforced sheath will be correspondingly larger.

Dilator lumen (inch) Standard sheaths are usually compatible with 0.035 inch wires. Microsheaths for instance used in the pedal circulation may require an 0.014inch wire.

Length (cm) A typical vascular access sheath is about 15 cm long. There are also longer sheaths, which are usually used when additional support is needed.

Alarm: Do not forget to take the length of the sheath into account when choosing catheters, balloons, guidewires, etc.

Know what to ask for

You do not want to change horses midstream, so think about what equipment you are likely to need to introduce, e.g. angioplasty balloons/stents, and choose a sheath large enough to allow this.

In general, use the shortest sheath that will do the job but there are occasions when a longer sheath can be helpful, e.g. when working over the aortic bifurcation. A long sheath can also be used for angiography by injecting through the sidearm.

Consider a reinforced sheath whenever kinking is likely to be an issue.

Know how to use it

Preparation for use: The sheath is flushed with heparinized saline via the sidearm.

Assembly: The sheath is then assembled by inserting the dilator. This usually 'clicks' into place.

Insertion: The sheath is advanced over a guidewire in the case of a vascular access sheath; this is usually up to the hub.

Removal of the dilator: The hub is then held in place while the dilator is removed, either together with the short guidewire or simply backed off over a longer wire.

Sheath flushing: Sheaths have a large dead space and should be flushed regularly. This is easily overlooked when focusing on the catheter and guidewire some distance away. Open the tap and aspirate until flowing blood is obtained, then flush with clear saline. Remember you cannot flush while the dilator or equivalent diameter catheter is in situ.

Passing a wire into the sheath: This should be easy, after all that is what the sheath is for, but the haemostatic valve can sometimes cause a problem.

Troubleshooting

The wire will not advance into the sheath Did you remember to use an introducer, if so the problem is either:

- **The introducer is not through the haemostatic valve**: you can confirm it is in far enough as there will be back bleeding. If not, simply push it further in.
- **There is a kink in the sheath**: this is most likely in an antegrade puncture. Try applying gentle traction to straighten out the kink. If this fails, reinsert the dilator with the wire until you are past the block. You may need to exchange for a reinforced sheath.

The sheath will not aspirate/flush You will recognize the former when nothing except air bubbles appears in the side-arm. Stop and do not flush it; there is some form of blockage, either:

The tip of the sheath is abutting the vessel wall, embedded in an occlusion or wedged in a small vessel: pull it back a few millimeters at a time and try again.

There is a kink: most sheaths are thin walled and will kink if the sheath enters the vessel at a steep angle, e.g. antegrade puncture in an obese patient. Kinking is almost inevitable if the abdominal fold was retracted during arterial puncture.

- Fluoroscope to try to identify the problem. The situation may be clearer if you use an oblique projection and you advance a wire until it stops at the kink.
- Try straightening out the sheath by flattening it against the abdomen.
- If this fails, advance a guidewire into the sheath until it stops. Carefully reinsert the dilator to the point of obstruction, then apply traction to straighten the sheath; the guidewire will generally advance. Try to aspirate again. This may be a temporary fix.

  If the sheath kinks repeatedly and does not readily respond to the above, then either replace with a reinforced sheath or find another access site.

 Tip: To prevent kinking, try to puncture at a shallow angle; or if a steep puncture is essential, then consider using a reinforced sheath from the outset – these have a larger outer diameter. This is one indication for considering alternative access, e.g. the contralateral or even the ipsilateral proximal SFA.

There is a blood clot in the sheath: this was the main reason not to flush; the clot tends to lodge in the haemostatic valve. Once you have ruled out both of the above, try aspirating with a 20 mL and then a 50 mL syringe. Sometimes the clot will suddenly come free into the syringe and you will again be able to aspirate freely.

  If this fails, ask yourself what would happen if you flushed the thrombus out? Generally this is a very bad thing to do, however, if you are in a vein, a tiny blood clot embolus is unlikely to cause much harm unless the patient has severe pulmonary hypertension or a right to left cardiac shunt.

- Assuming it is not safe to flush, if there is still a guidewire through the sheath, then the simplest action is to exchange the sheath for a new one.

- If there is no guidewire through the sheath, then apply suction with a 50-mL syringe and insert a straight wire and exchange for a new sheath. This carries a very small risk of distal embolization and should be used cautiously, particularly for patients with diseased run-off.

 Tip: You can re-use the same sheath. Put the sheath dilator back on the guidewire about 30 cm from the sheath. Remove the sheath, hold the wire and press to stop bleeding. Get your assistant to flush the sheath thoroughly, then reinsert using the dilator.

 Tip: Prevention is better than cure and if you have a sheath in situ for a long complex case and there is space between the catheter and sheath, consider using a pressurized heparinized saline bag to constantly flush the sheath via the side-arm.

Peel away sheath

Purpose

The peel away sheath is used when introducing indwelling devices such as tunneled central lines and pacemaker wires, which cannot be used with a conventional sheath.

Description

Peel away sheaths are thin walled plastic sheaths that are designed to split along their midline (Fig. 14.2) akin to peeling a banana. A few incorporate a haemostatic valve and side-port and have limited function of a conventional vascular access sheath. The majority of peel away sheaths do not have haemostatic valves.

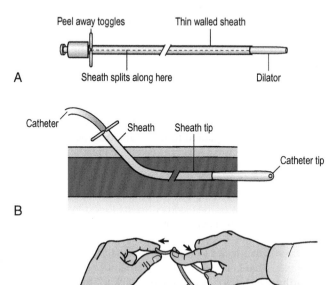

Fig. 14.2 ▪ Peel away sheath. (A) Sheath and dilator assembled. (B) Dilator and wire are removed to allow passage of the device. (C) Hold the catheter in place with a finger, then pull the hub to split and remove the sheath.

Measurements

- Diameter (French size): these start at around 7Fr
- Dilator lumen (inch): 0.018–0.038 inch wires
- Length (cm): a large variety of devices are available.

Know what to ask for

Fortunately most items which require the use of a peel away sheath include an appropriate device bundled as part of the kit. When this is not the case or if you have dropped the original device, just request an equivalent size and length peel away sheath.

Know how to use it

Preparation for use: In most cases, insert the supplied dilator and flush it. If the sheath has a side-port then flush and assemble much as you would a conventional sheath.

Insertion: The peel-away sheath and dilator are inserted over a guidewire.

Removal of the dilator

Alarm: When using in the vascular system, e.g. central veins, remember that, as most peel away sheaths do not have a haemostatic hub, this can lead to torrential bleeding and air embolism.

To safely remove the dilator: Use fluoroscopic guidance and pull the wire back until it is in the dilator. Then pull out the dilator and wire together leaving the sheath empty and the end open.

If you are working in central veins, ask the patient to hum while you do this; the positive intrathoracic pressure prevents air aspiration. Put your finger over the end of the sheath to stop bleeding and allow the patient to breath normally. If you did not pull out the wire, you cannot do this!

Inserting devices through the sheath: hold the device ready to insert close to the sheath hub. If you are working in the central veins, it is time for the patient to hum tunelessly again. Take your finger off the end of the sheath and introduce the device. Let everyone breathe normally again.

Tip: There may be a lot of back bleeding when removing the dilator and inserting devices. Place some swabs strategically to catch the blood or expect to find the floor and your clogs covered. In any case this is much better than air embolism.

Splitting the sheath: Once you have delivered the device to its target destination, the sheath splits by pulling apart two proximal toggles. That is the easy bit, the remainder of the sheath has to be split and removed without pulling the device out. There is a trick to this: first, maintain some forward pressure on the device with a forefinger, now hold the split ends close to the skin and start pulling back the sheath (Fig. 14.2). The sheath splits as you pull it back. You will need to reposition your fingers each time you have split a few centimetres. When the sheath has been fully split you will be left with two strips of plastic. This can be quite fiddly, so if you are struggling ask someone who understands the procedure to assist by performing the splitting while you remain responsible for keeping the device in place.

Guide-catheters

Purpose

These are large bore catheters and their principal role is to provide a safe and stable conduit for a conventional catheter from the puncture site to the target vessel. Because of their large lumen, they are sometimes used for thrombus aspiration. Guide-catheters are most frequently used during stenting procedures when the extra rigidity and increased bail-out options are a reasonable trade-off against the increased puncture site size. Occasionally, a guide-catheter can be very useful to take up the torque from tortuous iliac vessels and therefore allow selective visceral catheterization.

Description

These are large bore catheters, which come in a variety of shapes including straight, hockey stick and renal double curve (RDC).

Measurements

Outer diameter (French): these are catheters, hence the size refers to the outer diameter.

Alarm: It is essential to recognize that this describes the size of sheath the guide-catheter will pass through and not the diameter of the catheter lumen!

Inner diameter (inch): these are catheters, hence the lumen diameter is in inches.

Alarm: These are very wide bore and they will not sit snugly on a guidewire.

Length (cm): this is the working length from hub to tip.

Shape: OK, this is not a measurement but do not forget that guide-catheters come in a variety of shapes. Just like conventional catheters, you should pick a catheter which is likely to point you in the right direction and afford a stable position once it has reached its destination.

Know what to ask for

This depends on:

The intended destination Choose an appropriate length and shape. Remember to factor in the length of the guide-catheter when choosing catheters, balloons and stents to use with it.

What you intend to pass through it This is where life gets tricky, as you have a lumen diameter measured in inches and usually a French catheter size or stent size. You could do some maths to convert the French size to inches:

Diameter in inches = Fr size/25π

In practice, you will probably work on the basis that you need the guide-catheter your boss tells you will work, or one that is 2Fr sizes larger than the device you want to introduce.

Tip: If in doubt, test the compatibility *outside* the patient.

Know how to use it

Because of its large inner diameter, the guide-catheter does not sit snugly on the wire; this has three important ramifications:

1. It must be introduced through a sheath of the corresponding size.
2. You will need to put a removable haemostatic hub or Tuohy–Borst adapter on the end or there will be continual bleeding around the wire. Once the hub is in place they are prepared and flushed just like a vascular sheath.
3. They are intended to be taken to the target vessel ostium rather than rammed through a stenosis; conventional catheters and guidewires should be used for more distal catheterization.

Introducer guides

Purpose

Introducer guides (IG) combine the functions of sheath and guide-catheter.

Description

These are essentially guide-catheters with a side-port and a dilator. This allows them to be introduced like a sheath, while retaining the steerability and support function of a guide-catheter.

Measurements

These are guide-catheters, hence the French size refers to the outer diameter as described above.

Alarm: Introducer guides (IG) vs long sheaths. IGs are sized according to their lumen diameter in inches; sheaths are sized according to their lumen diameter in French. A 6Fr introducer guide will not accommodate a 6Fr guide-catheter/stent.

Know how to use it

Unsurprisingly, these are:

- Prepared for use like a vascular sheath
- Introduced like a vascular sheath
- Flushed like a vascular sheath
- Steered like a catheter.

15

Essential equipment: Taps, hubs and connectors

Taps

Purpose

Just as with domestic taps, these are turned on and off to control flow and there is even a mixer version.

Description

Only two types of tap are of importance but there are some important caveats:

Two-way taps These taps have two positions – on and off – they are often used on the end of connecting tubes.

Two-way taps come in two styles:

- Rotating valve: this is a standard form of tap and is almost ubiquitous.
- Sliding switch: this allows the tap to be turned on and off very quickly; this is particularly useful for CO_2 angiography.

Three-way taps Most vascular sheaths have a three-way tap attached to the side-arm. It will come as no surprise that three-way taps have an additional side-port. The tap acts as a selector allowing you to choose which of the ports are connected. The long arm of the tap is 'off', simply point it towards the port you wish to close.

Three-way taps permit:

- Air bubbles to be flushed out when a syringe is connected. This is the primary function of the tap on the side-arm of a vascular sheath.
- Two syringes to be attached together. This allows one to be used as a reservoir, e.g. during particulate or liquid embolization.
- The system to be calibrated to atmospheric pressure in pressure measurement circuits.
- Connection of pressurized saline flushing systems (Fig. 15.1).

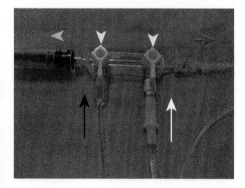

Fig. 15.1 ▨ 'Traffic light' system. Two interconnected 3-way taps (yellow arrowheads), with pressurized inflow of contrast (black arrow) and heparinized saline (white arrow). Adjusting the taps allows filling of syringes (turquoise arrowhead) and flushing of catheters/sheaths (red arrow).

Measurements

These do not strictly apply but not all taps were created equal and there are two important considerations.

Fitting Slip fit is fine for the ward but has no place in interventional radiology; only use taps with Luer lock fittings.

Pressure Most taps will be fine connected to a pressurized bag of saline used to flush a coaxial system. However, not all taps have been designed to allow high-pressure, high-flow rate injection using a pump injector. If you want to avoid an exploding tap treating everyone to a contrast shower, make sure you ask for a high-pressure tap.

 Tip: The same caveat applies to connecting tubes. If you are using a pump injector for arteriography you need a high-pressure connector and tap capable of allowing the planned pressure and flow rates.

Know what to ask for

In general, stick to the simplest tap which will do the job. If you are working in arteries or intend to use a high-flow pump injection then make sure that you have a suitable high-pressure tap.

Know how to use it

Just make sure you know the on and off positions. The commonest mistakes are leaving a tap open and finding a puddle of blood, trying to inject against a closed tap or injecting out of the side-port of a three-way tap.

Haemostatic seals

Purpose

These are seals designed to:
- Prevent blood and other fluid leaking from catheters and coaxial systems, such as sheaths, while you are thinking about something else.
- Allow the introduction of catheters and wires.

Description

There are two designs in common use; although they have similar functions they require different preparation and so are discussed separately.

Haemostatic hubs

These are ubiquitous on vascular sheaths but are also found as standalone devices. Unlike those used on IV cannula, they come with a wide bore built-in side-arm. Removable hubs are great if you are using guide catheters, as this effectively converts them into sheaths. A membrane like diaphragm stops back bleeding.

Measurements
Fitting Most removable hubs have Luer lock fittings, a few will be slip fit but these tend to be insecure.

Tip: The only time you might want a slip-fit hub is when performing thrombus aspiration.

Size It is safe to assume that a sheath hub will accept a catheter of at least the same size as the sheath. If you are using a removable hub, you may need to scrutinize the packaging to check what it will accommodate.

Know what to ask for

A removable hub. If there is doubt state the French size you want to use, ask your assistant to check whether you need this or a Tuohy–Borst adapter.

Know how to use it

Introducing and removing catheters and wires These are simply pushed through the diaphragm. Actually, that is not quite true, angled hydrophilic and floppy tip wires are normally introduced through a cheater (a tapered tube). Not only does this make things easier, it also avoids inadvertent mangling of the tip before you have even started. The cheater is pushed into the diaphragm to open the valve and the wire introduced, then the cheater is removed. You have probably realized that opening the diaphragm will lead to a jet of blood, so have some gauze ready and remember to flush the sheath again afterwards.

 Tip: You can usually avoid the need for a cheater if you are introducing a catheter and wire together. Then, simply keep the wire tip just in the catheter and advance through the diaphragm together.

Injecting contrast and flush Just use the side-arm. Unfortunately, the seal from the diaphragm is not 100% reliable and there is often some leakage when injecting forcibly around a guidewire or simply a drip around fine/stiff guidewires/catheters. This can be really frustrating but do not despair, there is a device available to save the day coming up next.

Haemostatic valves are also available with a screw-type iris and side-arm for flushing, which can be attached to any catheter and largely take away the need for the more complex Tuohy–Borst adaptors.

Tuohy–Borst adaptors

This invaluable, but slightly fiddly, Y-shaped device not only allows a haemostatic seal to be formed but will also grip guidewires/catheters snugly, helping to retain their position (Fig. 15.2). In addition to preventing a puddle of blood on the floor, contrast or drugs can

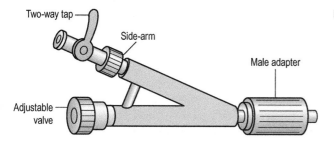

Fig. 15.2 ▪ Tuohy–Borst adaptor.

Two-way tap

Side-arm

Male adapter

Adjustable valve

be injected through the side-arm of the Tuohy–Borst around the wire without the annoying leak, which can occur with a haemostatic hub.

Measurements
Fitting Most Tuohy–Borst adapters have Luer lock fittings to allow a two-way tap to attach to the side-port.

Size Tuohy–Borst adapters are available in a range of sizes. Most, but not all, will close completely so there is not usually a minimum size compatibility problem. In contrast, there may be an upper limit to French size, so check this before assuming that a 9Fr catheter will pass through.

Know how to use it

Rotating the hub of the Tuohy–Borst adapter opens or closes an iris. Those familiar with plumbing will recognize that this is simply a compression joint; tightening securely will prevent even the smallest leaks around the narrowest of wires.

Preparation for use Tuohy–Borst adapters have a large dead space, learning to flush the device properly will place you ahead of many of your colleagues:
1. Connect a two-way tap to the side-arm.
2. Open the tap and attach a syringe containing heparinized saline.
3. Open the adaptor valve (anticlockwise).
4. Place a finger over the tip of the adapter.
5. Flush with saline, this will expel air through the valve.
6. Close the valve (clockwise).
7. Remove your finger from the tip and flush again, this will flush the rest of the system.
8. Close the tap. The system is ready to use.

  Remember to repeat this each time the adapter is removed and reconnected. If the adapter fills with blood while attached, simply modify this sequence omitting step 4.

Introducing and removing catheters and wires To use the Tuohy–Borst, the catheter is passed over the guidewire until it stops at the valve. Loosen the valve sufficiently to allow the wire to exit and then tighten it so that it forms a snug haemostatic fit but allows the catheter to slide on the wire. There will inevitably be some back bleeding as the valve is opened, so once the catheter has been inserted flush the system again.

Connectors

Purpose

Connectors are simply hoses. They should also be used during hand injection to reduce your radiation exposure.

Description

High-pressure connectors

These are non-compliant tubes used to connect the catheter to the injection pump. They are designed for use at high pressures and with high flow rates. Most incorporate a two-way tap.

Low-pressure connectors

Just like their high-pressure cousins but made from compliant tubing. These are not suitable for use in the arterial system and may fail dramatically if used with a power injector.

Measurements

Connectors come in different lengths. Longer connectors are sometimes required due to the set-up of the room but remember that they have a larger 'dead space'.

Know how to use it

Attach a two-way tap as required. The tubing is simply flushed and the tap closed and they are ready to use. There are a couple of additional factors to bear in mind.

Radiation protection Once you have attached the connector, move away from the X-ray tube. Remember the inverse square law, even a small increase in distance results in a significant dose reduction. Get in the habit of taking a step backwards before performing an angiogram.

 Tip: Do not forget to look before stepping back – this avoids a slapstick fall!

Dead space This refers to the volume of fluid required to fill the tube. The longer the connector the greater the dead space, this can be several millilitres. Bear this in mind when injecting contrast, particularly by hand injection with a 10-mL syringe, as most of the contrast may remain in the tubing. This is a waste of time and radiation. The way to avoid this is to preload the connector by inject contrast under fluoroscopy until it starts to exit the catheter.

Dead weight These tubes are heavy; the longer the heavier. Remember to attach your catheter/connector assembly to the drapes before letting the connector take the strain. This is particularly important when connecting to a pump injector, as the operator will not be thinking of keeping your hard-won catheter position.

 Tip: To anchor the catheter and connection tube, make a fold in the drapes behind the hub of the connector and use a clip or towel forceps to fasten this sufficiently tightly that the tubing cannot be pulled back.

 Alarm: This tip only works if the drapes are securely attached to the patient. If not, you will not only remove the catheter and tube but also expose the patient.

Pin-vice This device is used to grip and steer guidewires and is particularly helpful when using hydrophilic and 0.018-inch wires. The device is threaded onto the wire and the 'nose cone' rotated to tighten onto the wire. Remember to check that the device you use is the correct size for your wire; a standard pin-vice may not grip a 0.018-inch wire.

16

Essential equipment: Pump injectors

Purpose

Even the strongest angiographer cannot hand inject rapidly enough for aortic runs. Pump injectors are used to deliver a rapid controlled bolus of contrast while you stand back and reduce your radiation dose.

Description

These are really syringe pumps on wheels for rapid injections. Pump injectors often integrate with the fluoroscopy table, which means that the pump will fire at a pre-set time after the run has started.

Know what to ask for

Really *when* to ask for it It is slightly variable depending on the individual patient haemodynamics and how strong you are. Essentially, if you are in the aorta above the renal arteries – you definitely need a pump injector. A pump injector will often be required in other territories, e.g. internal iliac or visceral injection.

Know how to use it

The settings may seem confusing at first but there are *only* six parameters to consider:
1. **Volume:** this is the total volume of contrast that will be delivered.
2. **Injection rate:** the flow rate in mL/s. Volume/injection rate determines the duration of the bolus.
3. **Maximum pressure (psi):** the peak pressure the pump will generate during injection.
4. **Pressure rate rise:** the time to peak pressure. In practice, it seems permanently set at 0.4 s.
5. **Inject delay:** delays the injection of contrast to allow mask images to be acquired. This is necessary when contrast will reach the target vessel immediately after injection, e.g. imaging the aorto-iliac segment.
6. **X-ray delay:** delays the X-ray exposure. This avoids unnecessary images prior to the contrast arriving at the area of interest, e.g. injecting in the aorta and imaging the feet.

Tip: Parameters 2–4 are limited by the catheter. Details of the maximum permissible pressure are displayed on the catheter hub (Fig. 16.1) and information about flow rates is on the catheter packaging. The maximum flow rate is only achievable at the maximum pressure (psi).

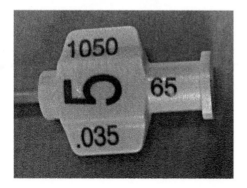

Fig. 16.1 Close-up of a catheter hub indicating: French size 5, length 65 cm, guidewire 0.035 inches and injection pressure 1050 psi.

A general guide to approximate injection rates in a variety of territories is given in Table 16.1.

Table 16.1 Flow rates and volumes for a variety of anatomical sites

Catheter position	Catheter type	Contrast volume and flow rate
Aortic arch	Pigtail	40 mL @ 20 mL/s
Non-selective abdominal aorta	Pigtail	20 mL @ 10 mL/s
Infrarenal aorta	Pigtail	15 mL @ 8 mL/s
Superior mesenteric artery	Multi-sidehole selective catheter	28 mL @ 6 mL/s
Iliac artery	Multi-sidehole straight catheter	15 mL @ 5 mL/s

These are guides and should be tailored for the patient in front of you, e.g. an 85-year-old patient will usually have a lower cardiac output and need less volume and flow rate.

Essential equipment: Snares

Purpose

Snares are essentially wire loops, which are used to capture/manipulate/remove wires, catheters and various other 'foreign bodies'.

Description

All snares are variations on the good old cowboy lasso, in other words, they have a loop that can be rotated and manoeuvred onto a target and then tightened by advancing a catheter to close the loop.

Simple single-loop lasso design

The nitinol Amplatz GooseNeck snare is probably the best-known snare and several other snares share a very similar design (Fig. 17.1). The snare is supplied with its own catheter, the GooseNeck catheter has a radio-opaque end-marker. This catheter can be shaped, if necessary, to increase manoeuvrability.

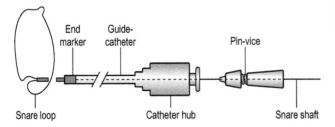

Fig. 17.1 An Amplatz GooseNeck snare.

Measurements

There are three relevant measurements.

Delivery catheter

1. Delivery catheter length in cm: you need to make sure that this is long enough to reach the target.
2. Delivery catheter diameter (Fr): This describes the sheath required to introduce the snare.

Tip: If you are removing something, e.g. a broken catheter, you need to consider its diameter (possibly folded in two) when choosing an appropriate sheath.

Snare

3. Snare loop diameter (mm): the diameter of the lasso. The GooseNeck comes in diameters of 2–25 mm.

Multi-loop design

An example of a multi-loop design is The EN Snare (Merit Medical). It is constructed with three pear-shaped snare loops (Fig. 17.2) but otherwise functions in much the same way as the GooseNeck snare. This design can be a distinct advantage when working in a confined space or when it is difficult to turn a conventional snare.

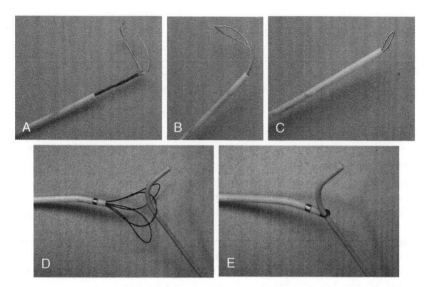

Fig. 17.2 (A–C) An Amplatz GooseNeck snare fully open, partially open and closed. (D,E) An EN Snare with catheter open and closed.

Measurements

Delivery catheter As for GooseNeck snare, above.

Snare working diameter Each snare has a range of working diameters, e.g. 2–4 mm, 4–8 mm, up to 27–45 mm (see Fig. 17.1).

Know what to ask for

The snare should be matched to the target vessel size.

Conventional lasso snares The GooseNeck snare shape changes rapidly from a circular loop to a narrow ellipse as it is tightened. To maximize your chances, ask for a snare diameter that is a little smaller than the vessel diameter in which you are expecting it to work. This will ensure that the snare is maximally open but still able to rotate if needed.

Multi-loop snares The snare loops are pear-shaped, which affords the greater range of usable diameters. The lower diameter should be less than the diameter of the vessel to allow rotation.

Tip: It is handy to have an idea of the typical sizes of vessels (Table 17.1) to allow the correct size to be chosen effortlessly.

Table 17.1 Snare diameters for use in common sites

Artery	Approximate diameter (mm)	Vein	Approximate diameter (mm)
Aorta	18–25	IVC	18–30
Common iliac artery	8–12	Common iliac vein	10–20
External iliac artery/CFA	6–8	External lilac vein	6–10
Superficial femoral and popliteal	4–6	Femoral and popliteal	5–10
Calf	2–3	Calf	2–4
Pulmonary artery	25	SVC	15–20
Subclavian artery	8–12	Internal jugular	8–12

Know how to use it

Using a snare in eight easy steps:

1. First position a guidewire adjacent to the object to be removed; if you cannot manage this, then you will not be able to remove it!
2. The guide-catheter is passed along the guidewire in the normal fashion and the guidewire removed.
3. The snare is compressed within an introducer and then advanced into the catheter.
4. As the snare loop emerges from the catheter, it opens like a lasso.
5. Allow the snare loop to open; it should fill most of the vessel lumen. The snare loop can be rotated, advanced or withdrawn to position it over the target.
6. Once the target is in the loop, keep the snare still and advance the guide-catheter over it. This progressively tightens the snare and grips the target (Fig. 17.2).
7. The snare and its prey can now be pulled back to the access site.
8. The prey is either removed, parked somewhere safe or, in the case of a large object, held onto until the vascular surgeon can remove it safely.

18

Essential equipment: Angioplasty balloons

Purpose of equipment

These are mostly used to dilate blood vessels but can be equally useful for strictures in other systems.

Description

Although there is a huge variety of different angioplasty balloons, they all boil down to a straight catheter with an inflatable balloon at the distal end. All angioplasty balloons have a channel for a guidewire and a separate channel to allow balloon inflation/deflation.

There are two principal constructions:

Over the wire balloons Most workhorse peripheral angioplasty balloons are constructed like this; the guidewire runs the whole length of the catheter from the hub to the tip (Fig. 18.1).

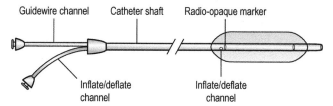

Guidewire channel   Catheter shaft   Radio-opaque marker

Inflate/deflate channel   Inflate/deflate channel

Fig. 18.1 ▬ Typical angioplasty balloon construction. Note the balloon length refers to the distance between the markers over which the balloon is of its rated diameter. The catheter shaft comprises the guidewire lumen and the inflation channel. Smaller shaft sizes can be achieved with thinner materials and smaller inflate/deflate channels.

Monorail – rapid exchange The wire only runs through the distal 15–20 cm of the catheter. Hence, the catheter shaft is only the inflate/deflate channel (Fig. 18.2). Monorail systems allow the use of shorter guidewires and catheter exchanges are much simpler and quicker. In addition, monorail systems tend to have a lower profile.

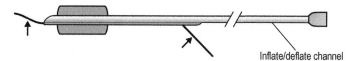

Inflate/deflate channel

Fig. 18.2 ▬ Schematic view of a monorail angioplasty balloon. The guidewire (arrows) enters the catheter at the tip and exits after about 15 cm. The remainder of the catheter shaft is the inflate/deflate channel.

Modern angioplasty balloons are designed to minimize the balloon profile and therefore the size of the access sheath required. They will dilate the majority of lesions but every now and then, you will come across a resistant stenosis. The choice is then usually either a high-pressure balloon or a cutting angioplasty balloon. High-pressure balloons are made of a thicker material to sustain higher inflation pressures and often need a larger sheath.

A cutting angioplasty balloon is simply an angioplasty balloon with small razor blades/'angiotomes' incorporated into the balloon. These make shallow cuts into the fibrous tissue which is preventing the lesion from dilating. In general, cutting balloons have a much higher profile and are much more expensive than conventional balloons.

Measurements

There are seven measurements which you need to know. They are all usually on the front of the balloon packet.

Catheter dimensions

Catheter size (French, Fr) This describes the sheath size recommended for the balloon.

Alarm: You may be able to squeeze a pristine balloon through a smaller sheath but removing it once it has been used is a different matter.

Catheter length (cm) This is usually the tip to hub measurement but beware, the construction of some balloons will specify a working length and a total length. The working length is the value which determines whether your balloon is long enough to reach the target. The total length to the distal hub is the value which determines whether your guidewire is long enough to allow the balloon to be introduced and removed. There is usually a diagram showing the relevant lengths on the packaging.

Catheter lumen (gauge) This describes the diameter of wire the catheter will accommodate. Most peripheral workhorse balloons are 0.035. Low-profile balloons often use 0.018-inch wires and monorail systems typically 0.014-inch.

Balloon dimensions

Working from straightforward to the more esoteric but very important these are:

Balloon rated diameter (mm) There is a huge range of sizes from 2 mm to massive balloons >25 mm, designed for use in the thoracic aorta. The diameter is usually given on the packaging and also the hub of the balloon.

Balloon length (cm) The length along which the balloon will reach the rated diameter. This is usually denoted by two radio-opaque markers on the catheter shaft. Monorail systems may have a single marker in the midpoint of the balloon.

Alarm: The balloon has to taper down on to the catheter at each end. Larger-diameter balloons may have surprisingly long tapers. This may have repercussions, e.g. when performing distal aortic angioplasty, the taper may extend into the iliac artery leading to mayhem! Balloon length is usually on the packaging and also the hub of the balloon.

Balloon rated inflation pressure (atmospheres) The balloon will be its rated diameter at this pressure. Some balloons are designed to be compliant, in which case there is usually a chart indicating how diameter will change with pressure. This sort of precision is popular in cardiology but is sometimes useful in day-to-day angioplasty.

Balloon maximum rated pressure (atmospheres) Also known as 'the burst pressure'. The vast majority of balloons will not burst if kept to this pressure; for purists, the manufacturer has 95% confidence that 99.9% of their balloons will not burst below this pressure. In practice, balloons can often be inflated to much higher pressures before they burst but you are on your own if you take this option – don't say we didn't warn you!

 Tip: If a stenosis is refractory to dilatation you are on much safer ground if you choose a balloon with a higher maximum rated pressure or use a cutting balloon. The penalty for this is usually increased sheath size and price.

 Alarm: Do not try this at home! Inflating an angioplasty balloon with saline and air until it bursts makes an impressive bang, and gives an idea of the damage it could cause in a blood vessel.

A note on dilating force Those of you with an interest in physics can Google Laplace and hoop strength. For everyone else, for a given pressure the dilating force increases with the diameter of the balloon; therefore, for the same pressure, a larger balloon will apply a greater force on the vessel wall. In practice, smaller balloons are usually inflated to much higher pressures than their larger cousins, e.g. 3-mm balloons are often inflated to 12 atm while 15-mm balloons only require a pressure of 4–6 atm.

 Alarm: Take great care when dilating large vessels such as the aorta, it is surprisingly easy to generate sufficient pressure to rupture the artery.

Know what to ask for

As a minimum you need to ask for a balloon that:

- is sized about 1 mm larger than the reference vessel diameter
- is long enough to cover the diseased segment but no more
- has a long enough shaft to reach the target
- will fit over your guidewire
- will fit through the sheath.

There are a couple of exceptions to these principles: when a short balloon cannot be held in a stable position during inflation. This phenomenon is akin to what happens when you pinch a lemon pip between your fingers and it shoots out. In these circumstances, a longer balloon length will add stability.

In refractory stenoses, you may need to consider a 'high-pressure' balloon or a 'cutting' balloon. A high-pressure balloon is the same diameter as the reference vessel. However, when requesting a cutting balloon, one way of keeping the sheath size down is to use a balloon sized for the stenosis rather than the reference vessel. Once the cuts have been made, simply use your original balloon to fully dilate.

In practice, there is a potentially bewildering range of equipment to choose from, ranging from everyday workhorses to thoroughbreds which will negotiate extremely challenging anatomy. How to make sure you saddle the correct horse is detailed in the section on how to perform angioplasty at different sites (Ch. 32).

Know how to use it

There are a few basic steps common to all angioplasty procedures.

Preparing the balloon It is important to purge as much air as possible out of the balloon. Air is more compliant than liquid and therefore less effective during inflation. In addition, if the balloon does rupture on calcified plaque it is better that it discharges fluid than air, which can act as an embolus! Attach a two-way tap to the hub of the inflation channel and aspirate using a syringe with a few mL of contrast in it. Hold the syringe upright and aspirate on the hub until some bubbles appear, then release the pressure and allow the space to fill with contrast. Repeat then close the tap.

Getting the balloon to the target This is always achieved using a previously positioned guidewire.

Conventional over-the-wire balloons Easy, these are advanced and withdrawn like standard catheters.

Monorail systems These are usually used in conjunction with a guide catheter or long sheath, both to support the balloon during its journey and to perform angiography. The balloon is threaded on to the guidewire and advanced into the sheath. Once the 15–20-cm section with the wire channel is in the sheath, the wire is held at the sheath hub while the balloon is advanced using the catheter shaft. This simplifies control of the guidewire.

Balloon inflation Balloons are inflated with a saline/contrast mix, usually in a 3:1 ratio. This mixture is opaque enough to see but less viscous and easier to aspirate than full-strength contrast. Balloons can be inflated by hand with a standard syringe or using a special inflation handle. Usually, the choice is made based on the target size and resistance. As a guide, balloons <3 mm or >10 mm usually get an inflation handle; between these sizes some operators will use a standard syringe and if defeated reach for the inflation handle. The inflator is simply connected to the inflation channel of the balloon. On a conventional balloon, this is the hub without the guidewire – this usually comes off the shaft or hub at an angle. On a monorail system, there is only one hub! Fluoroscope during balloon inflation to check that the balloon remains in position and that the balloon has completely 'de-waisted'. Try to feel how much pressure you are applying with the inflation device and regularly check the pressure gauge to ensure that you do not exceed the recommended pressures.

 Tip: Note that when the stenosis yields, the balloon pressure will fall and the balloon may need to be topped up further.

Balloon deflation Release the pressure on the inflation handle and pull it back fully. Contrast is viscous and will slowly trickle back into the syringe. Often aspirating the balloon as completely as possible using an empty 20-mL syringe is quicker and more effective. Perform check fluoroscopy to confirm the balloon is really empty before attempting to remove it.

 Tip: Do not fluoroscope while the balloon is emptying – this is wasted radiation. Wait until no more fluid is coming out or there is a short rush of bubbles. If this is not obvious, wait 30 s before screening to check deflation.

Before removing the balloon If you have a long sheath or guide catheter in situ or have performed an antegrade puncture then do a check angiogram. If the stenosis has not responded fully, you can dilate it again without having had the bother of removing and reintroducing the balloon.

To retrieve the balloon Over-the-wire balloons need to be backed off gradually over the wire, taking care to keep the guidewire in position. If in doubt, perform continuous or intermittent fluoroscopy over the wire tip to confirm that it is safe.

Monorail systems simplify introducing and withdrawing the catheter, as the wire is controlled from very close to the hub of sheath. To remove a monorail system, the guidewire is fixed by the hub. The catheter can then be pulled back until it stops at the point at which the wire channel exits. After this, the last portion is handled in the same way as usual.

Removing the balloon through the sheath With modern balloons this is usually straightforward. If there are obvious wings on the balloon, clockwise rotation of the balloon during withdrawal will help wrap the wings onto the catheter shaft and reduce the profile.

If the balloon is reluctant to come out of the sheath – **STOP** – do not impact the balloon as it will cause the sheath to concertina. Try to aspirate the balloon again, if necessary with a 50-mL syringe, and confirm on fluoroscopy that the balloon is fully deflated.

 Alarm: When removing balloons and catheters, always keep an eye on the sheath to make sure that it is not heading for an early and bloody exit. If it is moving with the catheter, ask your assistant to hold it in place while you concentrate on controlling the catheter and wire.

19

Essential equipment: Inflation handles

Purpose

The only way to be certain a balloon is being used at the correct pressure is to use an inflation handle with a pressure gauge (Fig. 19.1). Besides precision, the inflation handle allows you to effortlessly generate and sustain high pressures without hurting your skilled hand.

Description

These are modified syringes, the plunger is driven into the syringe barrel with a screw thread leading to a progressive and controlled increase in the balloon pressure. There is usually a release mechanism to disengage the thread, allowing the plunger to be pulled back for balloon deflation. In reality, the rate-limiting step is flow through the balloon's inflate/deflate channel.

Measurements

These are usually 'one size fits all' devices; most are based on a 20-mL syringe.

Know what to ask for

An inflation handle.

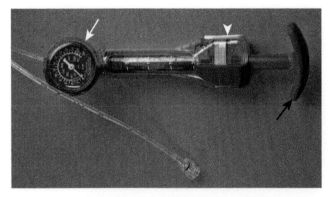

Fig. 19.1 ▪ Inflation handle. The balloon is inflated by screwing the handle (black arrow) clockwise until the gauge (white arrow) shows the appropriate pressure. Pressing the button (arrowhead) releases the screw thread; the handle can then be pulled back to deflate the balloon. Further aspiration with an empty 20-mL syringe may be needed to empty the balloon completely.

Know how to use it

Inflation Use approximately one-third strength contrast to inflate the balloon. Remember to check those inflation pressures before starting and to keep an eye on the gauge as well as fluoroscopy of the balloon. Pressure rises surprisingly quickly, especially in small balloons.

Deflation You will need to check how to release the screw thread on your particular device.

Once you have mastered this, simply pull the handle back and wait for the contrast to trickle out. As for standard balloons, an empty 20-mL syringe is usually faster and more effective.

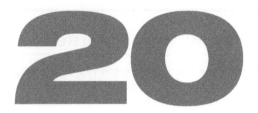

Essential equipment: Stents

Purpose

Stents are scaffolds used to maintain luminal patency in many systems, e.g. vascular, biliary, gastrointestinal and tracheobronchial. They act by exerting an outward radial force to overcome stenoses/occlusions and elastic recoil after angioplasty. Stents may also reduce the likelihood of distal embolization during angioplasty by trapping plaque/thrombus against the vessel wall.

Description

Stents comprise a metal strut latticework, they have a high expansion ratio allowing them to be compressed to a small diameter for introduction into the patient and then expanded to many times that diameter. There are two principal stent types relating to how they are deployed.

Balloon-expandable stents Most of these come premounted on an angioplasty balloon. As the balloon is inflated the stent expands to the same diameter.

Self-expanding stents These come mounted, constrained on a delivery catheter. The stent is progressively unsheathed and opens due to intrinsic radial force. Note that self-expanding stents will often require additional balloon dilatation.

Stent construction

This is a complex subject and every manufacturer will try to tell you why their device is the best. Here is a simple guide, which is really all you need to know.

Material Almost all stents are made from alloys of stainless steel or nickel and titanium (nitinol), some have finishes/coatings or properties such as drug elution or radioactivity intended to reduce thrombogenicity and restenosis. There are even novel stents designed to be resorbed once their work is done.

Nitinol If you want to impress your boss you should know that nitinol is an acronym for Nickel Titanium Naval Ordnance Laboratory. Virtually all new self-expanding stents are made of nitinol for the simple reason that it has thermal 'shape memory' and 'superelasticity'. This means that once the stent is made it can be deformed into one shape at a low temperature but will magically 'spring' back to its original shape when warmed. In practice, the stent is cooled and compressed for mounting on the delivery catheter but expands to its original shape at body temperature. Nitinol's properties make it particularly suitable for applications requiring flexibility and motion.

What about patients with nickel allergy? No need to worry there, although nitinol is 50% nickel, the polished surface forms a stable titanium oxide coating. Do not forget that nickel it is also present in significant amounts in stainless steel and other alloys and in fact, these tend to release nickel faster!

Structure

There is generally a compromise between stent designs which favour radial force or flexibility, so there is no magic stent which will fulfil every therapeutic need. Self-expanding stents are either laser cut from nitinol or braided from overlapping wires.

As a general rule:

- **Closed-cell structure stents** (think trellis fence) in which every cell is linked to all adjacent cells tend to have greatest radial strength at the cost of reduced flexibility and trackability.
- **Open-cell structure stents** have fewer links between cells. This increases flexibility and trackability but reduces radial force. In addition, open cell stents cover less of the vessel surface.

This nomenclature applies to both balloon-mounted and self-expanding stents.

Measurements

Stent dimensions

Stent diameter (mm) There is a huge range of sizes from 2 mm to stents up to >40 mm designed for use in the thoracic aorta. Remember that self-expanding nitinol stents can expand up to their rated diameter, while balloon-mounted stents can often be dilated beyond their rated diameter simply by using a larger balloon. Stent diameter will be on the packaging and usually also the hub of the balloon. Aim for a stent that is 1 mm greater than the target vessel.

Stent length (cm) This is where things can be confusing; this refers to the length at the expected diameter. For most nitinol and balloon-expandable stents, expect the stent length to be what it says on the packaging. However, some stents shorten as they expand. This is particularly true of braided stents, such as the Wallstent and some closed-cell balloon-expandable stents, such as the Palmaz stent. This is not necessarily a problem but the shortening needs to be taken into account when selecting, positioning and deploying the stent.

Catheter dimensions

Catheter size (French, Fr) This describes the sheath size recommended for the stent. Most modern stents up to about 12 mm will pass through a 6Fr sheath, some will even pass through a 5Fr sheath and a few smaller stents pass through a 4Fr sheath.

Catheter length (cm) Balloon expandable stents follow the same rules as angioplasty balloons. Self-expanding stents have a very wide range of delivery systems; the working length (whether the stent delivery system will reach the target) is often much shorter than the catheter length (which determines the length of guidewire required), so do not be surprised to be reaching for 260-cm long wires. There is usually a diagram showing the relevant lengths on the packaging.

Tip: When considering which wire to use it is better to err on the long side.

Catheter lumen (gauge) This describes the diameter of wire the delivery catheter will accommodate. Most peripheral artery stents are 0.035. Low-profile stents often use 0.018-inch wires and monorail systems may use 0.014-inch wires.

Know what to ask for

Here are the key questions to ask:

Do I need a strong stent? Closed-cell designs tend to exert the greatest radial force and many operators will opt for a balloon-mounted stent in these circumstances. Remember that strength comes at the expense of flexibility and conformability.

Alarm: A stent will not help if you are unable to dilate the lesion with balloon angioplasty.

Is precise positioning essential? If this is the case, it is all about how precisely the stent can be delivered and many operators will reach for a balloon-mounted stent but, in practice, a nitinol stent can usually be deployed with similar accuracy (Fig. 20.1). There are some stents to avoid in these circumstances and it is best to avoid a stent which may shorten unpredictably, hence the Wallstent should not be your first choice.

Will there be challenges reaching the target site? This is where trackability, flexibility and crossing profile come into the equation.

Trackability is how well the device follows the guidewire, hence it can usually be improved by using a stiffer wire. Some devices have less column strength and inherently track less well, this is all to do with the delivery system; the actual stent is pretty much irrelevant.

Tip: Most nitinol self-expanding stents are usually constrained within an outer catheter; this helps tracking and crossing.

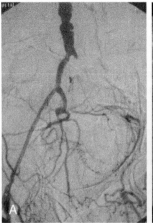 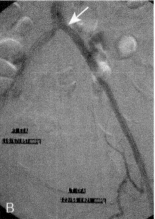

Fig. 20.1 (A) Typical long iliac occlusion. (B) Two overlapping stents have been deployed from the contralateral approach. Note the proximal stent position at the iliac bifurcation (arrow) and the distal at the inguinal ligament. Unilateral stents can be used to treat these patients, provided the stents are accurately deployed and do not cover the contralateral iliac artery origin.

Flexibility is necessary if the stent needs to perform calisthenics, such as crossing the aortic bifurcation. This relates to the delivery system and the stent. This is not the time to choose a rigid closed-cell design. While the majority of stents with an open-cell design are sufficiently flexible to pass over the aortic bifurcation and conform to the vessel anatomy allowing deployment in the contralateral iliac system (Fig. 20.1), this may not be sufficient to track around a tortuous mesenteric artery.

Crossing profile is important if the stent has to pass through an occlusion or a severe stenosis, especially if it is calcified. Balloon-mounted stents do not have a covering, so unless you introduce them through a guide catheter or long sheath they may be a victim of friction or worse, the stent may start to open or come off the balloon as it tracks around a bend.

Is the target site of uniform diameter? This is where the ability of the stent to conform to the vessel wall is key. Conformability is also important when the vessel is tortuous. The archetypal example is when treating both the common and external iliac arteries the diameter will need to be larger proximally and smaller distally. When it comes to conformability, the self-expanding stent is king. Within limits, open-cell nitinol stents and braided stents, such as the Wallstent, will both accommodate a range of diameters along their length.

Alarm: Remember, if you choose a nitinol stent, it must be sized for the maximum diameter. Balloon dilatation is futile, as it will simply spring back to its rated size!

Balloon-expandable stents can be made to conform but obviously this requires more than one balloon. Choose a size matched to the smaller diameter and then use a larger balloon to tailor where the greater diameter is required.

Alarm: Remember if you choose this approach that the stent may only be anchored over a short distance and could be dislodged when introducing the larger balloon.

Is the target site straight or tortuous? If it is straight, there is no problem. If the vessel is tortuous, conformability is important again. Remember that although the vessel will straighten transiently during balloon inflation (or if you have used a ruthlessly stiff guidewire), it will resume its normal shape afterwards. Therefore choose an open-cell stent self-expandable or balloon-mounted stent. A rigid stent will probably just simply create a kink just beyond the stent in a blood vessel and this will lead to thrombosis if left untreated.

Is there a risk of stent compression post-deployment? If so, avoid balloon-expandable stents and think hard whether you really want a stent at all. Balloon-expandable stents will be deformed and potentially occluded by external compression, e.g. in the carotid, subclavian and popliteal arteries. In these circumstances, a self-expanding stent is better but even these may be damaged by repeated flexion/compression. If the stent fractures, it is likely to lead to occlusion; this has been a bugbear of treating the distal SFA.

Will imaging be required in the future? If you are using ultrasound for follow-up vascular imaging, this is not an issue. However, magnetic resonance angiography (MRA) is increasingly used either as part of your plan for follow-up or to investigate another problem. In this case, stick with nitinol; the latest designs will cause minimal artefact. Forget about using a stainless steel stent, the susceptibility artefact will obscure the vascular detail and the adjacent soft tissue.

Tip: Experience is usually required when choosing a stent for particularly challenging anatomy so ask your boss or phone a friend before you start. This is so much better than calling your boss for help when you are faced with a partly open balloon-expandable stent wedged over the aortic bifurcation.

What about drug-eluting and bioabsorbable stents? Well, although these are commercially available, they are expensive and have not yet been proven, hence they should probably be used only in the context of clinical trials or in special circumstances, e.g. recurrent stenosis where there is no option but to stent.

Know how to use it

Balloon-mounted stents

The basic rules of angioplasty balloons apply. Stents are typically oversized by 1 mm to ensure secure fixation when deployed. Most stents come ready mounted on the balloon catheter. This is generally the best option, the stent and balloon have been chosen to work together and this minimizes the chance of the stent and balloon parting company with the stent going walkabout inside the patient. The only downside is that this does require holding a range of sizes in stock.

Self-expanding stents

There are a huge variety of deployment systems for self-expanding stents. Fortunately, they all share the same underlying principles, as they have basically to achieve the same function. All self-expanding stents are held in a compressed state on the delivery catheter by an outer sheath. Regardless of construction, the deployment system works to progressively uncover the stent, allowing it to expand in a controlled fashion at the target site (Fig. 20.2).

Contemporary pusher and sheath systems

The only difference from above is that the entire stent, pusher, sheath combination is integrated into a single delivery catheter.

The stent is mounted on a central catheter shaft which incorporates the tip of the delivery system. This central shaft corresponds to the pusher. The stent is held in place by a movable

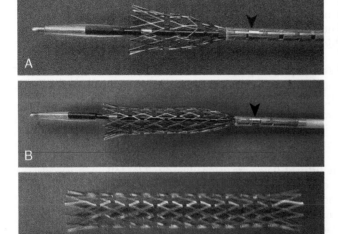

Fig. 20.2 ■ A self-expanding stent opening as the outer sheath is retracted. Note that the distal marker (arrowheads) moves back with the sheath but the stent remains in the original position.

outer sheath, which should join the catheter tip with a smooth transition. The central shaft is longer than the outer sheath and the proximal end is often a relatively rigid metal shaft over which the sheath can slide. Most systems incorporate a mechanism or safety catch to prevent premature deployment. To deploy the stent, the central shaft is held stationary while the outer sheath is manually pulled backwards over it (Fig. 20.3). These systems are tried and tested. As long as you remember which hand to keep still and which to move, you are likely to succeed.

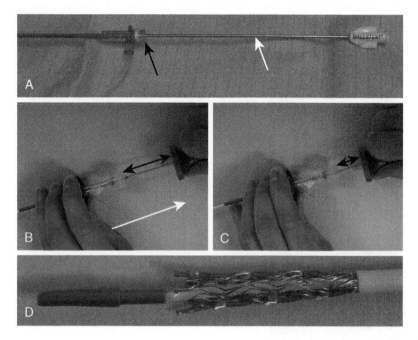

Fig. 20.3 ▪ Deploying a stent using an integrated pusher and sheath delivery system. (A) Delivery sheath (black arrow) and pusher (white arrow). (B, C) The pusher is fixed and the sheath pulled back (white arrow) until the stent is deployed. (D) Stent opening as it is unsheathed.

'Trigger' and 'screw' systems A modification of the pusher and sheath and they incorporate either a trigger mechanism or a screw mechanism to gradually unsheath the stent. Trigger systems can be operated one-handed, and less coordination is required to deploy them.

Markers

Almost all delivery systems incorporate radio-opaque markers to help positioning. Unfortunately, these are not standardized; markers may be on the delivery system, the stent or both. Some markers move with deployment as the sheath is retracted, others stay still. You need to be familiar with the markers on the stents you use or malpositioning is inevitable.

 Alarm: Self-expanding stents tend to creep forward during initial deployment, particularly for larger nitinol stents; deploy slowly initially and watch those markers.

A note on the Wallstent The Wallstent was one of the first self-expanding stents. The Wallstent has a closed-cell structure formed by braiding multiple Elgiloy wires, just like a braided hose. This results in significant shortening during deployment. The final deployed length of the

Wallstent is variable and depends on diameter. A chart on the back of the packaging helps you predict how long the stent will be, e.g. a 10 × 68-mm-long Wallstent is roughly 95 mm long when constrained, and it will shorten to 83 mm long at its minimum recommended diameter of 7 mm. It is 77 mm long at 8 mm and 69 mm at 9 mm. Hence, the markers at the end of the Wallstent delivery catheter bear little relation to the final position of the stent (Fig. 20.4). The critical marker lies closer to the proximal end. This indicates the limit to which the stent may be deployed and still be re-sheathed. It also corresponds roughly to where the proximal end of the stent will shorten when unconstrained. Because the constrained length of the Wallstent is so much greater than the deployed length, it is not suitable for use in situations where there is little space beyond the target.

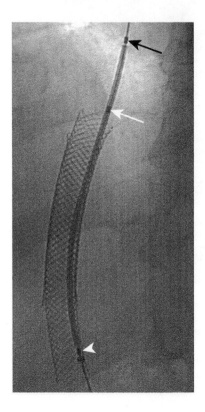

Fig. 20.4 ▪ Wallstent markers shown during a TIPS revision. The distal marker (white arrowhead), the proximal marker (black arrow) and the 'critical marker' (white arrow), which indicates roughly the point to which the stent will shorten and the limit of deployment for re-sheathing.

Tip: It is common practice to start with the distal end of the Wallstent well beyond the target site. When the stent has partially opened, it can be pulled back until the 'critical' marker is in position. This is fine in superior vena cava obstruction (SVCO), but is best avoided in an occluded iliac artery, unless you are intending to embolize the run-off.

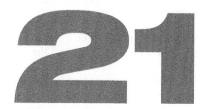

Essential equipment: Stent grafts and covered stents

Purpose

Covered stents provide an impermeable conduit and are used in both the vascular and non-vascular system. In the vascular system, they are called 'stent grafts'.

Vascular The most important indications are treating aneurysms and arterial rupture. Other indications are TIPS and in certain circumstances to manage stenotic and occlusive disease.

Non-vascular Outside the vascular world, they tend to be called 'covered stents'. In the majority of cases, they are used in the context of oncology to prevent tumour ingrowth and manage fistula, particularly in the trachea, oesophagus and bile duct.

Description

These are simply stents incorporating graft material; this makes them larger and more expensive. As with stents, stent grafts can be balloon-expandable or self-expanding.

Stent graft terminology

Stent grafts come in a range of shapes and sizes from simple tube grafts, via modular bifurcated devices for endovascular of abdominal aortic aneurysm (AAA) repair (EVAR) onto complicated fenestrated and branched devices for treating thoracic and complex abdominal aneurysms. Only those working in high-volume, tertiary centres will need to use the full gamut of device types.

Straight Straight grafts are most commonly used in iliac artery aneurysm or to repair post-traumatic false aneurysm or arterial rupture.

 Tip: You need to be familiar with at least one such device and be able to deploy it in an emergency.

Tapered Tapered grafts are needed when there is discrepancy between vessel diameters at the proximal and distal anchorage sites, e.g. in aorto-uni-iliac grafts.

Bifurcated Bifurcated stent grafts are the most commonly used devices to repair abdominal aortic aneurysms. They extend from the abdominal aorta into the common iliac vessels. They divide into two limbs: the ipsilateral limb is typically combined with the larger-diameter body (like a tapered graft) and the contralateral limb plugs into a 'socket' in the body.

Fenestrated Fenestrated grafts are custom-made and have notches fabricated in the sides, corresponding to the position of branch vessels that need to be preserved, e.g. the renal arteries. Fenestrated grafts are suitable in aneurysms in which the neck is short but of normal calibre.

Branched This is the next step in the evolution from fenestrated grafts intended for use in the thoracic aorta and in AAA, with ectatic and aneurysmal necks. Here, the branches are used to bridge the gap between the stent graft and the vessel to be preserved.

Construction

This is a rapidly changing area with a vast range of devices vying for your attention in a crowded market. Design and construction differ in many respects, including stent material and design, graft fabric (material, thickness, attachment to stent) and incorporation of anchorage features to prevent migration (hooks/barbs, which may be combined with proximal or distal bare stents). There is a drive to reduce the profile of delivery systems and as a result, the graft material is thinner than a conventional surgical graft.

As with stents, there is no standardization of marker systems and the differences between delivery systems can be quite bewildering. As a result, most operators will actually become familiar with a limited range of equipment.

Measurements

For tubular covered stents, the measurements catheter size, length and lumen, stent-graft diameter and length are basically the same as stents, but expect eye-watering Fr sizes for the largest devices.

Rather more tricky are the measurements of modular devices, where the relationship between the patient anatomy and nuances of the individual system come into play. In addition, each manufacturer has specific guidance that you need to refer to during graft sizing.

Know what to ask for

Stent grafting is not dissimilar to stenting but the margins for error are fewer. For a stent graft to be effective, it must fit precisely within the target vessel. An undersized graft will allow blood to flow between it and the vessel wall. Oversized devices will have creases in the graft material, which may adversely affect flow and promote thrombosis. Stent grafts that are too long or mispositioned may occlude vital side branches.

Stent grafts are used in two different sets of circumstances.

Spontaneous and iatrogenic arterial rupture

One of the most important indications for using stent grafts is the treatment of vessel rupture during angioplasty – classically iliac artery rupture. **All catheter laboratories should keep one or two stent grafts in reserve specifically to treat this eventuality.** Your patient and their lawyer will expect you to know how to use it!

Use similar principles for choosing a stent for occlusive disease. Choose a device that is long enough to cover the defect in the artery wall and is an appropriate diameter (i.e. oversized by at least 1 mm). Remember that it may be necessary to increase the size of your arterial sheath; most stent grafts require at least an 8Fr sheath. Choose the stent graft that is simplest to use and most likely to do the job effectively.

 Tip: You are attempting to fix a hole. The graft is usually either the same size as the balloon or 1–2 mm greater in diameter. Choose a length at least as long as the balloon or longer if you can deploy without covering anything important.

Three devices to 'get out of jail free'

You must have the equivalent of at least one of these on your shelf and know how to use it, unless you want to support a lawyer.

- **Balloon-mounted** (e.g. Atrium, Maquet) – basically just like a balloon-mounted stent. Great when the target site is of uniform diameter.
- **Self-expanding** The Viabahn (e.g. Gore Viabahn) is flexible, trackable and very simple to deploy by simply pulling a ripcord once the device is in position – there are several alternatives (e.g. Fluency, Bard) which are effectively like deploying a Nitinol stent.
  Remember, if you choose a Nitinol-based stent you really need to make sure you deploy the correct size as you cannot simply balloon it up – the Nitinol recoils.
- **Wallgraft** – a variation of the Wallstent – if you can use the Wallstent you can use this. Tends to shorten like the Wallstent. Not the number one choice if working close to critical branch vessels (Fig. 21.1).

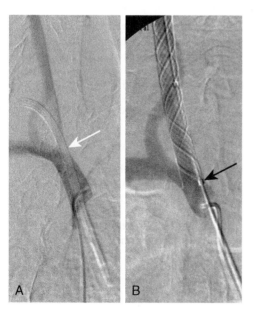

Fig. 21.1 ■ The great escape. (A) A 13.5Fr dialysis catheter has been placed in the right common carotid artery. The low puncture (arrow) would necessitate a thoracotomy to repair surgically. (B) Following placement of a Wallgraft (Boston Scientific), the dialysis catheter was removed without bleeding after the graft was placed. Note the end of the graft (arrow) overhangs the origin of the subclavian artery. Covering the hole was much more important than the potential for arm ischaemia.

Planned elective repair of aneurysmal disease

This is covered in more detail in the section on treating aneurysmal disease (Ch. 33). Clearly AAA rupture can be treated by stent grafts and the rules regarding sizing are similar to elective repair.

 Tip: Make sure that this is reviewed at the safety check and is available before starting the case. Otherwise you will find that someone used it for the unscheduled aneurysm yesterday.

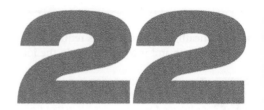

Essential equipment: Inferior vena caval filters

Purpose

Inferior vena cava (IVC) filters are placed to prevent pulmonary embolism. They are most often used when there is a contraindication to anticoagulation. Despite the name, they are occasionally used in the superior vena cava.

Description

IVC filters use a form of wire lattice, often umbrella-shaped, to catch large blood clots, while allowing flow through the inferior vena cava. They are introduced in a constrained state and expand when released (like a self-expanding stent). IVC filters are designed to anchor to the IVC wall using a combination of radial force; most have additional barbs/feet, which pierce the wall. Some designs incorporate secondary struts to help centre the filter within the IVC.

Measurements

Filter

Orientation This is not a measurement but is vitally important. Remember, this relates to whether the filter is intended to be deployed from above (e.g. jugular vein) or below (e.g. femoral vein).

Diameter (mm) A range of IVC diameters of the device can be safely deployed. This varies significantly between devices. Consult the instructions for use of the device.

 Alarm: If you choose too small a filter, you will find yourself wondering whether cardiothoracic surgery assistance is needed to extract it from the heart or pulmonary artery?

 Tip: If you find yourself asking this question the answer is yes!

Length (mm) There is usually plenty of space to allow filter placement but, in some cases, space will be at a premium, e.g. in the rare SVC deployment.

Delivery system

Diameter (French size) This dictates the sheath size required.

Length (cm) This determines whether the device will reach the deployment site from your access point and also how long a guidewire you will need.

Guidewire size (inches) In practice, almost all devices are designed for use with a 0.035-inch guidewire.

Know what to ask for

There are only three considerations:

Diameter of the IVC You must ensure that the device you choose is suitable for deployment in the patient's IVC. Consult the instructions for use of the device.

Permanent or retrievable?
Retrievable filters are placed to cover a period of risk (e.g. hip surgery in a patient with previous pulmonary embolism). They are deployed with the intention of removing them when the risk has abated.

 Alarm: Some retrievable filters can only be removed for a specified time, after which they risk incorporation in the IVC wall and have become permanent.

Permanent filters are intended to be left in place for life. Many retrievable filters have been designed to be left permanently in place if the situation changes, e.g. they have caught a large thrombus.

 Alarm: Some filters cannot be retrieved. These are by definition permanent.

Which approach? The vast majority of IVC filters are placed from the right internal jugular vein, this is a simple straight route and can be used in patients with extensive deep vein thrombosis.

 Tip: Before asking for the filter your boss prefers, make sure you have assessed whether it is suitable for the patient-specific scenario. Then simply ask for a jugular or femoral filter.

Know how to use it

The IVC is the commonest deployment site. If possible, the filter should be placed below the level of the renal veins. Remember to check the IVC diameter is appropriate for the planned device. Most devices are deployed as a variant of the familiar pusher/sheath system.

- The deployment sheath is placed below the planned deployment site.
- The compressed filter is inserted and pushed to the end of the sheath.
- The sheath is withdrawn and the filter deployed.
- Most systems have an attachment mechanism that is then released. However, each type of filter is deployed differently and there may even be differences for a single type of filter, depending on whether the jugular or femoral route is used. Read the instructions carefully before use; if you do not understand them, **seek help!**

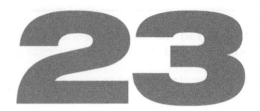

Essential equipment: Embolization

Essential equipment

Embolotherapy is the deliberate blockage of blood vessels; embolization may be lifesaving when used to stop haemorrhage. Embolization is increasingly used as an adjunct to surgery and in the treatment of a variety of benign and malignant tumours. Many embolic agents are available to block vessels of different sizes, from large arteries to capillaries. The choice of the agent used depends on the individual circumstances of the case.

Embolic agents are usually divided into:

- Mechanical occlusion devices: coils and vascular plugs
- Particulate agents: polyvinyl alcohol (PVA), Gelfoam and autologous blood clot
- Liquid agents: sclerosants, adhesives and Onyx.

Most embolization procedures use permanent embolic material, however there is one 'temporary' agent available, 'Gelfoam', which can be invaluable in particular circumstances.

Coils and plugs

Purpose Coils and plugs are permanent embolic agents and are used when you need to block a few feeding vessels or pack small aneurysms.

Action Coils and plugs have three effects:

- They damage the intima leading to release of thrombogenic agents.
- They provide a large thrombogenic surface.
- They cause mechanical occlusion of the lumen.

The first two factors are the most important; even the tightest-packed coils will not effectively block a vessel without thrombus. Some coils have fibres to increase thrombogenicity.

Coils are pushed through the delivery catheter with a guidewire or a dedicated coil pusher.

 Alarm: Friction between the coil and the lumen of the catheter progressively damages the lining and this can cause considerable problems when multiple coils are required. If you notice increasing resistance to coil introduction, change the catheter before a coil jams in the lumen and blocks the catheter leading to loss of your hard-fought-for position!

Units of measurement There are many types of coil available; all have three size parameters:

Diameter of the coil wire This is equivalent to guidewire diameter and varies from 0.014 to 0.038 inch diameter. Use a coil that is the correct diameter for your delivery catheter – too big and it will not fit; too small and it may jam with the pusher in the catheter.

Unconstrained length Measured in centimetres (cm). This varies with the type of coil but, in general, increases with the coiled diameter. Shorter coils are much easier to manage. Very floppy coils often come in very long lengths due to their ability to pack very tightly into almost any shaped space.

Diameter of the formed coil Measured in millimetres (mm). Coils come in a large range of diameters from 2 mm to over 20 mm. There are even 'straight' coils for blocking tiny vessels, e.g. in the colonic mesentery. Coils should be slightly oversized relative to the diameter of the target vessel, as this allows them to grip the vessel wall and to be closely packed (Fig. 23.1).

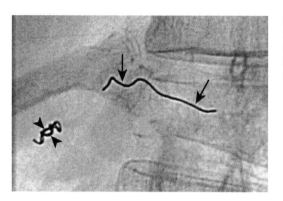

Fig. 23.1 ▦ Embolization of a vertebral artery for renal metastasis. The effect of coil size: 3-mm coils (arrowheads) have packed tightly but a 4-mm coil has remained straight (arrows).

Know what to ask for

Judging coil size is more often practiced as an art rather than as a science. If possible, and particularly if you are inexperienced, measure from available cross-sectional imaging as a guide. Remember vessel diameters can change due to vasodilation/constriction and the decision at the time of embolization is the key. First, think about the catheter lumen – do you need an 0.018 (microcatheter) or an 0.035 (conventional catheter). Next, decide the target vessel diameter – oversize by at least 1 mm. Softer coils mean that you can oversize a bit more with an added safety margin. Finally, how much space do you have before the next non-target vessel (behind the point of embolization) – this determines the coil length. Eventually, this will all become second nature and you will find you have confidently uttered the words – 'could I have a 035/6 mm coil and what lengths do we have?' To complicate matters further however, there are different coil materials and geometry, though these are all far less important than making sure the size is right!

Know how to use it

This is a brief guide relevant only to coils, there is further information below.

Position the catheter Before even opening that coil, confirm that the catheter position is stable by passing the coil pusher/guidewire to its tip. If the catheter dislodges during this manoeuvre, it will definitely displace if you try to deploy a coil through it!

Introducing coils into the catheter Coils are held straight in a short cartridge, which is discarded after the coil has been pushed into the catheter. The tip of the cartridge is placed into the hub of the catheter and the coil is pushed into the catheter using the provided pusher or the stiff end of a straight guidewire. Make sure that you hold the cartridge and the catheter tightly together if you do not want the coil to deploy in the catheter hub!

Pushing the coils – standard 0.035 coil Once the coil is in the catheter, it is normal to use the reverse end of the guidewire to advance it 10–20 cm along the catheter. Coils can be pushed with conventional straight guidewires.

Pushing the coils – 0.018 coil The guidewires supplied with microcatheters can jam when used to deliver coils. Special microcoil pushers have a flexible plastic fibre tip on a stiff metal shaft. They are packaged separately and have to be requested. Use the back end of the wire until the coil is at least 30 cm into the catheter.

Extruding coils This is the stage when things are most likely to go wrong. Be careful to hold the catheter in position as the coil is pushed to its tip. Slowly start to push the coil out of the catheter; you may feel slight resistance as it starts to coil. Make sure that the catheter is not pushed back out of the target vessel. Continue slowly until the whole coil is out of the catheter. Following placement of the first coil, the catheter may have to be pulled back a few millimetres to make sufficient space to allow subsequent coils to be deployed.

 Tip: Note how much of the pusher remains outside the catheter when the coil is about 15 cm from deployment. Consider marking this position on the drapes. For subsequent coils, do not screen until you reach this stage.

After multiple coils have been deployed, it can be difficult to be certain the last coil has been completely deployed and is clear of the catheter; always use the guidewire against the coil to back the catheter off.

Completion angiography After a few coils have been deployed, perform an angiogram to assess flow. It is helpful to pull the catheter back a little and to inject gently in order not to dislodge a newly formed clot. When the flow is very slow, wait for a couple of minutes to see if the vessel thromboses. If there is still brisk flow, then more coils are needed. If the flow has stopped, you can stop too.

Vascular plugs

Purpose Vascular plugs are most often used where multiple coils would be needed or there is high flow and a particular risk of distal embolization. The Amplatzer vascular plug (AVP) is a self-expanding nitinol wire mesh used for occlusion of vessels from approximately 3–16 mm diameter. Microvascular plugs (MVP) are nitinol/polytetrafluoroethylene (PTFE) plugs, which will pass through a standard microcatheter.

Action The nitinol mesh is mounted on a delivery wire by a screw thread and inserted into a delivery catheter in a compressed form. The tip of the delivery catheter is positioned just beyond the deployment site. When the AVP reaches the target site, the plug is held in position while the delivery catheter is pulled back; this allows the plug to open. Correct sizing can be confirmed before the plug is detached. Thrombosis usually takes 5–10 min to occur.

Know what to ask for

There are a variety of different AVP devices (currently imaginatively numbered 1–4) available with different configurations. The primary decision is to decide the target vessel diameter and then oversize by 30–50%; there is a sizing guide available in the manufacturer's literature. The device lengths vary depending on the particular AVP type.

Know how to use it

Assess the target As with all embolization, imaging is the key. The size and length of the target vessel must be assessed. If the site is suitable, a device is chosen, which is 30–50% larger than the target vessel diameter.

Suitability The AVP must be delivered to the target site; this can be a real challenge in very tortuous vessels.

Access Choose a sheath size appropriate to the AVP/guide-catheter needed. Suggested catheter sizes are: 4–8-mm 5Fr; 10–12-mm 6Fr and 14–16-mm 8Fr.

Deployment The AVP comes constrained in a plastic tube to allow introduction into the delivery catheter. Feel free to push it out of the tube to see how it expands, as it is readily pulled back in. Do not pull it out, as you will need to backload the delivery wire into the plastic tube to constrain it again. Simply pop the outer plastic tube through the haemostatic valve and use the delivery wire to push the plug to its destination. It may need some determined pushing for the larger plugs but it usually gets easier. Once in place, the sheath is pulled back to allow the AVP to expand. If repositioning is needed, maintain traction on the wire and re-advance the delivery catheter to recapture the device.

Check angiogram Perform a check angiogram to confirm the position of the device. If it is in the correct place, then simply attach the supplied pin vice and turn the delivery wire anticlockwise to unscrew and release the AVP. You should wait 5–10 min before performing another check angiogram to confirm occlusion.

Particulate embolic agents

 Alarm: These agents are injected and great care must be taken to avoid inadvertent embolization. Hence, it is standard practice to prepare these agents on a separate trolley and, if possible, to use syringes of different sizes from those on the angiographic trolley.

Spheres and beads

Purpose Vascular occlusion; small- to medium-sized arteries. Some of these agents may be combined with drug-elution or radioactive particles.

Action The particles wedge in vessels of the corresponding diameter, where they either cause simple occlusion or local release of a therapeutic agent or localised radiotherapy.

Units of measurement Usually measured in micrometres (μm). Remember that particle sizes suitable for plain PVA embolization may not be safe for novel agents.

Know what to ask for

The first thing to ask is: 'why am I not using standard PVA? It's cheap, usually effective and the agent that has the most experience and evidence behind it'. Either you have a specialized application or are always on that optimistic edge that means new is better. The potential candidates are:

- Spherical PVA: More regular surface than conventional PVA and also more compressible; theoretical advantage of lower catheter occlusion but more distal embolization and increased necrosis. Rarely needed or used.

- Bead Block: A PVA hydrogel-based microsphere that comes preloaded in coloured syringes – it is still not radiopaque though, and needs to be mixed with contrast.
- DC Bead: A Bead Block variant that can be loaded with doxorubicin (needs to be done in your pharmacy), and is used in the treatment of hepatoma. Other drug–bead combinations are available, e.g. irinotecan.
- Embospheres: These are gelatin-based microspheres, which come in coloured pre-filled syringes and are mixed with a 50/50 contrast saline mix to visualize.
- Theraspheres/SIR spheres: These are glass microspheres that contain the radioactive material Yttrium 90, used in the treatment of liver tumours.

Know how to use it

The principles of embolization practice are the same as PVA, however for some of these specialized applications, e.g. radioactive microspheres, additional expert training and precautions are needed.

Liquid embolic agents

Liquid agents divide into two main categories: sclerosants and glues. The former includes absolute alcohol and sodium tetradecyl sulphate (STS). The use of tissue adhesives, such as cyanoacrylate, is increasing, particularly for AVM and trauma with impaired coagulation. The final category of agent is Onyx, a polymer that is injected dissolved in dimethyl sulphoxide (DMSO).

Liquid agents are the most difficult of the embolic agents to control and are the least forgiving. Liquids permeate to the smallest vessels and therefore can cause complete tissue necrosis. Their use is best restricted to expert hands and, therefore, only limited discussion is given here.

Sclerosants

Absolute alcohol

Purpose Permanent and complete vascular occlusion; most often used to treat vascular malformations and tumours.

Action Causes cell death by dehydration. Can cause perivascular necrosis and will cause local tissue necrosis if extravasation occurs.

Units of measurement Usually measured in millilitres (mL). Maximum adult dose is ethanol 1 mg/kg.

Know what to ask for This is not an agent for beginners, so the first thing to ask for is an expert. The second thing to ask for is often anaesthetic help. An absolute alcohol injection is often very painful and therefore suitable sedation/analgesia and frequently general anaesthesia, are needed.

Know how to use it Absolute alcohol is not visible fluoroscopically, it is mixed 1 : 1 with contrast. Establish a secure and safe position and a safe injection rate that does not cause reflux or extravasation with test injections of contrast. Balloon occlusion catheters or, where appropriate, tourniquets can be used to achieve better control. Frequent check angiography is mandatory to ensure that the situation does not change as thrombosis occurs.

If large amounts of absolute alcohol enter the systemic circulation, toxic effects including central nervous system (CNS) depression, haemolysis and cardiac arrest can occur. Systemic absorption may make the patients feel alcohol-intoxicated and it is worth warning them about this effect.

Sodium tetradecyl sulphate (STS)

Purpose Permanent vascular occlusion less potent than absolute alcohol; most often used in venous sclerotherapy and as an adjunct to coil embolization during varicocele embolization.

Action STS is a chemical irritant and damages vascular endothelium, which causes thrombosis. Anaphylactic shock has been reported.

Units of measurement Measured in millilitres (mL). Maximum adult dose 10 mL per treatment session.

Know what to ask for Most people will use either 1% or 3% STS. Higher concentrations are usually used for larger lesions.

Know how to use it There are two techniques for using STS:

1. Direct injection of liquid STS is most commonly used to occlude small tributaries during varicocele embolization. Usually distal coils have been deployed. A test injection of contrast is made to check distal occlusion and the volume of STS, which will be required to fill the desired section of the testicular vein. Ask for 3% STS and take particular care to avoid spill of STS into the epididymal veins, as this will cause epididymitis.
2. Alternatively, STS is made into a foam by mixing with air (foam sclerotherapy). Simply use a three-way tap, connect a syringe with 1 mL of STS to 3 mL of air. Mix back and forward until a foam is formed. STS foam displaces blood and can travel further than you think. Foam sclerotherapy is often used to treat varicose veins and progress of the foam is monitored and, if necessary, controlled by using real-time ultrasound. Intense venous spasm is common.

Glue

Purpose Glue (n-butyl-cyanoacrylate) is a permanent embolic agent, which can permeate into the smallest vessels or AVM nidus. It was initially used for arteriovenous malformations, particularly by neuroradiologists, however it is increasingly used for peripheral embolization.

Action Cyanoacrylate polymerizes when it comes into contact with ions (e.g. in blood or saline flush) forming a solid cast. The polymerization reaction is exothermic, which also induces a localized inflammatory response.

Units of measurement Glue usually comes in a 1-mL vial. Only small volumes, usually <1 mL, of glue are injected at a time.

Know what to ask for

N-butyl cyanoacrylate (NBCA): this is basically superglue for medical use. There are different preparations of NBCA available; these have slightly different polymerization properties. It is important to become familiar with the brand used in your local practice.

Lipiodol: this is usually added to the cyanoacrylate, as it both opacifies the glue and by varying the proportion, can be titrated to delay the polymerization. Catheters need to be prepared with a flush of 5% dextrose so that they do not contain ions or the glue will set in the catheter – nil points.

Know how to use it

This is another of these expert agents and there are no second chances if you over-inject glue. This section is brief as it is not an agent to learn to use from a book!

- Glue is always injected via a microcatheter, which should be close to the target but not so close that it will get glued in place. Lipiodol causes polycarbonate to disintegrate and it is important to make sure that your catheters, taps and syringes are compatible with this use.
- A three-way tap is connected to a 1-mL and 5-mL syringe.
- Practice injections are made to estimate the correct volume and injection rate to use; contrast via the 1 mL and flush with 5% dextrose via the 5 mL. It is vital to get the rate of both the initial injection and the flush correct.
- A solution of cyanoacrylate and Lipiodol is prepared. It is usually mixed between 1:1 and 1:4, which makes polymerization between 1–4 s, respectively, but note this is not exact!
- The microcatheter is flushed with 5% dextrose.
- The three-way tap is attached with a 1-mL syringe (glue) and a 5-mL syringe (dextrose).
- Everyone concentrates and injects as planned.
- When the opacified glue has exited the catheter the microcatheter is usually withdrawn as the dextrose is injected, to stop it being glued in place.

What could possibly go wrong … well it is possible to glue in the catheter, mis-time the polymerization with non-target embolization, etc. Definitely, one to learn from an expert colleague.

 Alarm: Following glue embolization, change the catheter. Never ever flush or perform angiography through a catheter that has been used for glue embolization, there is always some residual glue, which will result in disaster.

Onyx

Purpose Onyx is a novel permanent viscous liquid embolic agent with delayed solidification, which makes it more controllable than other liquid agents. It is used mainly in the embolization of AVM and endoleaks.

Action Onyx is comprised of EVOH (ethylene vinyl alcohol) copolymer dissolved in DMSO (dimethyl sulfoxide), and suspended in tantalum powder. The agent solidifies to form a solid cast after a period of about 10–30 min.

Units of measurement Onyx is supplied in 1.5/6-mL vials, and is mixed with the same volume of the solvent DMSO. Multiple vials of Onyx may be required for larger lesions.

Know what to ask for

Onyx is delivered via a microcatheter, which should be placed into the target lesion if possible. Preparation of Onyx has several key steps and the vials are kept on a shaker for at least 20 min to ensure proper mixing of the tantalum powder.

Know how to use it

Another expert agent, and while more controllable than many liquid embolic agents, the complexities of preparation and the need to titrate the volume of Onyx with the evolving angiographic picture mean that experience is needed. In outline:

- Onyx preparation usually starts before the microcatheter reaches its final destination.
- The microcatheter is placed in the lesion and check angiography performed.
- The microcatheter dead space is flushed with DMSO – slowly, as DMSO is painful and over-injection will cause vasospasm.
- One-mL aliquots of Onyx are injected over at least 40–60 s under continuous fluoroscopic guidance.
- Repeated injections may be required and repeat angiography and catheter repositioning are possible.

Onyx is certainly more controllable but the usual risks of embolization apply and it is an expensive agent if large volumes are required.

DMSO has a very characteristic aroma; it is important to warn the patient that they will smell of this for some time after the procedure.

 Alarm: Monopolar diathermy and Onyx do not mix, as the Onyx will ignite – important to inform that surgeon about to excise the AVM after embolization.

Temporary embolic agents

This is a short list of one, or at a stretch possibly two, agents. The most versatile of all embolic agents and an invaluable tool used is Gelfoam. Remember it is likely to be temporary but this is not guaranteed.

Gelfoam

Purpose Gelfoam is multipurpose and can cause vascular occlusion from capillary to medium-sized vessels, depending on the form (powder/sheet) and how you prepare it.

Action Gelfoam swells on contact with blood and causes vascular occlusion. It causes minimal inflammatory response and vessel recanalization can occur after several weeks and it is therefore defined as a 'temporary' agent.

Know what to ask for

Gelfoam comes in different forms with completely different uses:
- **Gelfoam sheet** is cut into 'pledgets' 1–2 mm in size, or larger 'torpedoes' 1–2 × 10–15 mm; these are used to block larger vessels; tissue infarction is rare.
- **Gelfoam powder** comprises small particles (40–60 μm); vessel occlusion occurs at the capillary level; hence tissue necrosis is likely.

 Tip: Stick with the Gelfoam sheet, it is much more forgiving. In reality, Gelfoam powder is rarely used.

Know how to use it

The usual embolization standards of selective catheterization and stable catheter position apply.

Gelfoam pledgets Simply prepared using sharp scissors to make parallel cuts about 1 mm wide across the Gelfoam sheet until it resembles a comb (Fig. 23.2). This is then trimmed at right

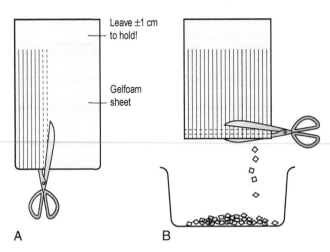

Leave ±1 cm to hold!

Gelfoam sheet

A   B

Fig. 23.2 ■ The Gelfoam comb. (A) Cut 1-mm longitudinal strips into the Gelfoam sheet. (B) Cut transversely across the Gelfoam comb. Do not forget to catch the pledgets in a gallipot.

angles to this to make 1 × 1 mm pieces. The pledgets are soaked in about 20 mL contrast for a few minutes to allow the Gelfoam to soften. Syringing the Gelfoam back and forwards in the gallipot will help soften the particles. When the pledgets become soft and slightly translucent, they are ready to use.

Using Gelfoam pledgets The soft pledgets can be drawn up into a 20-mL syringe. This should be connected to a 5-mL syringe via a three-way tap. The 20-mL syringe is the reservoir and the 5-mL is used to inject the pledgets. Pledgets can be injected through conventional angiographic catheters and guide-catheters. Microcatheters will tend to block. Gelfoam floats in contrast and therefore injection should be made with the syringe nozzle pointing upwards. Injection is made under continuous fluoroscopic guidance and continued until the flow in the target vessel is almost at a standstill. Check angiography shows a characteristic pruned appearance, with the main vessel and proximal portions of branches filling.

Gelfoam torpedoes These are made from the same Gelfoam sheet but cut into larger squares.

Using Gelfoam torpedoes The 5 × 5 mm stamps can be rolled and injected like large pledgets; use only with a very stable catheter position; 10 × 10 mm stamps are used dry and rolled tightly, they then can be pushed into a catheter or sheath; in this form they are excellent for plugging tracts (see Ch. 38).

Alarm: Gelfoam slurry can be completely mixed into an emulsion via the three-way tap system – be aware this is effectively liquid embolization and may reach capillary level and cause necrosis.

Autologous blood clot

Ah … nostalgia! This is now rarely used and is reserved for situations in which a short duration of occlusion is desirable, e.g. post-traumatic high-flow priapism. A sample of the patient's blood is withdrawn at the start of the procedure and allowed to clot in a gallipot. The clot can be macerated and aspirated into a syringe for injection into the target vessel.

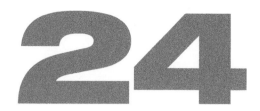

Essential equipment: Drainage catheters

Purpose

Drainage catheters allow fluid to be released from collections and structures.

Description

Virtually all drainage catheters are pigtail-shaped. The pigtail in some catheters is locked in position to provide anchorage.

Measurements

Drainage catheters are sized primarily by their diameter in Fr. The bigger the Fr size, the bigger the drainage holes and the thicker the material that will drain.

Know what to ask for

Think about the likely drainage contents or, even better, look at what was aspirated as you targeted the collection. As a guide: 8–10Fr for fluid/thin pus; 12–14Fr for thick pus; >16Fr for really turbid/semisolid collections.

Know how to use it

The mechanism to lock the catheter usually involves tensioning threads between the catheter hub and pigtail. As the locking mechanism varies between individual devices, familiarize yourself with the systems used in your hospital. Failure to unlock the catheter at removal will cause a large exit wound; intense screaming from the patient usually warns the alert operator.

 Alarm: During catheter removal, it is easy to accidentally leave the suture behind, which can cause a foreign body reaction. Check that the retention suture has come out with the catheter.

Essential equipment: Ureteric stents

Purpose

Ureteric stents are placed across ureteric strictures to relieve ureteric obstruction and restore anatomical drainage from the renal pelvis to the bladder/ileal conduit.

Description

All ureteric stent systems are hollow plastic tubes with a double-ended pigtail configuration (Fig. 25.1). There are differences in materials and delivery systems. Interventional radiologists are usually involved in antegrade stent placement via a nephrostomy. A pusher is used to deliver the stent into position over a suitably stiff guidewire. Some designs incorporate an inner plastic stiffener, which runs through the stent. Either the pusher plugs into the proximal end of the stent or a suture loop is present to allow stent retraction if pushed too far.

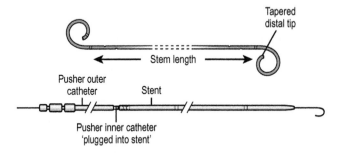

Tapered
distal tip

Stem length

Pusher outer
catheter

Stent

Pusher inner catheter
'plugged into stent'

Fig. 25.1 Ureteric stent system.

Measurements

There are two factors to consider: diameter and length.

Most departments use 8Fr diameter stents. The way manufacturers describe stent length can be confusing; some are described from tip to tip; others only describe the length of the stem component. Make sure you know which design your department favours.

Know what to ask for

An 8Fr 22-cm stem length ureteric stent.

Know how to use it

This is covered in more detail in Chapter 41.

Access Percutaneous via nephrostomy.

Insertion The stent is delivered over a suitably stiff guidewire; Amplatz superstiff with a 7-cm floppy tip is a popular choice.

Positioning The distal stent is advanced into the bladder and the guidewire retracted slightly to allow the loop to form in the bladder. The proximal end is fluoroscoped to ensure it lies within the renal pelvis and positioning adjustment made.

Deployment The wire is carefully withdrawn until the floppy part of the wire enters the proximal stent when the pigtail will start to form, skilfully and gently push forward on the pusher and the pigtail forms and you retain access as the wire will prolapse into the renal pelvis. If pushed too far forward, the stent can be retracted using retention sutures if present! Keep the pusher in situ until the retention suture has been cut and removed to avoid accidently misplacing the stent.

 Alarm: Sometimes advancing the stent is difficult – consider using a peel-away sheath advanced into the proximal ureter to reduce friction.

Section Three

Principles of intervention

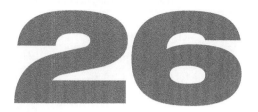

Principles of imaging guidance for intervention

A wide range of interventional procedures can only be safely performed with accurate imaging guidance. The aim of this chapter is to outline the basic principles of imaging-directed intervention. Ultrasound, computed tomography and fluoroscopy have complementary roles; individual circumstances dictate the optimal modality.

Ultrasound guidance

Ultrasound is ideal for many biopsy and drainage procedures and allows the procedure to be visualized in real-time. Use ultrasound if it clearly demonstrates the target and a suitable approach. Usually, this is achieved in solid organs or for larger abdominal collections. As a basic principle, use the highest-frequency probe that gives a good image from the skin to the target site. Use a 7.5-MHz probe for superficial structures and a 3.5–5-MHz probe for deeper structures. It is exceedingly helpful to have a probe with a small footprint, as this improves access.

Sterility All invasive procedures should be performed with aseptic technique. Sterile ultrasound probe covers and ultrasound gel are readily available. Sterile ultrasound gel is used outside the ultrasound probe cover, but ordinary ultrasound gel can be used inside the probe cover. A clean drape should be used to cover the probe cable. Attach the cable to the drapes with a towel clip to save dropping an expensive probe.

 Tip: If you do not possess a suitably sized probe cover, improvise with a sterile surgical glove. Cut the cuff off the second glove and use this as a 'rubber band' to attach the glove/drape to the probe.

Directing punctures The ultrasound image represents a slice of tissue only 1 mm thick; much less than the width of the probe. For effective guidance, the needle must pass along the scan plane, which runs directly along the midline of the probe; even a small degree of misalignment will mean that the needle is not in the scan plane (Fig. 26.1). The importance of this relationship cannot be overemphasized; this is the single most important factor in successful ultrasound guidance.

 Tip: If you cannot see the needle, look to check that the needle and probe are aligned correctly.

Many probes come with a needle guide that can be used for the majority of ultrasound-guided interventions; the alternative is to use the freehand technique.

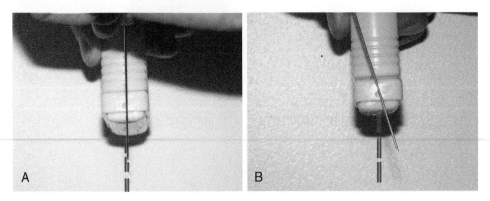

Fig. 26.1 ■ The importance of keeping the needle in the plane of the ultrasound beam. (A) The needle path will be in the focused ultrasound beam. (B) Despite starting in the middle of the probe, the needle is angled out of the beam and will not be visualized.

A needle guide is so simple to use that no experience is needed to manage it. The guide attaches to the probe and constrains the needle to a predetermined path. The needle trajectory is displayed as two broken parallel lines superimposed on the image. This usually has to be selected on the ultrasound machine itself. The probe is positioned so that the projected needle path crosses the target. The needle is then advanced to the target (Fig. 26.2).

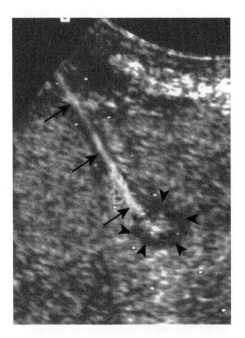

Fig. 26.2 ■ Biopsy of a small hepatic metastasis using a needle guide (arrowheads). The white dots showing the projected needle path are clearly visible and the needle (arrows) can be seen entering the lesion.

In reality, almost all interventionalists use the freehand technique, as it allows greater flexibility in approach because you are not constrained to the path of the needle guide. In addition, with the freehand technique, there is no needle guide to unclip before proceeding with intervention. As the name suggests, the needle is advanced along the scan plane with one hand, while the probe is fixed with the other. The most common problems are due to angulation or rotation of the probe relative to the path of the needle. Remember that wafer-thin ultrasound beam and work within it. Spending time and practice on ultrasound phantoms or other models to become efficient at ultrasound-guided puncture is highly recommended.

Tip: When the needle tip is not clearly seen, gently oscillating the needle backwards and forwards greatly enhances its visibility.

Computed tomography guidance

CT is used to guide biopsies and drainage of areas that cannot be seen on ultrasound, e.g. the lung, mediastinum, bone and areas of the abdomen obscured by bowel gas. There are several disadvantages to using CT compared with ultrasound:

- Needle passage cannot be viewed in real-time.
- The patient must be brought in and out of the scanner for each needle pass.
- It is time-consuming and exposes both patient and operator to radiation.

The principles of CT guidance are simple, although the procedure can be technically challenging. When performing procedures in the chest and abdomen, it is important to explain to the patient the necessity to try to take the same size breath during each scan and needle pass.

Patient positioning The diagnostic scans are reviewed and a suitable needle path is chosen. The patient is positioned either supine or prone, depending on the position of the target. Remember that, although angled needle trajectories can be used, it is simplest to judge a vertical needle pass.

Tip: Sometimes, it can be helpful to tilt the CT gantry as this allows the needle to be angulated cranially or caudally while remaining in the scan plane.

The simplest way to mark the puncture site is to use a reference grid placed over the region of interest. Grids can be purchased or can be readily made from some thin plastic tubing (Fig. 26.3).

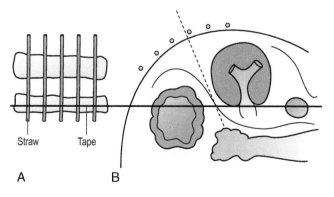

Straw   Tape

A   B

Fig. 26.3 (A) A CT grid can be readily made using plastic tubing and adhesive tape. (B) The optimal approach is determined by the markers.

CT guidance: a step-by-step approach:

1. The grid is positioned with the markers oriented perpendicular to the scan plane.
2. The patient is rescanned with the grid in place.
3. Select the slice that shows the optimal approach to the target and return the patient to this position.
4. Identify which of the grid lines corresponds to the best approach.
5. Turn on the light beam and simply mark where it intersects the chosen grid line.
6. Move the table to bring the patient out of the scanner gantry.
7. Clean, drape and anaesthetize the skin.
8. Advance the needle along the anticipated trajectory.
9. Re-scan the patient.
10. Repeat steps 8 and 9 as necessary.

If you are lucky, your unit will have a CT fluoroscopy module. Do not get too excited though, as it is not quite as dynamic as real fluoroscopy, but it does speed the procedure up significantly. Exact designs vary but, essentially, this system allows the operator to control the X-ray exposure at the table-side, doing a very small number of cuts at your chosen level. Some systems have motor-driven movement to the chosen position.

Tip: If you are uncertain about judging the approach, then use a 22G needle to verify the approach. A second needle is positioned alongside the first and its position checked again.

A common pitfall is for the needle to pass obliquely through the scan plane. This can be demonstrated by performing one or two cuts above and below the target plane. If the needle tip is still in a satisfactory position, proceed as normal; if not, reposition the needle, compensating for the incorrect angle.

If a drain is planned, most operators will acquire a short acquisition after the guidewire has been inserted to ensure enough wire is in place and coiled appropriately and also after the drain has been placed. It is very easy to contaminate the wire on the CT gantry – take care when re-positioning and weigh the wire down using, e.g. wet swabs.

Fluoroscopic guidance

Fluoroscopic guidance is used principally to guide percutaneous nephrolithotomy and biliary drainage and increasingly rarely to biopsy pulmonary masses and bones. Whenever possible, use an X-ray machine with a C-arm, and avoid machines with over-couch explorators. Remember the basic principle of radiology: two views are necessary for localization.

Position the patient for the procedure and fluoroscope to identify the target lesion. Centre the field on the lesion and mark the position with a pair of sponge forceps. It is nearly always possible to choose an approach that allows the needle to be advanced perpendicular to the skin. For pulmonary biopsy, ask the patient to suspend respiration. Advance the needle part-way to the target and then fluoroscope to confirm that the tract is passing in the correct direction. Rotate the C-arm through 90 degrees and fluoroscope again to determine the position of the needle tip relative to the target. Advance the needle until it reaches the target and re-confirm the position on the original projection.

The situation is slightly different during biliary drainage and nephrostomy, as an oblique approach is required for catheter and guidewire manipulation. When aiming at a specific duct or calyx, it is essential to know whether the needle is passing anterior or posterior to the target duct. This is resolved by rotating the C-arm (the patient can be rotated but remember there is a long needle sticking in them) and observing the movement of the needle relative to the target. If the needle is posterior, when the C-arm is rotated, the needle moves in the same direction as the C-arm rotation; if it moves in the opposite direction, it is anterior to the target. Remember that the reverse is true if you are turning the patient. When you think that you have grasped this concept, just wait until you try it in practice.

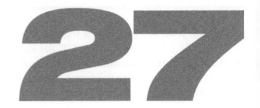

Principles of good fluoroscopy and radiation protection

Many interventional radiology procedures remain dependent on X-ray guidance. It is important to have good technique in order to minimize the radiation dose to the patient, yourself and the staff.

Fluoroscopy

Fluoroscopy or screening Real-time imaging is essential for catheter and guidewire manipulation. Whenever using fluoroscopy consider how to balance image quality with radiation dose. There are several factors which will come into play and different stages of the procedure may have different imaging requirements.

There are a couple of issues to bear in mind, the most important and perhaps least remembered is: it is easy to lapse into a fugue state with your foot on the pedal while considering what to do next, only screen when necessary.

 Tip: Get into the habit of regularly taking stock and considering the parameters you are using and ensuring you are optimizing them.

Image quality

There are only two settings to consider here:

Continuous fluoroscopy (high dose) Used when optimal image quality is required, e.g. embolization therapy with particles/liquids.

Pulsed fluoroscopy (lower dose) Used when less detail is required, e.g. when screening over-sensitive organs such as during fibroid embolization. Radiation dose is reduced as X-ray production is intermittent; the image from each pulse persists on the monitor to give an impression of continuity. At fewer than 7 pulses/s, the image is rather jerky (think dancing in a strobe light) and only suitable for crude catheter positioning, e.g. positioning a pigtail catheter. Whenever possible, use fluoroscopy rather than DSA runs, as this keeps the dose to a minimum.

Collimation/image area

This is a case of 'less is more'; pay attention and keep the X-ray beam collimated to the region of interest, this minimizes the patient dose. This will also reduce scatter, will improve image quality and reduce your radiation dose.

Image intensifier position

Always keep the image intensifier (II) as close to the patient as possible. This again reduces radiation dose and produces the sharpest quality image. There is sometimes a need to work close to the primary beam, e.g. during biliary intervention, particularly early in the procedure. Sometimes moving or angling the II will reduce your dose.

Many procedures will involve moving either/both the II and the patient. Try to do this without continually screening and only fluoroscope to fine tune.

Your position and standard radiation protection

Remember the inverse square law and stand as far from the X-rays as possible. If you have to work close to the primary beam, then make sure that you use standard radiation protection:

- Keep screening to a minimum and use the lowest dose that will suffice
- Try to keep your fingers out of the beam – collimation and tube angulation
- Protective glasses: these should be non-negotiable and if necessary insist on prescription glasses
- Thyroid shield
- Lead screens on the X-ray table
- Glass screens
- Use connection tubes.

Consider additional protection as long as they do not impair you

- Radiation protection gloves
- Additional lead strips. These can be wrapped in sterile drapes and will help to protect from scattered radiation.

Review your position regularly and move back as soon as it is possible to work with longer catheters and wires.

Store key images for reference

Last image hold The last fluoroscopic image is automatically stored on the monitor. Most systems have the facility to save these images so if you spot something important, stop screening and keep the image. In systems with two monitors, this image can be transferred to the reference monitor and used for guidance.

 Alarm: Do not just wear the radiation badges but make sure you know your radiation dose – it is a great incentive to improving radiation protection.

A guide to good fluoroscopy

Radiation protection is so important here is a guide to good fluoroscopy Aim to keep everyone's radiation exposure to a minimum. You are the person most at risk!

- Keep the image intensifier close to the patient.
- Centre over the area of interest.
- Try to move the table to the position of interest before screening when changing position or using oblique views.
- Use collimation.

- Use pulsed fluoroscopy if available – there is little dose reduction at >7 frames/s (FPS).
- Keep your hands out of the field – you may need your fingers in years to come.
- Use angiographic runs to sort out anatomy and pathology – do not perform repeated fluoroscopic injections.
- Keep your foot off the pedal unless you have a reason to screen and you are actively looking at the fluoroscopic image.

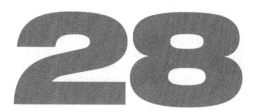

Principles of vascular access

Vascular access is the starting point for all diagnostic and interventional arterial and venous procedures. Common principles apply regarding choice of access site and equipment but there are significant differences between puncturing arteries and veins.

Choice of puncture site is dictated by the planned procedure; think what you need to achieve, consider the site of the lesion, and the size of sheath and catheter required.

The basic technique, first described by Seldinger, has three components:

1. Vessel puncture
2. Passage of the guidewire
3. Introduction of the catheter.

In general, arteries are pressurized and have thick walls, veins are at very low pressure and have thin walls, and this affects the puncture techniques, hence they are discussed separately.

Arterial puncture

Puncture sites are points where the artery has a consistent position, is relatively superficial, immobile and compressible against bone to obtain haemostasis. The most commonly used site is the right common femoral artery (CFA). However, many factors such as the upholstery of the patient, strength of the pulse and the site of the disease will influence the decision. The shortest, straightest route is nearly always best.

 Alarm: It is important to be familiar with the vascular anatomy at the chosen puncture site, as most arteries are accompanied by veins and nerves.

 Arterial puncture: a step-by-step guide

1. Check the patient is appropriately consented for the procedure. The main complications of arterial puncture can be readily remembered as the three **B**s: **bruising**, **bleeding** and **blockage** of the vessel; <1% of patients should need either a blood transfusion or an operation to put things right.
2. Choose the optimal puncture site; take time to find the pulse; clean and drape the area.
3. Palpate the pulse.
   If there is a weak or absent pulse or a thrill:
4. Use ultrasound to check what is happening.
5. Perform puncture using ultrasound guidance.

Tip: Have a low threshold for using ultrasound guidance when obtaining arterial access, especially in esoteric sites and in the larger patient. However, for day-to-day retrograde CFA access, you will hit the artery much more often than you will miss.

If there is a good pulse:
6. Feel for the point of maximum pulsation.
7. Infiltrate from skin to artery with 1% lidocaine. Many operators place a finger to either side of the point of maximum pulsation and infiltrate in between. Disconnect the syringe but leave the needle in situ to mark where to make the skin incision.
8. Make a skin incision appropriate to catheter/sheath size.
9. Place gauze swabs to absorb blood.
10. Insert the needle at 45 degrees to the skin, aiming towards the point of maximum pulsation. Pulsation transmitted to the needle increases as the needle tip approaches the artery wall but falls as the wall is punctured. There is often a change in resistance felt at the arterial wall and on entry to the vessel lumen.

Alarm: A crunching sensation indicates either heavy calcification in the wall or that you are in bone. In the former case, consider using ultrasound to look for a window in the plaque. In the latter case … pull the needle back and start again.
11. Free pulsatile backflow indicates that the needle tip is in the lumen.
12. Poor flow is seen below a high-grade stenosis or occlusion or if the needle is abutting the artery wall.

Alarm: There will be little flow when using a 21G needle.
13. The needle position is usually quite stable; it does not need to be held with a vice-like grip.

Tip: You will occasionally transfix an artery as the needle is introduced. This occurs most often in young thin patients with compressible arteries. Always pull the needle back slowly after a puncture, you may get a second bite at the cherry.

Fluoroscopic guidance If by chance either ultrasound is not available or the views are suboptimal, then fluoroscopy may help. However, fluoroscopy is far inferior to ultrasound, not least because of the proximity of your fingers to the beam. The presence of vascular calcification can be an additional aid to localizing the vessel. Very rarely, a roadmap image from another catheter can be used. If you cannot get access at your preferred site, use an alternative approach; remember to include the original access site in the subsequent angiogram to clarify the situation.

Passage of the guidewire

The 3-mm J-wire is the most frequently used initial guidewire. Arterial sheaths often come with a short guidewire with straight and J-tips (at the opposite ends); the straight end is useful in small vessels. Use the introducer to advance the J-wire into the needle. If the introducer is not immediately available, which usually means it has migrated to the floor, it is possible to straighten the J-wire by applying tension to the inner mandrel (Fig. 28.1). The wire should advance smoothly and without resistance when held loosely between finger and thumb. There is a very characteristic feeling when a guidewire is passed through a needle or has a catheter passed over it – you will learn to recognize it but it is still best to use fluoroscopic guidance to ensure that the wire follows the expected path without buckling or deforming (Fig. 28.2). It is better to put plenty of wire in the vessel rather than too little!

Alarm: Never use force on a guidewire; something is wrong; **STOP** and **CHECK**. Use fluoroscopy to check wire passage. Force is **never** necessary and **always** harmful.

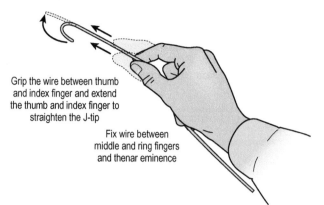

Fig. 28.1 Straightening the J-wire. Fix the wire between the middle and ring fingers and the thenar eminence. Grip the wire between thumb and index finger and extend the thumb and index finger to straighten the J-tip.

Fig. 28.2 A 0.018-inch guidewire has kinked at the end of the catheter (arrow). Further pressure has caused a subcutaneous loop to form (arrowheads). The wire was pulled back and straightened to allow the catheter to be advanced.

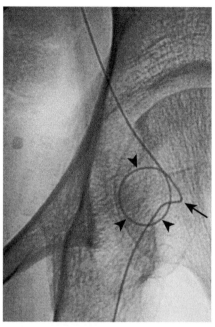

Troubleshooting

The wire will not advance beyond the needle tip

- It is not intraluminal – usually the needle has been advanced too far and is in the far wall of the vessel. Remove the wire and verify pulsatile backflow; reposition as necessary.
- The needle tip is abutting plaque – alter the angle of the needle; flattening towards the skin is often helpful (Fig. 28.3). Try straightening the wire tip and re-directing.

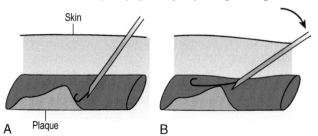

Fig. 28.3 Flattening the needle against the skin will often allow the wire to negotiate plaque adjacent to the puncture site.

Still no progress? If there is good backflow, gently inject some contrast under fluoroscopic guidance to confirm intraluminal position. This may be all that is required to resolve the problem but if more detail is required then consider an angiographic run. If the needle position is relatively stable use a connecting tube, but check you can still aspirate freely after connecting and before injecting. A roadmap may help you to navigate the wire. Use tight collimation; keep your fingers out of the main beam.

Alarm: Never omit the gentle test injection under fluoroscopy; this can avoid an unsightly splurge or even dissection of the artery.

Try another wire Many sheath wires have both a 'J' and a straight tip. The straight end will often pass when the 'J'-tip will not advance. The Bentson wire often finds its way past plaque (Fig. 28.4) that the J-wire will not negotiate.

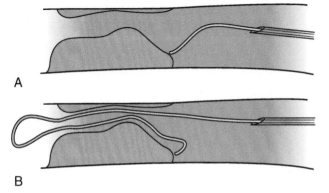

Fig. 28.4 ▪ The very floppy tip of the Bentson wire will negotiate plaque with minimal risk of dissection.

A

B

Alarm: Never use a Terumo wire through the cutting bevel of the needle because the hydrophilic coating may shear off.

If there is still no success, obtain haemostasis and try again or consider another approach.

The wire stops after a short distance

- Fluoroscope to confirm that the wire is taking the expected route and is not in a branch vessel. Re-direct as necessary.
- Make sure blood can still be aspirated from the needle.
- Insert a 4Fr dilator (see below) to secure vascular access.
- Make sure blood can be aspirated from the dilator.
- Using fluoroscopy, gently inject contrast to confirm intraluminal position.
- Perform a hand-injected angiogram to identify the problem; this is usually a tortuous vessel, unexpected stenosis or occlusion.
- Use a roadmap and steerable hydrophilic wire to negotiate diseased and tortuous vessels.
- If all fails, try again using a shaped catheter (e.g. Cobra II).

Alarm: Make sure that you have plenty of wire in the artery before exchanging the dilator for a catheter. If necessary, replace the hydrophilic wire with a standard wire for stability.

Introduction of a dilator, sheath or catheter

The choice of what to insert depends on the procedure but the simple rule is that the catheter follows the wire and not vice versa. If the guidewire is held straight under slight tension, the catheter should slide smoothly along it. In a scarred groin, it often pays to use a dilator and consider changing for a stiffer guidewire. Use the following basic rules:

- Always insert plenty of guidewire, as this increases safety in case you inadvertently pull it back or kink it; in addition, there is a greater weight of wire in the patient so more support when you advance the catheter.
- The guidewire should be held out straight and under slight tension.
- The catheter should be held initially close to its tip, always within 1–2 cm of skin/sheath.

 Alarm: Do not try to advance the catheter from the hub, it does not work and may result in pulling the wire out! The only exception to this is when you are assisting and the first operator is fixing the wire close to the skin.

- Push the catheter to advance it.
- Feel the catheter slide freely along the wire. If you encounter resistance try rotating it from side to side.

 Alarm: If the catheter seems to stick and pulls on the wire as it is advanced then the wire has kinked. STOP. Use fluoroscopy to show the problem (Fig. 28.5).

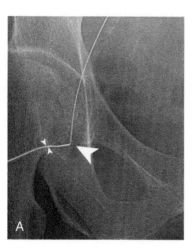

Fig. 28.5 (A) If the catheter (small arrowheads) is difficult to advance through the skin, the wire may have kinked (large arrowhead). (B) Schematic view. (C) The wire is pulled back until the kink lies outside the skin.

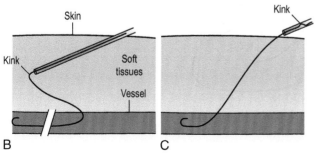

Solution: This was why you put in lots of wire! Pull back the catheter and wire until the kink is outside the skin (Fig. 28.5). Try again, using a 4Fr dilator and then change the wire that has been damaged.

The catheter tip is often difficult to see, especially when using 3Fr catheters in obese patients. Pull back the guidewire until it takes the shape of the catheter tip; J-wires can be felt to engage the catheter tip. The position is now readily seen on fluoroscopy. Use a test injection of contrast to confirm intraluminal position before flushing the catheter or performing a run. If the catheter is extraluminal, an extensive dissection will be avoided!

Commonly used arterial puncture sites

Common femoral artery The CFA runs over the medial half of the femoral head (Fig. 28.6). You can readily check your position on fluoroscopy but if in doubt there is no substitute for ultrasound guidance. Always aim to puncture the artery at the level of the midpoint of the femoral head, whether for retrograde or antegrade puncture (Fig. 28.7). This is usually the point where the pulse is most readily palpated.

 Alarm
- Puncturing too high, above the inguinal ligament, increases the risk of bleeding into the pelvis. Unlike a groin haematoma, this may remain undetected until the patient collapses.
- Puncturing too low, i.e. superficial or profunda femoral artery puncture, increases the risk of false aneurysm and arteriovenous fistula (Fig. 28.7).

The wire generally does not need any steering to enter the external iliac artery; however, occasionally a plaque may deflect the wire into the deep circumflex iliac artery, which comes

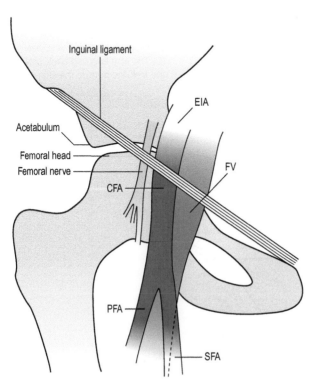

Fig. 28.6 ■ The femoral anatomy. Note the femoral vein (blue) lies medial to the artery (red) in the groin but then passes deep to the superficial femoral artery (SFA). CFA, common femoral artery; EIA, external iliac artery; FV, femoral vein; PFA, profunda femoris artery.

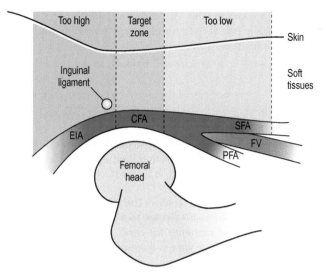

Fig. 28.7 ■ Target puncture zone in the common femoral artery (CFA). Puncture at sites too low or high cannot be effectively compressed. Puncture above the inguinal ligament is especially dangerous. EIA, external iliac artery; FV, femoral vein; PFA, profunda femoris artery; SFA, superficial femoral artery.

off the CFA at approximately 10 o'clock. This is usually easily appreciated on fluoroscopy; take care in this vessel as it is prone to severe spasm, which will retain the wire in a vice-like grip. The spasm usually responds to vasodilation with nitrates and the passage of time.

Antegrade puncture This (Fig. 28.8) is more difficult and carries increased risk as dissection flaps tend to be elevated by the flow and may occlude the vessel lumen. In practice, antegrade puncture is now almost always undertaken with ultrasound guidance. The point of skin puncture is always higher than you expect, especially in well-covered patients. Remember to aim to hit the artery at the level of the midpoint of the femoral head. In some obese patients, abdominal folds may overhang the groin. Do not struggle alone, ask your assistant to hold back the abdominal folds. The downside of this is that when they release, everything will revert to its normal position and your previously straight trajectory may end up curving back on itself. In extreme cases, the folds will need to be held back during every catheter and wire exchange.

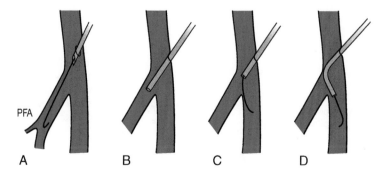

Fig. 28.8 ■ Antegrade common femoral artery (CFA). (A) Wire repeatedly enters profunda femoris artery. Insert a 4Fr dilator. (B) Perform an angiogram in the profunda oblique to confirm puncture is proximal to superficial femoral artery. (C) Carefully pull back the dilator to CFA and try to direct an angled hydrophilic wire down the superficial femoral artery. (D) If still unsuccessful, exchange for a Cobra catheter and use this to direct the wire into the superficial femoral artery. PFA, profunda femoris artery.

The profunda femoris artery (PFA) arises posterolaterally. This is in line with the needle; hence, the guidewire tends to pass preferentially into it. When this occurs, several manoeuvres will help you catheterize the superficial femoral artery (SFA):

- Flatten the needle and point it towards the SFA. If the wire still passes into the PFA, try steering by straightening the wire tip.

  If this fails:

- Put a 4Fr dilator into the PFA. Withdraw it slowly into the proximal PFA, injecting contrast to show catheter position.
- Obtain a roadmap image in the profunda oblique projection (ipsilateral anterior oblique 25 degrees). Inject hard so that contrast refluxes into the CFA and then opacifies the SFA.
- Confirm that the puncture site is proximal to the SFA origin. If it is not, start again using ultrasound guidance.
- Try using an angled hydrophilic wire or a 15-mm J-wire to select the SFA. Do not exchange over a hydrophilic wire; pass the dilator into the SFA and change to a safer wire.
- No luck? Pass a J-guidewire deep into the PFA and exchange for either a 4Fr Cobra or RDC. The catheter is pulled back into the CFA and the wire is directed into the SFA.
- Still no luck? Time for an alternative approach.

Alternative arterial access These divide into those sites which are not used on a daily basis and those which are positively esoteric and only rolled out on special occasions.

Popliteal artery (Fig. 28.9) This is sometimes used to access the SFA and CFA when angioplasty via the CFA has failed. Long SFA occlusions may be easier to traverse from below, especially in the presence of collaterals. Balloons up to 8 mm can be used through a 4Fr sheath. Some operators think nothing of using a 6Fr sheath for stenting; others prefer to cross the lesion from below using a 4Fr platform and then rendezvous with 6Fr access from another site to perform the stenting. With the patient prone, use ultrasound guidance to puncture the artery at the level of the patella.

Superficial femoral artery This is occasionally used for both antegrade and retrograde approaches. However, the SFA is relatively mobile and not readily compressed against bone; in addition the distal SFA lies deep in the thigh. This makes the SFA a more challenging vessel to puncture and also to obtain haemostasis. In practice, most procedures will be performed using a micropuncture set under ultrasound guidance and use of a closure device is the norm.

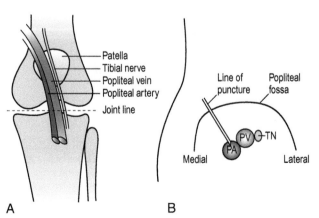

Fig. 28.9 ▨ The popliteal fossa. (A) The popliteal vein (PV) lies superficial and lateral to the popliteal artery (PA). (B) Puncture at the level of the patella, medial to the popliteal vein and tibial nerve (TN).

Arm approaches

Brachial artery (Fig. 28.10) This is used when the femoral approach is precluded; it may be the most stable route for upper limb angioplasty and stenting and also for fistulography. The left brachial artery is the preferred approach as it is usually the non-dominant arm and this route crosses the fewest cerebral vessels. The brachial artery is a small muscular artery and is prone to spasm. To prevent spasm, use a micropuncture set and straight guidewire, and administer prophylactic intra-arterial glyceryl trinitrate (GTN). Consider a surgical cutdown for sheaths larger than 7Fr.

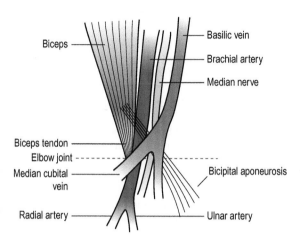

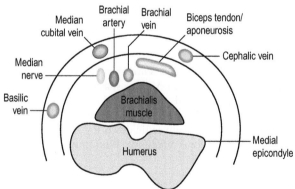

Fig. 28.10 ■ Anatomy of the antecubital fossa. The brachial artery is punctured in the antecubital fossa above the elbow joint; it lies medial to the biceps tendon.

 Tip: The guidewire tends to pass into the ascending aorta from the arm. To catheterize the descending aorta use the left anterior oblique (LAO) 30-degree projection and a Cobra or Berenstein catheter to direct the wire into the descending aorta.

 Consent issue: An additional risk of the arm approach is causing a stroke as the catheter passes across the great vessels of the arch. Patients should be reassured that the risk is low (1%) but even that will be too high for some.

Esoteric arterial access sites

In the past 15 years, the authors have needed to use the translumbar, radial and pedal arteries on a few occasions but have never required the axillary artery. Our advice is to keep an open mind and be prepared to try novel approaches if they will solve a particular problem.

Radial artery This alternative route is now favoured by cardiologists for coronary intervention. It is more fiddly than other approaches but has advantages for haemostasis. Bedrest is not necessary, so it is well suited to outpatient procedures. Use a micropuncture set, a 4Fr sheath and prophylactic GTN. For diagnostic angiography, a 120-cm-long catheter is needed, which restricts flow rates to 6 mL/s. Long-term rates of thrombosis are not known.

Alarm: Before starting, perform Allen's test to confirm the ulnar arterial supply to hand. Alternatively, place a pulse oximeter on the middle finger. Compress the radial and ulnar arteries: desaturation will occur. Release the ulnar artery; resaturation confirms dual blood supply to the hand. The reverse Allen's test involves release of the radial artery to confirm its contribution to supply.

Pedal arteries This access site is getting more popular in the treatment of critical limb ischaemia, as it can be simpler to traverse a calf artery occlusion from a retrograde puncture of the dorsalis pedis or posterior tibial artery. Use a pedal access set and consider making a separate antegrade puncture with a through-and-through wire to perform angioplasty.

Translumbar aortic puncture The translumbar aortogram has long been superseded by non-invasive approaches. With the advent of endovascular aneurysm repair, it is occasionally helpful to puncture the aneurysm sac to treat an endoleak. In this case, CT is usually used to target the actual leak, rather than a blind puncture into the aorta.

Axillary artery Puncturing the mobile axillary artery can be difficult and haemostasis no easier. There is a significant risk of brachial plexus injury secondary to haematoma. This approach is less safe than brachial puncture.

Venous puncture

The principles of venous access are similar to arterial access, but remember that veins are low pressure, thin-walled, highly compressible and prone to spasm. Venous spasm is readily provoked by injudicious catheter and wire manipulation. This can be a real catheter-gripping affair. Do not be tempted to start a tug-of-war – completely avulsing part of the venous system is seldom a satisfactory outcome. STOP and let the vein settle down for at least 5 min. If this does not work, try either GTN via the catheter or oral nifedipine. Blood pressure monitoring is advisable.

Venous puncture: a step-by-step guide

1. Check the patient is appropriately consented for the procedure.
2. Choose the optimal site depending on the planned procedure. Preliminary ultrasound assessment can be invaluable.
3. Consider using a tourniquet, Valsalva or Trendelenburg manoeuvres to distend the vein.
4. Clean and drape the area. Infiltrate the skin with 1% lidocaine. Leave the needle in situ to mark where to make the skin incision.
5. Make a skin incision appropriate to the catheter/sheath size.
6. Select an appropriate puncture needle; mini-access systems can help avoid spasm.
7. Attach a 5-mL syringe to the puncture needle. Advance the needle at 45 degrees to skin, aspirating as you go – a change in resistance may be felt on entry to vessel lumen.
8. Confirm intraluminal position by aspirating blood. If the tip is not in the vein, aspirate as the needle is slowly withdrawn. Flush the needle between attempts.
9. Guidewire passage and catheterization are the same as for arterial puncture.

Ultrasound-guided vein puncture Ultrasound guidance is invaluable and should be used if possible. It is particularly important to use ultrasound guidance if:

- the vein is not visible or palpable. Ultrasound should be used for all elective central venous access and also other superficial veins and visceral veins, such as the portal vein
- there is any difficulty or when there is a contraindication to arterial puncture, e.g. coagulopathy
- access options are limited; even just one failed entry to the venous system is usually enough to cause a haematoma that will compress the vein and make subsequent puncture difficult.

 Tip: Watch the needle advance to abut the vein wall and then advance quickly to puncture. If you advance the needle slowly you are likely to see the vein compress.

There are several signs on ultrasound that suggest a downstream stenosis or occlusion, especially with jugular vein puncture:

- Thrombus in vein
- Spontaneous contrast, swirling echo pattern from slow-moving blood
- Presence of collateral veins
- Abnormal distension
- Loss of pulsatility or respiratory variation.

Only absence of the vein precludes puncture; the rest should make you anticipate trouble and consider an alternative approach.

Commonly used venous access sites

The approach chosen depends on the objective of the procedure.

Common femoral vein The CFV lies medial to the CFA (see Fig. 28.6). Palpate the CFA and infiltrate local anaesthetic 1–2 cm medial to it. Aim to puncture the vein at the level of the midpoint of the femoral head. The right femoral vein is preferred to the left as it has a straighter course to the inferior vena cava (IVC).

 Tip: Remember veins are easily compressed. Do not palpate over the vein during puncture because this just flattens the vein. Always aspirate as the needle is withdrawn, since sometimes a compressed vein has been transfixed during puncture and opens as the needle is pulled back.

Internal jugular vein The IJV is one of the most important venous access points; it is used for central venous catheterization, hepatic venous intervention and IVC filter insertion. The right IJV provides a straight path to the right atrium and IVC. The left IJV detours via the (left) brachiocephalic vein; this angled course can limit its utility for interventional procedures. The vein is punctured 1–5 cm above the clavicle guided by ultrasound. Guidance makes the procedure simpler, safer and sometimes quicker than using anatomical landmarks.

Ultrasound-guided jugular vein puncture A 5–7.5-MHz ultrasound probe offers the best combination of resolution and depth for guidance. Turn the patient's head away from the side to be punctured and scan the neck to identify the vein lateral to the carotid artery and infiltrate local anaesthetic. It is usually easiest to position the probe transversely unless your probe has a very small footprint. Position the transducer 1–2 cm caudal to the skin puncture site and line up the vein with the midpoint of the probe head. Slowly advance the needle into the scan plane and onto the anterior vein wall. The vein is easily compressed and should be punctured with a quick stab. Free aspiration of blood confirms intraluminal position.

Subclavian vein and axillary vein These are also punctured under ultrasound guidance. The subclavian vein is usually punctured approximately two-thirds of the way along the clavicle and 1 cm inferior to its inferior margin. The axillary vein is punctured at a point just lateral to the first rib.

'Blind' central vein puncture In the UK, the National Institute for Health and Care Excellence (NICE) has recommended that all central venous punctures should be made with ultrasound guidance. You are expert at this and have access to ultrasound, so there is little justification for blind puncture.

Median cubital vein This is the medial superficial vein in the antecubital fossa (Fig. 28.10); it drains into the basilic vein and is most commonly used during fistuloplasty and may be punctured antegradely or retrogradely when managing stenoses in either the venous outflow or arterial inflow.

Cephalic vein This can also be used during fistuloplasty and is particularly useful when managing central cephalic vein stenoses, which can be impossible to access from any other approach.

Esoteric venous access sites

These sites are not used in daily practice but may be useful for some forms of intervention and also in cases where there are no options left.

External jugular veins These lie posterolateral to the IJV and drain into the subclavian veins and are occasionally required for access.

Anterior jugular veins These lie anteromedial to the IJV and also drain into the subclavian veins and are a port of last resort for access.

Inferior vena cava The IVC can be used for long-term central venous access. It is punctured using fluoroscopic guidance from a posterior approach to the right of the spine. If possible, place a pigtail catheter in the IVC below the renal vein; this provides a target to aim at and also helps to hold the vein open during puncture.

Hepatic vein The hepatic veins are another approach for long-term venous access and may also be used for intervention in Budd–Chiari syndrome. The target vein is punctured peripherally under ultrasound guidance. Colour Doppler is essential to clarify that the vein is patent and that it is not a portal vein radicle. The mini-access set is very useful in these circumstances. The initial puncture uses a 21 G needle, which is relatively atraumatic.

Portal vein Portal venous access is required for preoperative portal vein embolization and also to treat post-transplant stenosis. The transhepatic and trans-splenic approaches can both be used. It is also possible to access mesenteric radicles via a mini-laparotomy.

Renal vein Rarely used for placement of a dialysis catheter in a defunct native kidney.

Collateral veins These are a useful last resort for central venous access. They are usually identified and punctured with ultrasound guidance. Preliminary venography will help plan the path through to the central veins. Even using hydrophilic catheters and wires, it can be very difficult to navigate through these small tortuous vessels.

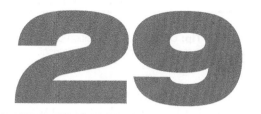

Principles of diagnostic angiography

Angiography is a team sport and a successful angiogram depends on cooperation between the patient and the angiography staff (radiographer, nurse and doctor). A little understanding of the basic principles of angiography can vastly improve the standard of the final study. This chapter reviews the key areas in image acquisition and manipulation.

Digital subtraction angiography: basic principles

Digital subtraction angiography (DSA) uses a computer to subtract an image without contrast (mask) from a series of subsequent images acquired after contrast injection. Assuming that everything remained in exactly the same position, the resultant images show only the opacified blood vessels. These are clearly seen in high contrast as the underlying bone or soft tissue is not displayed. Unfortunately, any movement between the mask image and the contrast image will result in image degradation; bone edges and bowel are the worst offenders.

Most DSA examinations are performed with positive (iodinated) contrast media; however, negative (CO_2 gas) contrast can be used.

Digital subtraction angiography techniques

Although non-invasive modalities are rapidly replacing diagnostic catheter angiography, the techniques underpinning peripheral angiography are still important.

Multi-position DSA (MPDSA) Angiography is performed in discrete sections, each with its own contrast injection. In peripheral angiography, this usually gives the best results at the expense of a slight increase in radiation dose.

Stepping table DSA Rarely used, as computed tomography angiography (CTA) or magnetic resonance angiography (MRA) are used for diagnostic purposes. Five positions are usually needed to cover from the abdominal aorta to the feet. Mask images are obtained in each position. The table or C-arm moves to each of the positions in a series of overlapping steps to keep pace with a single contrast bolus. A skilled radiographer is needed to trigger the table movement to the next station when the vessels in the current position have been demonstrated. The technique only works well with a patient with broadly symmetrical disease.

Supplementary runs are frequently necessary, particularly of the crural vessels. MRA is basically stepping table DSA with pre-programmed movement of the table and using MR instead of X-rays.

Tip: Consider multi-position digital subtraction angiography (MPDSA) if symptoms or pulses are markedly asymmetrical.

Rotational angiography and angiographic CT These are variations on MPDSA; the C-arm is rotated in an arc around the patient while masks are acquired. The rotation is repeated during the injection of contrast. The mask is matched with the image acquired at the same tube angulation. Modern data reconstruction algorithms allow the angiographic image to be reformatted into a 3D reconstruction akin to a low-resolution CT scan.

Rotational angiography is most useful when multiple oblique projections are required, e.g. renal transplant angiography, intracranial aneurysm. Angiographic CT may be useful when performing hepatic chemoembolization and at completion of endovascular aneurysm repair (EVAR) to demonstrate the origin of subtle endoleaks.

Reaching the target: catheter guidance

For all but the simplest catheterization procedures, it helps to have a mental map of the relevant anatomy backed up by some non-invasive imaging. This will enable you to select the appropriate tools to reach your destination. However, when it comes to more complex navigation, nothing beats an angiographic route map to guide you to your desired target.

There are two adjuncts to fluoroscopy, which will help.

Roadmap (non-subtracted fluoroscopy) Once you are in more or less the right area but are starting to need some assistance, simply perform a DSA. This image is superimposed on the normal fluoroscopic image (Fig. 29.1A). The transparency of the superimposed image can be adjusted to suit the application. This is particularly useful in the chest and abdomen as the

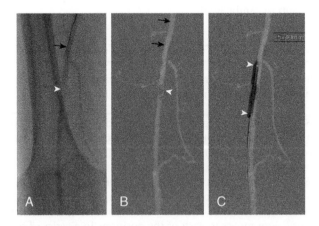

Fig. 29.1 ■ The principal techniques for guiding catheters and guidewires shown during superficial femoral artery (SFA) angioplasty. (A) Fluoroscopy fade: an image of the vessel is superimposed on the standard fluoroscopic image; the guidewire (black arrow), stenosis (white arrowhead) are clearly seen, as is the femur. (B) Roadmap: the background is subtracted, as is the guidewire (black arrows); the tiny channel passing the plaque is clearly shown (white arrowhead), making it easier to traverse the lesion. (C) The lesion has been crossed and a 5-mm balloon (white arrowheads) inflated. Note that the balloon and wire are now seen, as they were not present on the original image. Despite slight movement, it is clear that the balloon is in the correct place and appropriately sized.

superimposed image does not move with respiration. Confusingly, this is called by a different name by each of the manufacturers, e.g. on a Siemens' machine, it is called 'fluoroscopy fade'.

Roadmap (subtracted fluoroscopy) In this mode, a subtracted fluoroscopic image is obtained after a few seconds of fluoroscopy. Contrast is injected to opacify the vessels, and fluoroscopy stopped. The next time screening is activated, the catheter and guidewire will be seen superimposed on the subtracted image of the blood vessels (Fig. 29.1B). This is used particularly to navigate strictures and avoid branch vessels and also can show that angioplasty balloons are correctly sized (Fig. 29.1C).

 Tip: Subtracted roadmapping is not effective in the chest and abdomen, as respiration and peristalsis interfere with the subtraction and degrade the image.

Dose reduction

When imaging for guidance rather than diagnosis, consider using roadmap imaging and conventional fluoroscopy with last image hold; this can reduce dose by an order of magnitude.

Archives and imaging

The best study in the world can be sabotaged by careless and inadequate hard copy/archival/post-processing. Most images are now stored digitally to a picture archiving and communication system (PACS).

Unlike CT/MRI where all of the data are retained, it is not uncommon for some of the study to be discarded almost immediately after acquisition. Vital information may be lost irretrievably if we fail to convey to radiographic staff the essential objectives of the study. In particular, complex or unfamiliar studies should be reviewed at the console with the radiographer, to ensure that no important imaging is lost.

Suboptimal imaging is most often due to elementary errors. Try to apply the following basic guidelines:

- Consider whether it is desirable to image all phases of the run: arterial, capillary and venous. If so, make sure that you do not stop too early.
- Optimal image density is a level of grey that allows overlying vessels to be discriminated from each other. This requires contrast of the correct strength and appropriate window levels. Too black an image will obscure pathology (Fig. 29.2).
- Include non-subtracted images to show landmarks.
- Annotate views with relevant information, e.g. tube angulation when it has been difficult to obtain a suitable oblique projection.

 Tip: While it is always worth trying to blame the radiographer, no amount of radiographer ingenuity can make up for images that were never there – always review the study on the console before removing the catheter.

Pixel shifting If there is no movement between the mask and the run, then a single mask image will suffice. In reality, most patients do not keep completely still, especially if a large volume of contrast has been injected. If there has only been slight movement, then the resultant image can often be markedly improved by pixel shifting (Fig. 29.3). This entails realigning the chosen mask with the image to allow effective subtraction. Pixel shifting is not

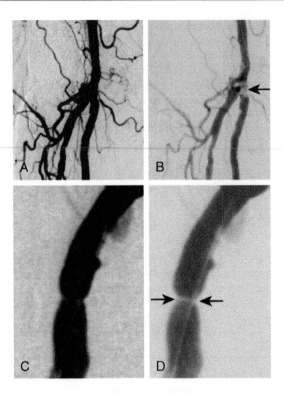

Fig. 29.2 ■ Effect of incorrect window settings. (A,B) Profunda oblique view: the large posterior plaque (arrow) is obscured by narrow windows. (C,D) Subtle 'web-like' stenosis (arrows) in a vein graft is only appreciated on correct settings.

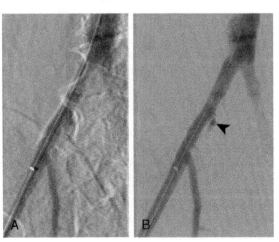

Fig. 29.3 ■ This patient experienced pain during iliac angioplasty and stenting. (A) Movement has severely degraded the angiographic image. (B) Choosing an appropriate mask and pixel shifting has improved the image and now contrast extravasation (black arrowhead) is clearly seen at the angioplasty site.

as helpful when there is considerable movement such as respiration, or when there is rotation.

 Tip: If you notice that the patient moves during a run, consider continuing imaging after the contrast has passed and use a late image as the mask. If the patient keeps moving, then this is futile.

Masking Some patients cannot stop breathing for the duration of image acquisition, especially if a long sequence is involved. In this case, the solution is multi-masking. Multiple masks are made over several respiratory cycles before injecting contrast. Normal respiration is continued throughout the run. A dedicated radiographer can match images from the run with a mask in the same phase of respiration, allowing subtraction.

 Tip: No amount of pixel shifting and re-masking can compensate for bowel peristalsis. Paralyse the bowel with hyoscine butylbromide (Buscopan) or glucagon.

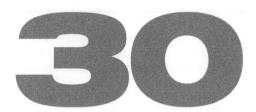

Principles of using catheters and wires

Knowing the equipment is a great start but it comes into its own if you know how to use it. Remember wires go first, and the initial step of most procedures is to establish safe guidewire access to the target zone.

 Alarm: Exceptions to the catheter follows the wire are: manoeuvring a pigtail up and down the aorta and moving catheters up and down the aorta to allow them to engage a branch vessel – even then, take care in a diseased aorta.

Achieving a selective position or negotiating complex anatomy usually requires catheters and wires working together.

 Using guidewires and catheters together: a step-by-step guide:

This section is about the use of guidewires and catheters together to navigate from A to B. This assumes that you have already managed to pass a wire through the puncture needle (Ch. 8) and then achieved access with a sheath (Ch. 14). Guidewire and catheter selection is discussed in the essential equipment chapter (Chs. 11 and 12). We are assuming here you know what to ask for but not necessarily how to use it – in fact: 'all the gear – no idea'.

Advancing the guidewire

Very often, a J-tip or steerable wire can be advanced to close the target site without need for a catheter. J-wires tend to stay in major vessels but steerable wires, such as the angled Terumo, will often stray from the path, and readily enter branch vessels.

As the guidewire is advanced, pay attention to detect any resistance to the passage of the wire. Learning to feel an increase in resistance as soon as it occurs is a key skill in intervention. This is an adjunct to using fluoroscopy.

 Alarm: Use fluoroscopy to keep on track and detect deviation before causing a problem.

Troubleshooting

The wire does not go where you expect it to This happens when it enters a branch or collateral or is no longer in the lumen.

- If the wire is moving freely, then simply pull the wire back, rotate the shaft of the wire and advance under fluoroscopy.

- If the wire repeatedly takes the same (wrong) path: advance a catheter over the wire and carefully aspirate to make sure there is backflow. Use a gentle contrast injection to determine your position. If in a branch vessel, pull back into the main vessel and rotate the catheter when advancing the wire to avoid the offending branch.
- If there is no backflow then you are either wedged or extraluminal. Pull the catheter back aspirating as you go until there is backflow and then check again.

Advancing a catheter over a guidewire

The catheter follows the wire when it is being introduced and advanced except during proximal vessel selective catheterization.

- Hold the wire close to the skin.
- Ask your assistant to load the catheter onto the wire until it reaches your fingers.
- Extend the wire so that it is in a straight line and hold the wire close to the catheter hub keeping it under tension.
- Start to advance the catheter into the sheath a few centimetres at a time. Always manipulate it just a few centimetres away from the sheath.
- Keep the wire fixed in position with your right hand.
- As the catheter gets further in, reposition your hand to maintain tension in the guidewire.
- Fluoroscope over the wire tip when you advance the catheter and try to maintain a constant position.

Troubleshooting

The catheter sticks on the wire before it reaches the sheath This is most likely with a hydrophilic wire that has become dry. Use a wet sponge to wet the wire. Catheters can stick on conventional wires usually when there is a blood clot or a piece of gauze stuck to it. Clean as above. If the catheter still will not advance, try to take it off the wire, flush it and clean the wire.

The catheter does not advance once it is in the patient Fix the catheter and wire and ask the radiographer to pan the C-arm down from the wire tip while screening. Try to see if there is an obvious cause such as a kink or loop in the catheter. The reason may not be obvious in the case of a very tight stenosis.

- If there is a kink, you will probably need to exchange the wire for a new one. Consider whether a stiffer wire would be more appropriate.
- If there is a loop, it is normally necessary to pull the catheter and wire back together until they straighten out.
- If there is a known tight stenosis, e.g. you are planning to treat it, then if possible keep the wire across it. If there is room, insert some more wire to improve stability and try again. If this fails, you may need to change to a low profile system.

Maintaining your position

- When you are not manoeuvring, keep a hand on the catheter/wire close to the access site.
- Remember that hydrophilic wires are incredibly slippery when wet and sticky when they dry out. Keep the wire lubricated and make sure you are still holding it. Take care when 'letting go' of a dry wire, as it may be attached to your glove.

 Tip: Always assume that your assistant is determined to pull the guidewire out during catheter exchanges. Get a grip!

Catheter and guidewires: advanced techniques

Wires come in a variety of diameters, lengths and stiffness. There are occasions when even a stiff wire is not enough to support the device or will not advance to the target. In these cases, adjunctive methods of providing additional support can be very helpful. Two techniques stand out for this:

Through-and-through wire (body flossing) This involves two separate vascular access points and is fully described in Chapter 36. In essence, a long wire is introduced through one sheath and brought out of a second site. The wire can then be held under tension, affording considerable support like a tightrope! Body flossing is used when the wire runs directly across the target site.

Buddy wire This is used in situations where body flossing is impossible, e.g. when the target vessel is an end artery (e.g. the renal artery). As the name implies, this requires two separate guidewires.

The 'buddy wire' is a stiff wire; the first step is to place it deeply in a vessel close to the target. This allows a guide-catheter or sheath to be brought in proximity to the target. The first wire effectively acts as an anchor for the guide-catheter and provides a stable platform to allow the target vessel to be catheterized with the second wire.

 Alarm: The observant will have noticed that the sheath must be large enough to accommodate the buddy wire and whatever catheter/delivery system is required for the target vessel. Using an 0.018-inch wire keeps size to a minimum but this will still require a sheath 1–2Fr sizes larger than normal.

Catheters

Flushing and aspirating catheters

The aim of flushing is to fill the catheter lumen with heparinized saline solution rather than alternatives, such as air or blood clot. At best, these will block the catheter, at worst, the next run you perform will fire off a distal clot or air embolus. If you have not performed a run or flushed the catheter for a few minutes, check for backflow and flush again. Multiple sidehole catheters should be flushed vigorously to ensure adequate flow through both the catheter tip and sideholes. As in many toilets, there are full flush and light flush options.

Double-flush technique Used in the cerebral circulation, where injection of even a small thrombus or air bubble could be disastrous. A syringe with saline is attached to the hub of the catheter and aspirated until blood flows freely into the syringe. This syringe is discarded and the catheter is then flushed with a syringe containing clean saline meticulously prepared to exclude air bubbles.

Single-flush technique This is appropriate outside the cerebral circulation. The objective is to demonstrate that the catheter is free of clot and then to fill it with heparinized saline. Slowly aspirate the catheter with a syringe containing saline until a small bead of blood flows into the syringe. If you hold the syringe at 45 degrees to the horizontal, the blood pools near the syringe nozzle at the bottom and any air bubbles rise to lie against the syringe plunger at the top. Now inject saline to flush the catheter; with care, the air bubbles and the blood will stay in the syringe. If the blood mixes with the saline, simply discard the syringe and double flush.

Troubleshooting

If you are unable to aspirate blood freely from a catheter, then one of the following applies:

- The tip is stuck against the vessel wall (endhole catheters only): try rotating or withdrawing the catheter until free flow resumes, then flush as normal.
- It is blocked: in this case flow will not resume. Presume that you need to remove the catheter and flush its contents outside the patient. UNLESS you are able to sacrifice the territory supplied by the vessel the catheter lies in, e.g. during embolization.
- It is wedged in a small vessel: there is usually a giveaway 'sucking' sound when you remove the guidewire. Slowly pull the catheter back until flow resumes.
- It is kinked: use fluoroscopy to check for kinking. Usually a kinked catheter will need to be removed and exchanged, as wires and embolization coils will tend to stick.

Selective catheterization: keys to success

Choosing your weapon

The most important factor in catheter choice is the angle at which the target vessel arises from the parent vessel. Review the pre-procedure imaging and then choose logically; if the vessel points downwards, then even the most skilled angiographer will struggle with a forward-facing catheter, such as the Vertebral. Use Fig. 30.1 to aid your catheter choice and choose the simplest shape that will bring the tip close to the target and point it in the correct direction. Most catheters adopt their shape as soon as they are in a blood vessel of sufficient size; do not expect a 15-mm pigtail to form in a 6-mm external iliac artery. Similarly, other catheter shapes and effectiveness are affected by the size of vessel you are using them in.

Approximate positioning

- Get your catheter into roughly the correct area for the target vessel, e.g. renal artery L1/2.
- Perform a flush angiogram to demonstrate the target.
- Consider oblique views.
- Consider using roadmapping to guide you.

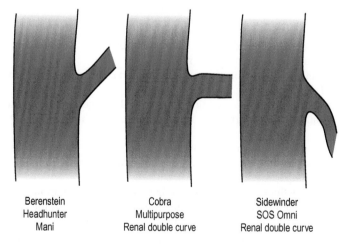

Berenstein	Cobra	Sidewinder
Headhunter	Multipurpose	SOS Omni
Mani	Renal double curve	Renal double curve

Fig. 30.1 ▦ Choose an appropriately shaped catheter for the target vessel.

Catheter manipulation

- Keep the catheter shaft straight. Using the hub, turn the catheter towards the target. If the catheter does not turn readily, then either it is catching on aortic plaque or most of the torque is being taken up in tortuous iliac vessels.
- If trying to catheterize an anterior vessel, make sure the catheter tip is facing anteriorly by rotating anticlockwise – if the catheter tip rotates the same way it is facing anterior.
- Most shaped catheters are pulled backwards towards the target vessel. If the aorta is relatively free of disease then the catheter can also be pushed forwards. Remember to be gentle, as the catheter can be an effective plough and dislodge plaque and thrombus.
- Deeper catheterization is achieved by pushing the catheter forwards, usually over a guidewire.

Reverse curve catheters

Reverse curve catheters work a little differently. The Sidewinder/Simmons/Sim is a little more complex to use; there are two stages: forming the reverse curve and using the formed catheter.

Forming a sidewinder shape catheter Reverse curve catheters (e.g. Sidewinder, SOS Omni) are straightened out by the guidewire during insertion. Those with a very short reverse curve will have space to adopt their working shape in the abdominal aorta. Catheters with longer reverse curve limbs need a little help. The techniques described for the Sidewinder catheter will work with other reverse curve catheters if required.

1. Over the aortic bifurcation: this is very safe. As it does not involve manipulation in the aortic arch, it is recommended in elderly patients and those with aortic arch disease.
   a. Catheterize the contralateral iliac artery, e.g. using either a Cobra or RDC catheter and hydrophilic wire.
   b. Advance the wire down to the CFA.
   c. Advance the catheter to the CFA and exchange for a J-wire.

 Tip: You can cut out step (c) and use the hydrophilic wire but this is safer until you get the hang of it.

   d. Exchange the Cobra for a Sidewinder catheter.
   e. When the shape forms over the aortic bifurcation, bring the wire back to the 'catheter knee'; this should be at the bifurcation.
   f. Push the catheter and wire together up into the aorta; the reverse curve shape should be preserved.
2. In the aortic arch: the arch and ascending aorta have the largest diameter, therefore this is used to allow the catheter to form. The 'quick aortic turn' technique (Fig. 30.2) is perhaps the simplest.
   a. Advance the catheter until the knee of the catheter is across the apex of the aortic arch.
   b. Simultaneously push the catheter forwards and rotate clockwise to re-form the reverse curve.
   c. Under continuous fluoroscopy, pull the catheter down into the aorta. The catheter may occasionally engage vessels on the way down. Remember to push the catheter in to disengage, then withdraw, rotating it slightly.

The aortic turn manoeuvre can be difficult in the unfolded aortic arch, so insert a guidewire to the level of the 'knee' of the catheter and try again.

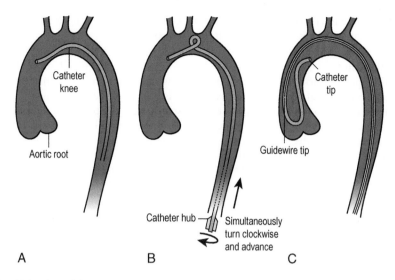

Fig. 30.2 ▥ Using the quick aortic turn to re-form the Sidewinder catheter.

An alternative is to pass a hydrophilic guidewire around the aortic arch; when it reaches the aortic valve, it will tend to double back on itself. Allow a large loop to form and then introduce the Sidewinder catheter until it forms adjacent to the aortic valve (Fig. 30.3).

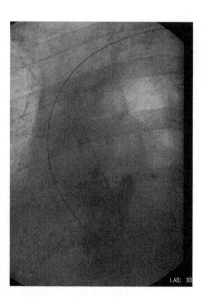

Fig. 30.3 ▥ Forming the Sidewinder using the aortic valve. A 260-cm hydrophilic wire is passed around the aortic arch until it doubles back on the aortic valve. The Sidewinder catheter is advanced over the wire and will form with its apex at the valve.

Alarm: There is a small risk of causing a stroke whenever a catheter is formed or manipulated in the ascending aorta or aortic arch.

3. In a branch vessel: this is similar to using the contralateral iliac artery but uses another vessel, such as the subclavian artery or renal artery. Once this has been catheterized and stable wire access obtained, exchange for the Sidewinder catheter. Carefully advance the

catheter into the artery as far as the apex of the curve, pull the wire back to the knee then push and rotate clockwise to disengage from the vessel.

Using the sidewinder Once the catheter has been formed, it is positioned above the target vessel and then pulled back down towards the target vessel. Take care doing this, the catheter tip will engage every vessel and plaque in its path. It is easy to get carried away and straighten the catheter out again, so make sure you use fluoroscopy. Steer the tip by rotating the shaft (Fig. 30.4). Once the tip is at the ostium, pulling it back further will result in the catheter engaging the artery. Once the knee of the catheter has reached the vessel ostium, further traction will start to pull the catheter out. At this stage, deeper catheterization can be achieved by advancing the catheter over a guidewire. This is easiest with an S3, possible for the gifted with an S2, and only for the divine with an S1.

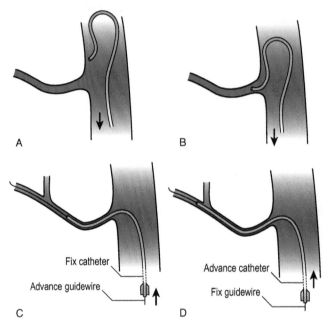

Fig. 30.4 ■ Using the Sidewinder. (A) Pull back to engage the catheter tip in the vessel ostium. (B) The catheter is advanced further by pulling back until the catheter is in as far as the knee. (C) For deeper catheterization, advance a guidewire into the vessel. (D) Push the catheter over the fixed wire.

 Tip: If the catheter loop is too large for the aorta, the tip of the catheter is held away from the aortic wall and will not engage branch vessels. Try introducing a guidewire around the apex of the catheter curve to straighten out the limb; if this fails, choose a smaller curve.

Catheter–guidewire interaction

Catheters and guidewires should work in harmony with each other. Initially, the wire leads the catheter into a large vessel such as the aorta or iliac arteries. The catheter then points the wire in the correct direction such as a branch vessel. The wire is advanced into this and then followed by the catheter. This principle applies whenever a catheter does not simply engage the target.

• Using fluoroscopy, point the catheter at the target and advance the guidewire smoothly and gently; steerable wires can be rotated to aid this process. If the wire starts to buckle or push the catheter back – **STOP** – do not try to force it. Retract the wire and then try advancing at a different angle.

- Get a reasonable length of guidewire into the target vessel. What is a reasonable length? There is no simple answer to this but, clearly, advancing a catheter across the floppy tip of the guidewire guarantees lost access, similarly, unless there is sufficient 'weight' (length) of guidewire in the artery both will 'spring-out'.
- Keep the guidewire absolutely fixed and under tension with the tip in sight when advancing the catheter.
- Advance the catheter smoothly and gently into the target vessel under fluoroscopy. If the catheter/wire start to buckle – **STOP** – the catheter and wire will spring out of the vessel. Try again, this time with more wire to increase stability or exchange for a different catheter.
- If the catheter backs out again, think about the anatomy and if you can get better stability by choosing a catheter that gets some support from the opposite wall. Failing this, you may need to think of using a coaxial system or buddy wire.

Coaxial systems

These include guide-catheters and microcatheter systems. If you are using a sheath, then you have already started. Coaxial systems use all the same basic principles as conventional catheters but are a little more fiddly until you get the hang of them. The key elements to consider are:

- Is everything compatible: no prizes if your working catheter will not fit inside the guiding catheter or is shorter than it!
- Guiding catheters (and introducer guides) are useful if the selective catheter is losing torque/stability on the way to the target – usually in tortuous iliac arteries. Remember, guide catheters have an even greater dead space for thrombus formation. They need regular flushing or, if working in a high-risk environment, such as the carotid artery, they can be flushed continually with heparinized saline using a pressure bag via a 3-way tap (Fig. 15.1).
- Keeping everything tidy: there is an additional catheter to consider. Try to keep the catheters in a straight line. Clipping the guide-catheter to the operative drapes will help hold it in position and free up a hand.
- In critical positions, ask your assistant to control either the guide-catheter or the working catheter/guidewire while you manipulate the other.
- The usual rules apply: keep everything out straight, fix the catheter, advance the guidewire, follow with the catheter and so on.
- On occasion, you will want to advance the guide catheter over the smaller inner catheter to give more support. This will only succeed if the guidewire is in place and the inner catheter sufficiently far into the target vessel. Fix the inner catheter/wire combination and use it like the wire for the guiding catheter.

Microcatheters

- Microcatheters are most often used to achieve distal catheterization. It is essential that a stable position has been achieved in the main target vessel (Fig. 30.5).
- Microcatheters are mainly steered with shaped guidewires. Angled-tip microcatheters are available and helpful for sub-selective catheterization but even the best of these catheters have very little torque.

 Tip: When using an assistant to fix catheters or wires, explain to them what you are planning to do and how they can recognize what is required of them, e.g. fix the wire so that the tip remains in the same place on the screen.

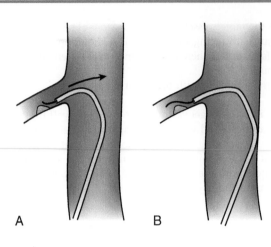

A   B

Fig. 30.5 ■ Achieving a stable catheter position. (A) The catheter backs out repeatedly, as it is not supported. (B) A catheter with a wider secondary curve sits against the contralateral aortic wall and maintains a stable position.

31

Principles of crossing stenoses and occlusions

Many interventional procedures have the primary aim of managing narrowings or blockages to restore flow of blood, urine, bile, air or even bowel contents. Once access into the appropriate lumen has been achieved, the basic principles of catheters and wires are used to navigate through the diseased segment. This chapter is concerned with the mechanics of getting across to the other side. Success is largely governed by:

- **Having a 'map' of the lesion:** this is a combination of pre-procedure imaging combined with per-procedure imaging, using contrast to outline the lesion and any key anatomical structures.
- **Choosing the right weapons:** a combination of sheaths, guide catheters, shaped catheters and guidewires.
- **Achieving a position of strength:** this usually means a stable catheter position ideally with mechanical advantage, just in case you need to push to cross an occlusion. Stability begins with the choice of access site and is supplemented by the use of sheaths and guide catheters.
- **Perseverance:** sometimes you can traverse the most difficult lesion in a matter of seconds. Try to look as though you are not too surprised at your luck when this occurs. However, success often takes time, this is much easier if you have prepared the patient for a longer procedure and ensured they have adequate analgesia.
- **Reassessing the situation:** if you have been trying without success for a while. Stop and think – is there anything you could be doing differently? It often helps to phone a friend at this stage, two heads can be better than one and sometimes a fresh approach is all that is needed.
- **Knowing when to stop:** OK, so this is normally associated with failure but there is a time to give up before causing any harm. Revisiting a case on another occasion is often successful, particularly when there has been chronic obstruction in a non-vascular system. A period of drainage can let oedema settle down and subsequent catheterization becomes much easier.

Crossing stenoses

Even the tightest stenosis can be negotiated with patience, a little skill and the right tools. Simple stenoses are readily negotiated with a guidewire alone: most operators will choose a steerable hydrophilic wire in the first instance but a Bentson wire can be used in conjunction with a curved catheter (Fig. 31.1).

Key steps

- Centre the image intensifier over the lesion and obtain a 'map' of the stenosis at appropriate magnification.

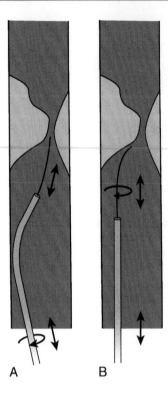

A   B

Fig. 31.1 ▨ Crossing a stenosis. Obtain a decent angiogram to use as a 'route map'. Use fluoroscopy fade or roadmap if available. (A) Straight wire and curved catheter. Turn the catheter to direct the wire through the stenosis. (B) Angled hydrophilic wire and straight catheter. Turn the wire, giving the wire space to rotate outside the catheter. You can practise this by trying to catheterize the nozzle of a syringe using different catheter/wire combinations.

- Start with the catheter 2–5 cm from the stenosis and advance the guidewire.
- Use your catheter and wire together to steer towards the apex of the stenosis.
- Take your time and do not use force. Hold the wire loosely, and gently probe with the tip until it engages.
- Use a pin-vice to steer the wire to advance through and across the lesion.

 Tip: A pin-vice makes it much easier to steer and control a hydrophilic wire. There is nothing macho about struggling without one, however, if none is to hand, dry the wire to allow you to grip it. Be careful! A dry wire will stick to your gloves and is easily pulled out!

This sounds simple but longer and more complex stenoses, especially those located on bends or at the origin of a vessel, can be very challenging. In longer lesions, the key is to steer through the narrow segment, using a shaped catheter and a curved hydrophilic wire.

Once you have crossed the lesion

Remember that the hydrophilic wire, which was great for crossing the lesion, is now a liability as it is readily pulled out. Exchanging for a conventional wire after negotiating the lesion is infinitely safer. To exchange the wire, fix it in position with the tip in sight. Advance a catheter through the lesion, remove the hydrophilic wire and inject contrast to confirm intraluminal position and then put in a suitable wire, such as a 3-mm J-wire or a stiffer wire, such as an Amplatz.

Troubleshooting

The wire crosses the lesion but the catheter will not follow This is particularly likely in heavily calcified lesions. Hold the guidewire as taut as possible and try to advance the catheter through the stenosis by rotating it from side to side as you push. If this fails, use the lowest-profile catheter available.

 Alarm: It is obvious when you think about it but make sure to use a catheter whose lumen is the same as the wire, e.g. do not try to advance a 0.035-inch catheter over a 0.038-inch wire.

Sometimes, it may be necessary to cross the lesion with a 0.014- or 0.018-inch guidewire. This is becoming more common when working retrogradely from an esoteric access point, such as a pedal artery. Once across the lesion with the low-profile wire, a microcatheter will usually follow and allow a more supportive wire, a low-profile angioplasty balloon can then be used to pre-dilate the lesion to 3 mm.

Crossing occlusions

Key steps

Crossing occlusions is more complex and requires a little more patience. Start with high-quality imaging and if possible, delineate both ends of the blockage – this may only be possible in the vascular system due to collateral flow.

- Look at the shape of the lumen at the point of occlusion.
- If the lumen tapers to a point – this is your target.
- Start with a straight wire and use a shaped catheter to direct it to the apex of the occlusion (Fig. 31.2). Sometimes the wire passes straight through the occlusion with minimal resistance. If you are treating arterial occlusion just make sure that you are dealing with a chronic process not fresh thrombus before angioplasty or stenting.
- If there is no obvious point to enter the occlusion, gently probe it near the centre using a straight wire with a shaped catheter to direct it. Once the wire enters the occlusion, proceed as above.

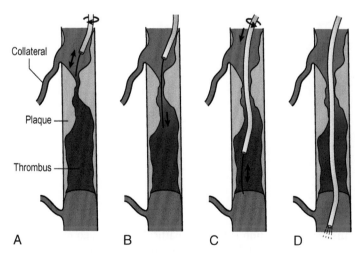

Fig. 31.2 Crossing an occlusion (see also Fig. 31.5). Occlusions occur where there is thrombus at the site of a stenosis. The thrombus propagates to the next collateral. (A) Gently probe the 'apex' of the occlusion with a straight wire, using a curved catheter to steer. (B) Typically, the wire will enter the thrombosed lumen with a slight give in resistance. (C) Advance the catheter into the occlusion to support and steer the wire through. (D) Perform an angiogram to confirm intraluminal position.

- If a standard straight wire does not work, then there are various options for escalation. First, try a straight and then a curved hydrophilic wire, remember that you are still trying to coax your way across the lesion.

Troubleshooting

- If the conventional wire starts to buckle, support the wire by advancing the catheter as you go; aim to have a maximum of only 2 cm of wire ahead of the catheter.
- If the hydrophilic wire starts to buckle, there is a good chance you will cause a dissection or perforation. Try to re-direct the wire before moving onto the more advanced techniques below.

Dissection If the wire starts to spiral down the artery, it is dissecting (Fig. 31.3)! Dissections occur in both vascular and non-vascular systems. If you have caused a dissection in a blood vessel, then you can continue the procedure as a subintimal angioplasty but remember not to propagate the dissection beyond the occlusion or the next major collateral as you may jeopardize the distal perfusion. In non-vascular applications, if you really cannot navigate beyond the dissection, then leave the system on free drainage for a few days and come back again.

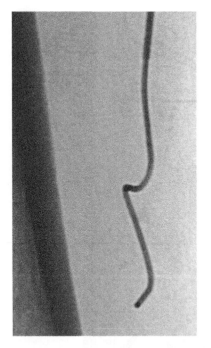

Fig. 31.3 Typical spiral appearance of a guidewire that is dissecting.

Perforation Guidewire perforation is not rare, particularly as we go more distally in the vascular tree (Fig. 31.4). What you do next depends on the system and any symptoms. In a blood vessel downstream of an occlusion, a perforation may well be self-limiting. Wait a couple of minutes and check. Some operators regard guidewire perforation as an occupational hazard of subintimal angioplasty. Causing a perforation in the biliary tree or urinary tract may require external drainage. Bowel perforation should be discussed with the surgical team and the patient will require close observation at a minimum.

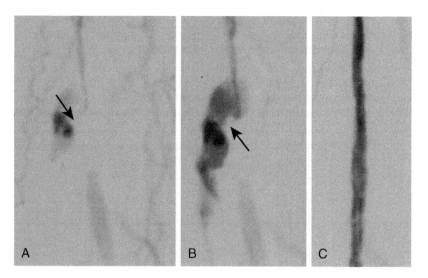

Fig. 31.4 ▦ (A,B) Guidewire perforation (arrow) of the SFA. (C) The extravasation resolved following satisfactory angioplasty.

Escalation

Despite all of your guile, you are not making progress. If you are planning to use a more 'forceful approach' before girding your loins and flexing your pecs:

- Consider whether there is an alternative technique, which might be simpler or even safer, e.g. endoscopic or surgical.
- Consider whether there is an alternative approach which is worth trying, e.g. contralateral in the vascular system, retrograde for the ureter, another duct or calyx, etc.
- Ensure that the patient has been consented for the risks of the procedure and that bail out equipment is available.

Once you are cleared for takeoff, do not reach straight for a 7Fr catheter and the back end of a stiff Terumo wire, gradually increase the force.

- Try a wire with a hydrophilic tip and a more supportive shaft, e.g. a Sensor wire or a stiff Terumo wire.
- Repeat the steps above.
- If the catheter backs off when you try to advance the wire, ask someone to fix it or increase the support by using a long sheath or guiding catheter.
- If the catheter still backs off try a more supportive catheter, e.g. a more auspicious shape, a braided catheter or a larger diameter (Fr size).

 Tip: If you are treating an iliac occlusion from the contralateral side, a reverse curve catheter such as a Sidewinder will offer more support than a forward-facing catheter.

If you have not made any headway This is the time to brace yourself and use alternative techniques.

Subintimal angioplasty

This is a technique best avoided in the early stages of an interventional career, especially when treating stenoses. In an occlusion, it is pretty much impossible to know what plane you are in within the artery wall and it is safest to regard this as 'who knows where you are angioplasty'. It is likely that many occlusions are traversed extraluminally without the operator knowing. There are two distinct strategies to extraluminal angioplasty.

1. Most commonly, an attempt is made to traverse the occlusion in the standard way but, after initially penetrating the occlusion, the guidewire does not make progress. If this happens, reach for your friend the Terumo wire and advance it until it stops. If you keep pushing, the wire will usually form a loop beyond the catheter tip (Fig. 31.5). If the

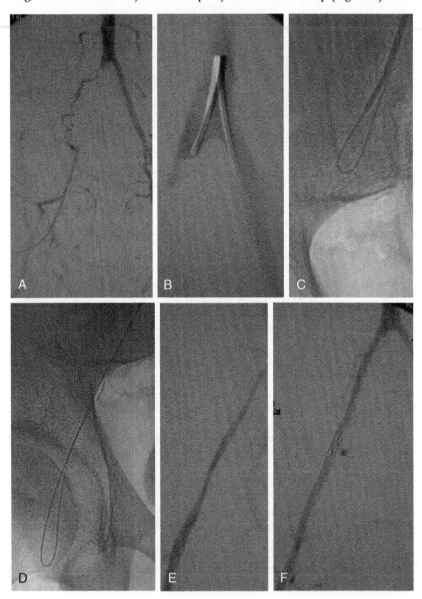

Fig. 31.5 Extraluminal angioplasty. (A) Complete right iliac artery occlusion. (B) A Sidewinder catheter is used to engage the origin of the CIA. (C) A loop has been formed in a hydrophilic wire and is advanced through the occlusion. (D) The loop has re-entered the arterial lumen in the CFA. (E) Injection around a 0.018-inch guidewire shows the extraluminal tract. (F) Completion angiogram following stenting.

loop can now be advanced with relatively little resistance, this is fine. It is important to remember where the occlusion ends and re-enter as close as possible to that point. Now comes the clever bit, re-entering the true lumen of the vessel! Frequently, the wire drops spontaneously straight back in; if not, this can take considerable time using a shaped catheter and wire or, rarely, a re-entry device.

2. The alternative is to deliberately enter the vessel wall above the occlusion. You will usually need a straight wire and a shaped catheter, such as the Berenstein to do this. Sometimes it is necessary to use the 'wrong end' of the wire to manage this. Do this with great care. Extraluminal position can be confirmed by injecting a small amount of contrast into the wall, this should show a localized dissection. If the contrast extends beyond the wall there is a perforation. This is one circumstance when this should not deter you; simply pull the catheter back and try again with a slightly different approach. Once the wall has been entered, a hydrophilic wire is advanced in a loop, as above.

The outcome of extraluminal angioplasty is akin to the false lumen in an aortic dissection. The channel communicates with the true lumen via tears at the entry and re-entry sites.

There are a few caveats to 'extraluminal angioplasty':

- Extraluminal angioplasty is seldom successful in heavily calcified vessels.
- Closely observe the diameter of the guidewire loop. If it starts to exceed the expected vessel diameter, you are at best 'subadventitial'. Success is highly unlikely. STOP before there is significant extravasation. Any further attempts are likely to follow the same path and you can always try again another day.
- Do not propagate the false lumen far beyond the point at which the vessel reconstitutes, or you risk losing important collateral flow and causing increased ischaemia if you cannot open the artery or if it re-occludes.
- Do not propagate the false lumen far beyond the point which compromises or changes the surgical options, unless this has been discussed and agreed with the patient and vascular surgical team.
- Consider using a stiff/supportive guidewire, e.g. the stiff Terumo, to help the catheter overcome friction when it is advanced.
- Consider using a low-profile angioplasty balloon catheter. They are excellent for dilating the lesion and can also be used to cross the lesion when a conventional catheter has failed.

Supporters of the extraluminal approach claim better long-term patency rates, particularly for long segment disease, because of the smooth subintimal lining. The downsides of the technique: it can be very difficult to re-enter; there is a higher incidence of vessel perforation and collaterals are occluded – important if the subintimal tract fails.

'Sharp recanalization'

This is definitely getting beyond the remit of a survival guide, as perforation is now much more likely and there is a risk of making false extraluminal channels. The first technique is to try the back of a standard Terumo wire. Confirm your position by imaging in two orthogonal planes before starting, as it is very easy to exit the lumen anteriorly or posteriorly. Aim for the centre of the lumen and try to advance the wire a few millimetres. Once you have achieved this, use the correct end of the wire again and see if you can advance; sometimes you will be surprised. In a blood vessel, this is a good time to form a loop in the wire and dissect (see subintimal angioplasty, above).

If this fails you really need to ask, 'Do I need to do this?' as you are moving into the realms of the dark arts. If yes, there are a raft of possibilities, which include radiofrequency guidewires, laser wires and diamond-tipped wires that drill through chronic total occlusions. These techniques need expert hands and do not always discriminate between the luminal pathway through the blockage and alternative routes through the wall of the vessel and adjacent soft tissues. Biplanar imaging is mandatory and the direction of travel should be reassessed every few millimetres.

 Alarm: Although there are reports of succeeding with these techniques, the complication rate is higher and in some cases more severe, e.g. cardiac tamponade when treating superior vena cava obstruction.

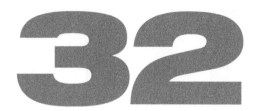

32

Principles of angioplasty

Angioplasty and stenting are cornerstone techniques in interventional radiology and have widespread non-vascular and vascular applications. The key skills and equipment choices remain largely the same, regardless of the site.

The main indication for angioplasty is the treatment of atherosclerotic plaque. Concentric plaque splits during balloon angioplasty and the intima and media stretch and tear (Fig. 32.1). When there is eccentric plaque, the tears occur at the interface between the plaque and the adjacent normal artery (Fig. 32.2). This often causes deep clefts and rarely results in distal embolization of part or all of the plaque. Balloon dilation stimulates nerve fibres in the adventitia, causing discomfort. Severe pain usually indicates that the vessel is being excessively dilated and at risk of rupture. Luminal gain occurs because progressive dilation irreversibly stretches the adventitia. Over a period of weeks, the damaged intima undergoes a period of 'remodelling'. This involves neointimal hyperplasia, which restores the smooth intimal surface. In non-vascular systems, the mechanism of plaque disruption triggering remodelling does not apply and balloon dilatation is usually used only to pre-dilate prior to stent placement

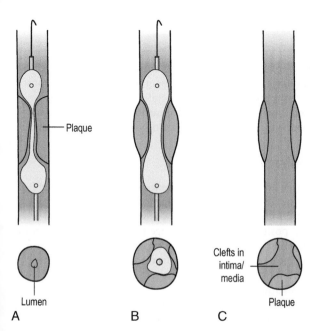

Fig. 32.1 ▥ Angioplasty of concentric plaque. (A) Balloon 'waisting' in stenosis before plaque rupture. (B) Balloon dilation – the plaque is ruptured but the plaque volume unchanged. (C) Balloon deflation – the luminal area is increased because of stretching of the media/adventitia and intimal clefts.

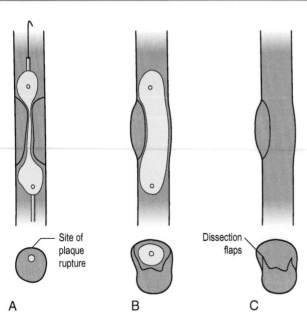

Fig. 32.2 ▤ Angioplasty of eccentric plaques. (A) Balloon 'waisting' in stenosis before plaque rupture. (B) Plaque has ruptured at its thinnest point – eccentric media/adventitia stretching. (C) Post-angioplasty dissection flaps in eccentric lumen. Plaque volume is unchanged.

Equipment

This is covered in more detail in the essential equipment section (Ch. 18). Choose the simplest balloon which you think will do the job, this is usually the workhorse over the wire device. To achieve an effective dilatation in the vascular system, use a balloon roughly 1 mm greater in diameter than the reference lumen diameter. Remember not to measure at a point where the lumen is dilated, e.g. beyond a tight arterial stenosis.

Key steps

By the time you are reaching for an angioplasty balloon you will already have established access and assessed the lesion, prior to navigating a passage across it. Remember the purpose of the guidewire now changes from steering to support. It is generally safest to exchange a hydrophilic guidewire for a conventional J-wire before trying to introduce a balloon. If you are performing vascular angioplasty you will normally give heparin before balloon dilatation.

Step 1: Position the balloon

- Image to delineate the lesion and store an image on the reference monitor, noting any key landmarks. Techniques which allow the live fluoroscopic image to be superimposed on a reference image are particularly useful for positioning.
- Failing this, inject some contrast and position some long sponge forceps over the midpoint of the lesion, then either apply a metallic marker, e.g. a towel clip on the drape or use a chinagraph pencil to mark the position on the screen. Confirm this is in the correct position with another contrast injection.
- **Remember:** Do not move the table after marking the lesion.
- Advance the balloon until the markers are centred on the target lesion.
- Fix the balloon and wire in position, paying attention to key landmarks.

Troubleshooting

Balloon will not cross the lesion This is particularly likely if the balloon has already been inflated. In this case, reach for a fresh balloon and try again. If this fails, pass a low-profile catheter across the lesion and exchange for a stiffer wire and try again. Still no luck – replace the low-profile catheter and place a supportive 0.018-inch wire; a low-profile over the wire balloon will almost always get through. Note that monorail systems are less likely to cross the lesion unless used with a guiding catheter, as the shaft is not supported. You can either pre-dilate or you may have the option of a low-profile balloon of the target size, in which case proceed directly to angioplasty.

Step 2: Inflate the balloon

- Ask your assistant to slowly inflate the balloon using an inflation device (you are busy with the balloon and wire).
- Fluoroscope throughout balloon inflation using the lowest-dose fluoroscopy, which allows you to see the balloon clearly.
- Make sure that the balloon does not migrate forwards or backwards as it inflates; this is particularly likely in short high-grade fibrotic lesions.
- Look for the waist at the site of the stenosis; the idea is to inflate until the waist disappears.
- If you are controlling the inflation (your assistant is holding the balloon and wire), regularly check the pressure gauge to ensure that you do not exceed the recommended balloon burst pressures.

 Alarm: Do not try this at home. Inflating an angioplasty balloon with saline and air until it bursts makes an impressive bang, and gives an idea of the damage it could cause in a blood vessel.

- Decide how long to leave the balloon inflated, the duration of inflation varies from operator to operator (depending on their attention span) and between lesions. There is no real science here but you will not go far wrong using the following principles:
  - For a stenosis, inflate for 1 min.
  - For a resistant stenosis, keep topping up the balloon to sustain the inflation pressure until the stenosis yields or you give in and get a cutting balloon.
  - For an occlusion, allow 2–3 min.
  - For a dissection flap, allow 3–5 min at low pressure.

Troubleshooting

The balloon migrates during inflation There are three possible solutions.

1. Inflate the balloon slowly and really focus on holding the balloon still; this might need you to apply a little counter-traction as the balloon tries to walk.
2. Use a long sheath or guide catheter to buttress the end of the balloon.
3. Use a longer balloon to allow it to grip on the adjacent wall.

The balloon bursts during inflation This is not uncommon with calcified plaque and is very likely if you ignore or exceed the rated burst pressure. Simply remove the balloon and try a new one. If this also bursts, then you need a tougher balloon or one rated to a higher pressure. Remember you may then need a larger sheath. If this still does not succeed it may be time to try a cutting balloon.

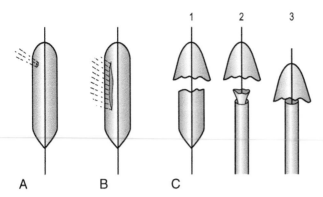

Fig. 32.3 ▧ Burst angioplasty balloons. (A) 'Pin-hole' tear: common and of no significance. (B) 'Longitudinal' tear: rare, but seldom a problem. (C) 'Circumferential' tear: very rare, but serious, as balloon will impact in sheath when it is withdrawn.

The stenosis will not dilate with the standard balloon Sometimes, being patient keeping the balloon inflated and maintaining the pressure will overcome the lesion. If this fails, it is best to reach for a high-pressure balloon or a cutting balloon. These do not always succeed and if the lesion still will not dilate, then it is time to stop.

Step 3: Deflate the balloon

Remember the inflation handle will usually not deflate the balloon completely. It is best to aspirate the balloon using an empty 20-mL or 50-mL syringe.

Troubleshooting

Very, very, rarely, a balloon will not deflate. Do not panic but simply puncture the balloon with a Chiba needle under fluoroscopic or ultrasound guidance. Often, the balloon will not deflate as there is a tap in the system turned the wrong way – remove all the taps from the balloon before reaching for that Chiba needle!

Step 4: Remove the balloon

You need to control the guidewire while doing this to ensure that you maintain access across the lesion at all times. Fluoroscope the wire tip as you back off the balloon to make sure that it is not advancing or retreating.

Troubleshooting

Sometimes the balloon will not easily pass through the groin sheath. Do not keep tugging. While determination is admirable, this will just impact the balloon in the sheath. Push the balloon back into the vessel and out of the sheath and aspirate again with a 50-mL syringe. Confirm on fluoroscopy that the balloon is deflated.

Occasionally, a balloon will burst with a circumferential tear; this turns the distal end into an open umbrella, which prevents it being brought back into the sheath (Figs. 32.3 and 32.4). Options here are to try to exchange for a larger sheath; you may need to cut the balloon shaft and keeping it on the guidewire, push it further into the patient. This will allow a new sheath to be placed over the wire; a snare is passed over the wire and used to capture the shaft and pull the balloon back. The alternative is to obtain access at a second site with a larger sheath. The wire is then brought out through the sheath and the balloon advanced into the sheath 'closing the umbrella'. Once again, the balloon will have to be cut to allow the shaft to be removed. When this has occurred, always check the retrieved fragments to make

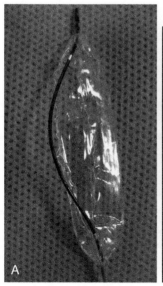
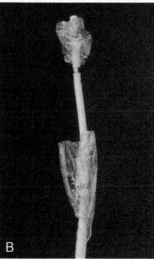

Fig. 32.4 ▣ Balloon tears. (A) Longitudinal and (B) circumferential. Balloons with longitudinal tears are easily removed. With a circumferential tear, the distal balloon crumpled up and wedged in place, as it was pulled into an 8Fr-reinforced sheath, and surgical removal was required.

sure that they add up to a 'whole balloon'. If not, the missing bit is still somewhere in the patient, either in the target artery or has migrated elsewhere with flow. It is essential to find this, as it will be an effective embolus and will need to be retrieved unless it is in an unimportant vessel/branch.

Step 5: Completion imaging

When dilating vascular lesions, assess the treated segment and the vessels distal to the angioplasty site – 'the run-off'.

Assessing the angioplasty site

Residual stenosis Less than 30% residual stenosis is the aim. Anything greater than this is a technical failure and symptomatic restenosis will be more likely. Residual stenosis can occur because the lesion has been under-dilated, secondary to elastic recoil or dissection.

• If possible, measure the pressure gradient across the lesion. If no gradient is present, stop.
• Many stenoses will remodel after angioplasty and if there is a 30–50% residual stenosis in a non-critical vessel, it may be appropriate to leave it.

Elastic recoil This describes the situation when the angioplasty balloon completely expands but the lesion recoils on deflation; often stenting is indicated. Do not stent lesions when it has not been possible to 'de-waist' during angioplasty, as you simply line a stenosis with a stent.

Dissection Short dissection flaps or intimal clefts are visible at many angioplasty sites; this is after all the consequence of plaque rupture. A dissection is only significant if it impedes distal flow (Fig. 32.5). Small non-flow-limiting dissections appear as linear filling defects with brisk flow. These will heal in time as the artery re-models. Occasionally, the intimal/medial interface has been very disrupted and the flap partially or completely occludes the lumen; this

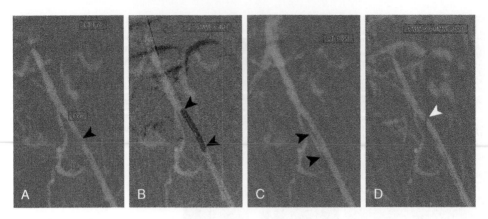

Fig. 32.5 ■ Managing flow-limiting dissection. (A) External iliac stenosis (arrowhead). (B) Inflation of appropriately sized balloon (arrowheads). (C) Very deep dissection cleft post-angioplasty (arrowheads) did not settle with prolonged balloon inflation. (D) Appearance following placement of a self-expanding stent (arrowhead).

is why you made sure the wire was still across the lesion. If a flow-limiting dissection is present, then:

- First, try a low-pressure balloon inflation for 3–5 min across the dissection flap. This often 'tacks' the flap back into position. If you restore brisk flow, you have succeeded.
- Persistent flow-limiting dissections can be readily treated by stenting across the flap.

Venous filling Venous opacification sometimes occurs, extending from the angioplasty site through venae comitantes into the adjacent vein. This is rarely of any consequence and can safely be left alone. A large arteriovenous fistula is a different kettle of fish! In this case, almost all the flow will shunt into the vein with little or no flow in the distal run-off. When this happens, the leak will sometimes close with prolonged low-pressure balloon inflation over the defect but, most likely, you will need a stent graft to repair the hole.

Extravasation This indicates disruption of all layers of the arterial wall and prompt action is essential. It is essential that you look for and can recognize extravasation (Fig. 29.3). Brisk haemorrhage can occur, particularly in the iliac segment and aggressive resuscitation may be required.

- Reintroduce the balloon and perform a low-pressure inflation proximal to the rupture to tamponade the bleeding. Sometimes this is sufficient to allow a small hole to seal.
- Have someone contact a friendly vascular surgeon and warn them you may need their skills.
- Put in a large drip and set up a saline infusion. Monitor the patient's pulse, BP and oxygen saturation. Take blood for a coagulation screen and cross-match.
- Time to get looking for a stent graft; think about the required diameter and length. It is far better to have confirmed this was available during the preoperative brief.
- Wait for 5 min, then repeat the angiogram. If extravasation persists, re-inflate the balloon to maintain haemostastic control.
- If expertise and equipment permit, a stent graft can be inserted (Fig. 32.6). This will not only rescue the situation but also prolong your increasingly tenuous friendship with the vascular surgeon! If nothing works, the patient will need immediate surgical intervention.

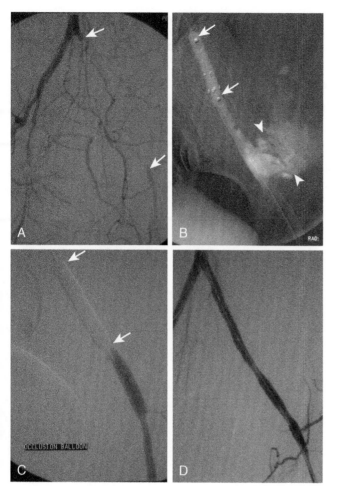

Fig. 32.6 ■ Managing iliac artery rupture. (A) Long iliac artery occlusion, which was traversed from the contralateral femoral artery. (B) Following stenting, there was severe pain during EIA angioplasty. The balloon was immediately inflated in the CIA (arrows). Angiography demonstrated EIA rupture with extravasation (arrowheads). (C) Balloon inflated to tamponade the rupture site. Brisk extravasation persisted despite prolonged inflation (arrows). (D) A stent graft has been deployed via the ipsilateral femoral artery. The occlusion balloon was pulled back to the CIA during deployment.

Assessing the distal vessels

Obtain good-quality angiograms to assess the run-off and the presence of any collaterals. Remember that collaterals often stop filling following successful angioplasty.

Distal embolization The signs of distal embolization are evidence of a new filling defect somewhere in the outflow circulation. In this case, assess the clinical status of the limb. If the limb is well perfused and the embolus is into a non-critical branch vessel, then further intervention is inappropriate. More worrying findings are marked slowing of flow or even stasis in the run-off vessels. In this case:

- Assess the clinical status of the limb to gauge the severity of the ischaemia.
- Let the patient know that there is a problem and what you will be doing to manage it.
- Arrange analgesia if required.
- Check coagulation status and give further heparin as required.
- Let Houston (the boss) know that there is a problem.
- Obtain ipsilateral access and perform clot aspiration (see Thrombosuction, Ch. 47, p. 319).

Tip: A useful technique that allows you to preserve guidewire access across a contralateral lesion is to inject around a 0.018-inch guidewire using a Tuohy–Borst adaptor and 0.035-inch lumen catheter when performing completion angiography.

General complications of arterial angioplasty

Complications related to specific sites are detailed in the chapters in Section 4.

For all angioplasty, the complications divide into:

- The 3Bs of arterial access: bruising, bleeding and blockage at the puncture site.
- Generic angioplasty-related: vessel occlusion, rupture or dissection, usually fixed by stent or stent graft, distal embolization 1–4%, often of no clinical importance. About 1% of patients will require surgery.

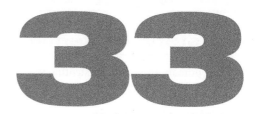

Principles of stenting and stent-grafting

Expandable stents are used to manage luminal narrowing in many systems from the aorta to the trachea. As with angioplasty, there is a common skill-set required for deployment, regardless of location but the indications and outcomes are very different so try to avoid a 'have stent, will travel' mentality. There is a simple basic concept regarding intent, which transcends most applications.

A procedure may be undertaken with the express intention of deploying a stent, so-called **primary stenting**, e.g. oesophageal stenting for tumour dysphagia and iliac artery occlusions (often primarily stented to reduce the incidence of distal embolization). Most angiographers will primarily stent ostial lesions of the visceral arteries without trying angioplasty because they really represent aortic disease, which will inevitably have elastic recoil.

A stent may be deployed to salvage an unsuccessful balloon dilatation procedure, e.g. recurrence of a benign stricture of the trachea. This **secondary stenting** is the commonest indication for using a stent in the vascular system, e.g. failed iliac angioplasty with residual pressure gradient, stenosis or flow-limiting dissection (Table 33.1).

Table 33.1 Indications for arterial stenting

Indication	Primary	Secondary
Failed angioplasty	✗	✓
Risk of embolization	✓	✗
Iliac occlusion	✓	✗
Ostial renal artery stenosis	✓	✗
Restenosis	✓	✗
Carotid artery	✓	✗

Equipment

This is covered in more detail in the essential equipment section (Chs 20 and 21). Choose the simplest stent which you think will do the job. Use pre-procedure imaging to gauge the size of stent you are likely to use (length and diameter) and make sure that you have a long enough delivery system.

 Alarm: There are no prizes for selecting a stent just to find it will only reach part of the way to the target.

Key steps in stenting

Whether primary or secondary stenting you will have imaged the target, achieved access, crossed the lesion and have a sufficiently supportive guidewire in place.

Position the stent

This involves the same elements as positioning a balloon for angioplasty and these are summarized below:

- Image to delineate and measure the lesion and mark the position either on the patient or on a reference monitor.
- **Remember:** Do not move the patient, image intensifier or table after marking the lesion.

  Alarm: If something moves, repeat the imaging to confirm position.

- Advance the stent into position so that the relevant markers are centred across the lesion and image again to confirm correct placement. This is the time to be sure that you know the significance of each marker (Fig. 33.1; See also Figs. 20.2 and 20.4).

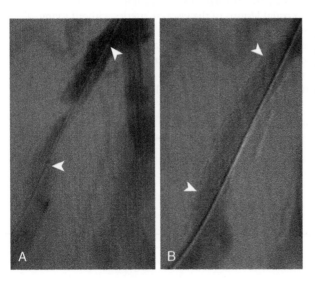

Fig. 33.1 ▦ Stent positioning and deployment in iliac stenosis. (A) Angiogram from the contralateral iliac, stent markers (arrowheads). (B) Post-deployment and angioplasty, stent position (arrowheads).

- Consider the implications of incorrect positioning, in particular the effects of covering vital vessels! If necessary, protect these with guidewires or balloons.

Troubleshooting

Stent will not cross the lesion This is most likely to occur in long high lesions, particularly if the stent is following a tortuous path. In arteries calcified occlusions are particularly problematic. There are several possible solutions:

- **Make sure you have a stiff enough wire:** this is usually the time to use an Amplatz wire or something of equivalent strength. When performing aortic stent-grafting use a Lunderquist or equivalent.

- **Pre-dilate the lesion:** Angioplasty with a 3–4-mm balloon is usually sufficient for arterial stents but scale things up for the oesophagus.
- **Pass a sheath across the lesion:** Sometimes the profile of the sheath and dilator is more favourable than the tip of the sheath catheter. The stent is subsequently introduced through the sheath and the sheath pulled back.
- **Try a different stent:** This is most likely to help if you can exchange for a stent that has better trackability and pushability. A low-profile self-expanding stent is more likely to cross the lesion than a balloon-mounted stent.
- **If all of the above fail, consider a rendezvous procedure:** Remember that if the guidewire is fixed in two places, you can apply considerable force, so proceed with great care.

The stent comes off the balloon This is commoner with operator stents hand-crimped onto the balloon and is pretty rare now we have manufacturer-crimped stents. It often occurs incrementally and the situation can sometimes be salvaged if recognized early. When things do go wrong, try to keep the situation in perspective. Remember not to cause more harm than necessary. It is often best to summon a more senior colleague or obtain surgical help.

- **The stent moves proximal or distal to the balloon markers prior to deployment** (Fig. 33.2): Do not attempt deployment if either end of the stent has moved outside the balloon markers. If there has been significant stent movement, asymmetrical balloon inflation will push the stent off the balloon.

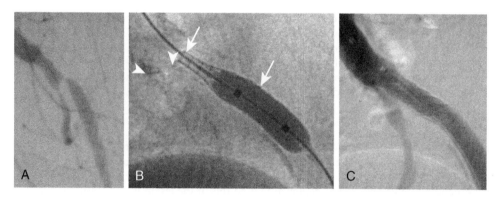

Fig. 33.2 ▨ (A) High-grade calcified EIA stenosis prior to femoropopliteal grafting. (B) During deployment, the balloon has 'been pushed out' of the stent (arrows); note the stent has not moved and remains perfectly placed in relation to the origin of the IIA (arrowheads). In this case, the balloon was deflated and repositioned to deploy the remainder of the stent. (C) Completion.

- **If the whole stent remains on the balloon:** Stay calm and slowly inflate the balloon with contrast, the ends of the balloon normally open first, leaving the stent in the middle in its compressed state. On fluoroscopy, this should resemble the shape of a dog bone. If this works it will usually help the stent to grip the balloon, allowing it to be positioned and deployed. If balloon expansion is asymmetric, stop and take stock.
- **The stent begins to migrate off the balloon:** Things are taking a turn for the worse, deflate the balloon and gently try to recapture the stent. This is safest and most likely to succeed if the stent is held in the stenosis with the balloon being advanced into it. If you are in a vessel like the renal artery, take great care if you are pulling the balloon back as the stent is likely to be dislodged and come completely off the balloon catheter. As always, remember to keep the wire in position!
- **If repositioning is successful, slowly inflate the balloon. Deploy the stent as normal if it remains in position.

- In you are not succeeding and the stent is partly covering the lesion, then it is probably best to deploy it where it is. If this is unsafe or impossible, then try to move the stent to a safe site for deployment, such as the iliac artery.

If the stent has come off the balloon and is missing in action

- **First, find the stent!** Fortunately, it is usually on the catheter shaft or has stuck in the groin sheath. Some stents are poorly opaque and it may be necessary to take spot radiographs to locate them.
- **If the stent is on the catheter:** pull the balloon back and if necessary slightly inflate it to withdraw the stent into the sheath, then remove the sheath and catheter and insert a new sheath (use one that you have prepared earlier). Consider a different type of stent but if you need to proceed with the same one make sure you crimp it on this time. If it is in the sheath, the same applies.
- **If the stent has come completely off the balloon catheter:** with luck, it will still be on the wire. This is much harder! Pass a 4Fr straight catheter through the stent and exchange for a 0.018-inch wire. Try to capture the stent with a small-profile angioplasty balloon. Alternatively, pass a GooseNeck snare alongside the guidewire and snare the stent by lassoing the wire.

Deploying the stent

- Take your time and use continuous fluoroscopy while deploying the stent and constantly maintain the position as you deploy.
- Use an empty 20-mL syringe to completely deflate the balloon.
- Screen during withdrawal of the delivery system to ensure that the stent is not dislodged.
- Use angioplasty to 'tailor' the stent to the vessel wall. All stents, including self-expanding stents, need a balloon for complete deployment.

Troubleshooting

The stent starts to move off the target If the stent is only partly open and not yet opposing the wall, it can sometimes be repositioned by gentle traction or pushing. Once the stent has engaged, there is usually little that can be done. You can try gentle traction but self-expanding stents tend just to deploy as you do this. If the lesion is only partly covered, you can deploy a second stent to treat the remainder of the lesion.

Completion imaging

This is the same as following angioplasty, check the treatment site and the run-off.

Troubleshooting

The stent diameter is too small The main risk here is stent migration. What you do next depends largely on where you are. Stents in the gastrointestinal tract quite often migrate with surprisingly little consequence. Free-range stents in the vascular system are more problematic.

Balloon-deployed stent This can be easily rescued. Use a 50-mL syringe to deflate the balloon as much as possible. Continue to apply suction to maintain a low profile, then carefully withdraw the balloon from the stent. Screen during removal of the balloon if the stent is not opposed to the wall. It is all too easy to accidentally displace the stent. Make sure you keep the guidewire access in situ. Now insert an appropriately sized balloon and dilate the stent up.

Self-expanding stent This is a little trickier. You have two options, depending on how much space you have on either side of the stent. If you have space, you can deploy an overlapping larger-diameter self-expanding stent; this will secure the smaller stent, but the second stent seldom has enough strength to open out the initial nitinol stent further. If there is no space, then an alternative possibility is to insert a balloon-expandable stent within the self-expanding stent; the second stent will be strong enough to oppose the nitinol stent to the wall. It is best to pick a similar length of stent.

Covered stents

Stent-grafting is not dissimilar to stenting but the margins for error are smaller. For a stent graft to be effective, it must fit precisely within the target vessel. An undersized graft will allow blood to flow between it and the vessel wall. Oversized devices will have creases in the graft material, which may adversely affect flow, lead to endoleaks and promote thrombosis. Covered stents are used in three sets of circumstances.

To manage strictures Especially neoplastic strictures, where the covering prevents tumour in-growth. In the vascular tree, they are sometimes used for 'in situ' grafting to reline a vessel, usually when there has been re-stenosis.

To manage leaks This includes the treatment of fistula and traumatic and iatrogenic vascular injury.

To manage aneurysmal disease Vascular disease only this time.
   In the first two circumstances, the stent grafts are used in exactly the same way as a stent but remember that these are impermeable, so a malpositioned stent graft has greater potential for ramifications than a bare stent. Take great care at bifurcations, e.g. the tracheal carina or at major bronchial origins and also not to cover important collateral vessels.

Stent-grafting for aneurysmal disease: basic rules

Management of aneurysmal disease follows slightly different rules. Pre-procedure assessment is more rigorous and detailed than for either of the previous indications. In general, consider the following:

Computed tomography with multiplanar reformats is currently the method of choice and has largely replaced angiography using calibrated catheters. Computed tomography (CT) is able to accurately measure the diameters, lengths and angulation of the aneurysm, its neck and the iliac arteries (Fig. 33.3).

 Tip: Use suitably wide windows when reviewing the images to allow you to distinguish between calcification in the vessel wall and contrast enhancement in the lumen.

Magnetic resonance imaging (MRI) is not widely used to assess abdominal aortic aneurysm (AAA) due to limited availability. It can offer similar information to CT but with the disadvantage that calcification is not as readily appreciated. Remember that magnetic resonance angiography (MRA) only shows the flowing lumen and additional sequences are required to assess the true extent of the aneurysm and the vessel wall.

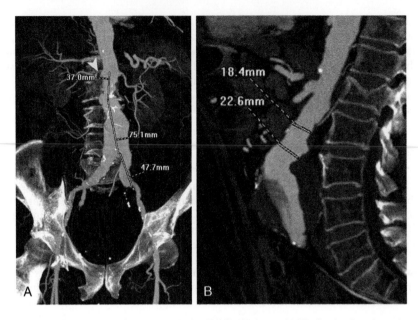

Fig. 33.3 ■ Use of CT to assess AAA suitability for EVAR. (A) Coronal MIP allowing lengths to be assessed. Yellow arrowhead indicates level of the renal arteries. (B) Sagittal MIP showing angulation of the neck.

Ultrasound can be used to assess peripheral arteries for tube graft repair, as only simple diameter and length measurements are needed. Ultrasound does not provide sufficient information for endovascular aortic aneurysm repair (EVAR).

Calibrated angiography is only needed when CT/MRI with reformats is not available.
Remember that individual devices will require different access diameters and have different recommended maximum and minimum diameters for treatment – these measurements are all available in sizing charts and the device instructions for use. For any aneurysm that we are trying to exclude with a stent graft, there are three factors to consider.

Access This is usually the common femoral and iliac arteries. Stent grafts can be very large devices, in excess of 20F, those needed to manage thoracic aneurysms are the largest to accommodate the stents and graft material. The access vessels need to be sufficiently large and straight to accommodate the device and to allow its passage through to the target deployment site. As devices evolve, contraindications are becoming technical challenges. Look out for:

Diseased puncture site Plaque is very common in the common femoral artery.

Too narrow Particularly iliac artery diameter. Another access issue occurs when the distal aorta is too small; this can prevent access for a contralateral iliac limb.

Tortuous vessels More than one ≥90 degree bend, especially if there is heavy vascular calcification, which makes the arteries rigid.

Solutions Look for alternative approaches and consider a cutdown onto the iliac arteries and placement of a temporary conduit. In some cases, angioplasty will suffice to treat a focal stenosis.

Anchorage sites

These are the points at which the stent graft makes a seal with the arterial wall. In occlusive disease, a stent will be in contact with the vessel wall over most of its length; conversely, a stent graft used to treat an aneurysm will be largely unsupported and only be in contact with the vessel in the non-aneurysmal sections. These must be of suitable diameter and length for the proximal and distal stents. In general, the stent-graft diameter should be 10–20% greater than the diameter of the implantation site.

Contraindications

- **Technical challenge:** the following make the procedure more difficult and more likely to go wrong: proximal neck length <10 mm, proximal neck angulation ≥60 degrees, conical neck (especially if enlarging distally).
- **Suboptimal surface:** extensive thrombus or atheroma within the neck makes achieving a seal less likely and migration more likely.

Solutions

In theory, issues with the proximal neck can be remedied by the use of grafts with suprarenal fixation (Fig. 33.4) or for very short necks – fenestrated grafts, which have greater contact with the wall or branched grafts and anchor proximally in the 'normal' aorta. In practice, consider whether this will be better for the patient than an open repair.

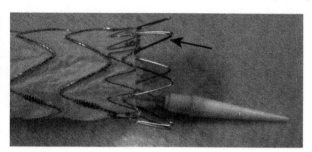

Fig. 33.4 Graft with anchor stent (arrow) proximal to graft material.

Tip: If the neck is short and angulated, then use reformats to assess the optimal obliquity to use for positioning angiography during graft deployment.

Alternative/adequate branch vessels

Branch vessels have important implications for stent-grafting and must be assessed on the pre-procedural angiograms. The stent graft must not cover vital branch arteries or the supply to the intestine, kidneys or brain, etc. Conversely, branch vessels may also carry blood back into the aneurysm and compromise treatment.

Contraindications

- **Aberrant vessels:** low renal artery origin. Aberrant branch vessels from the aortic arch
- **Essential vessels:** the inferior mesenteric artery (IMA) will be covered during stent-grafting; if the superior mesenteric artery (SMA) is severely diseased, bowel infarction may occur
- **Unwanted vessels:** branch vessels may adversely affect aneurysm exclusion, e.g. when treating an iliac artery aneurysm, retrograde flow through a patent internal iliac artery (IIA) would leave the aneurysm perfused.

Solutions

- **Aberrant vessels:** simply decide if the vessel can be sacrificed, e.g. a small accessory renal artery.
- **Essential vessels:** some aneurysms can be made suitable for stent-graft repair by performing extra anatomical grafting to prevent ischaemia, e.g. femoro–femoral cross-over. In other cases, the length of the anchorage site can be increased by more complex surgery, e.g. carotid subclavian bypass grafts, mesenteric/renal bypass or anastomosis of the carotid and subclavian arteries to a graft from the ascending aorta. Others can be treated with fenestrated or branched grafts.
- **Unwanted vessels:** in these circumstances, the artery should be embolized prior to deployment of the stent-graft to prevent type II endoleak, e.g. IIA. The same applies when the left subclavian artery is covered during TEVAR. The IMA and large lumbar arteries may be embolized pre-procedure.

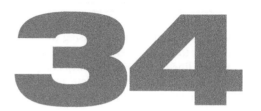

Principles of pressure measurement

Angiography, whether by computed tomography (CT), magnetic resonance angiography (MRA) or digital subtraction angiography (DSA) is not accurate at assessing the significance of a stenosis unless it is very tight or very inconsequential. Doppler ultrasound fares far better and can give excellent quantification of the haemodynamic significance of a stenosis but is not always practicable.

In practice, pressure measurements are not as scientific as they sound, and they are used in relatively few circumstances, i.e. during transjugular intrahepatic portosystemic shunt (TIPS) procedures to ensure appropriate reduction in portal vein pressure, and when there is uncertainty regarding the significance of aortoiliac arterial lesions pre- and post-treatment.

The key concept is that a pressure drop will occur across the stenosis if it is physiologically significant. Therefore, the pressure below the stenosis will be lower than above the stenosis. Small pressure drops are to be expected and most operators would regard a 10 mm mean pressure drop as significant across an arterial stenoses. It may be surprising, but these values will vary slightly between labs and trials.

Pressure measurements can be done in one of two ways:

- **Dual pressures**: simultaneous measurements from above and below the lesion. This needs two transducers and might seem more complex but is more accurate.
- **Pull-back pressures**: single transducer, so slightly simpler but less accurate, as it is subject to beat-to-beat variation in intra-arterial pressure and risks losing a hard-won position across the lesion.

Measuring pressures is simple but we have seen it made look very complicated, so **pay attention here**:

- You need to have access to both sides of the lesion; either you have crossed it with a wire or have access above and below the lesion, e.g. affected leg and contralateral leg for iliac intervention.
- The transducers cleverly do not need to be inserted into the patient but can measure the pressure from the standing column of fluid in a catheter.
- For dual-pressure measurements, a catheter is placed above the lesion and a catheter below the lesion. This is simple if you are using a femoral sheath for iliac intervention, just remember to use a sheath at least one French size larger than the measurement catheter.
- For pull-back pressure measurements, the catheter is inserted above the lesion and 'pulled back', while monitoring changes in the pressures.
- The pressure transducers are sterile and handed to the operator. One end attaches to the catheter. The other end has a plug that is given to your helper (who is not scrubbed) and is plugged into the monitor.
- The pressure transducers need to be calibrated or 'zeroed'. This is the step most often misunderstood. The transducer(s) will have a three-way tap; turn the tap so that the

transducer is open to air. If using two transducers calibrate both at the same time. Hold them at the same level and preferably about the level of the patient's right atrium (mid-axillary line in a supine patient). Ask your helper to press the zero button on the monitor and wait for the 'zero complete' message.

- Turn the tap so that the transducer is now reading from the patient – voila you have intra-arterial pressures!
- Get someone to write down the pressures and calculate the gradient – you will be too exhausted to remember them.

In iliac assessment, if there is a minor non-significant gradient, then some operators will perform a stressed gradient. The rationale is that while there is no significant gradient at rest, there may be a gradient when increased flow is required during exercise; this is simulated by the injection of a vasodilator. Who knows how physiological this measurement accurately represents exercise but at any rate, find out the practice in your unit for marginal pressure drops.

Tip: If using pull-back pressures, you can maintain a wire across a stenosis by using a standard catheter, a Y-adaptor and a 0.018-inch wire.

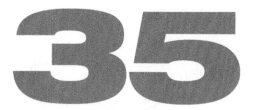

Principles of embolization

Embolotherapy is the deliberate blockage of blood vessels; it is usually performed to stop haemorrhage and may be life-saving in gastrointestinal bleeding and trauma. Embolization is sometimes used as an adjunct to surgery and in the treatment of a variety of benign and malignant tumours.

Many types of embolic agents are available to block vessels of different sizes, from arteries to capillaries. The choice of the agent used depends on the individual circumstances of the case.

General principles

The ideal embolization is a 'precision strike' to block the target vessel or target territory as selectively as possible to minimize 'collateral damage' to non-target structures. An understanding of the vascular anatomy combined with good-quality pre-embolization imaging is essential. Scrutiny of previous cross-sectional imaging can be invaluable in identifying arterial supply and variants.

 Alarm: Consider the consequences of ischaemia in the territory you are occluding and anywhere important that might be embolized should the embolic materials go astray.

Anastomoses between arterial territories are particularly important for two reasons:

1. Some lesions can potentially recruit supply from a number of different parent vessels. This situation is typified in the case of a gastroduodenal artery aneurysm, which will receive supply from both the hepatic artery and the superior mesenteric artery (SMA) via the pancreaticoduodenal arcade (Fig. 35.1). If you close the front door (the hepatic artery or gastroduodenal artery [GDA] proximal to the aneurysm), the lesion can still get supply via the back door route of SMA and pancreaticoduodenal arcade and this will be much harder to manage.
2. Blockage may affect adjacent arterial territory, sometimes with disastrous results, e.g. bronchial and spinal arterial anastomoses.

Level to block Occlusion can be achieved at any level from main artery to capillary level, depending on the agent. Decide at the outset whether you need to block a feeding vessel or an entire vascular bed. In general, to treat bleeding, only the source vessel needs to be blocked but to treat a tumour, the entire tumour circulation should be occluded.

Which embolic agent?

Ask the following questions:

1. Will temporary occlusion do the job? Some trauma cases can be satisfactorily treated with temporary occlusion using Gelfoam, particularly when there are multiple bleeding sites

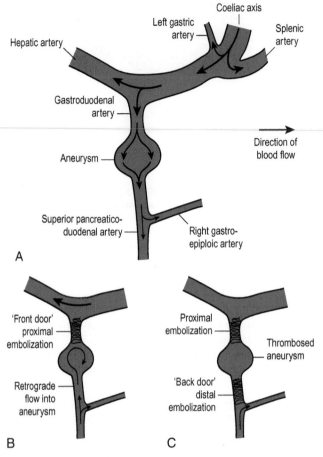

Coeliac axis

Left gastric artery

Splenic artery

Hepatic artery

Gastroduodenal artery

Aneurysm

Direction of blood flow

Superior pancreatico-duodenal artery

Right gastro-epiploic artery

A

'Front door' proximal embolization

Retrograde flow into aneurysm

B

Proximal embolization

Thrombosed aneurysm

'Back door' distal embolization

C

Fig. 35.1 ▨ Embolization of a gastroduodenal aneurysm. (A) Aneurysm supplied from the hepatic artery via the gastroduodenal artery. (B) Proximal embolization only closes the 'front door'. The aneurysm is perfused retrogradely via the pancreaticoduodenal arcade. (C) Proximal and distal embolization closes the 'front and back doors'. The aneurysm is no longer perfused and will thrombose.

off one parent vessel. Gelfoam occlusion lasts for between a few days and a few weeks and gives the vessel a chance to heal. Gelfoam is readily available, easy to use and prepare and is fairly safe.

2. What level of occlusion is required? If a permanent agent is needed, then determine the size of the target vessel; coils and plugs are used to occlude medium-to-small arteries; polyvinyl alcohol (PVA) particles are used to occlude multiple small arteries, arterioles and capillaries. Unless you are expert, avoid the use of liquid embolic agents.

3. Are adjuncts such as chemotherapy or radiotherapy needed, e.g. liver tumours?

4. Will repeat access ever be required? Generally for tumours or inflammatory conditions, blocking the parent vessel with a bunch of coils is less than helpful if re-treatment is required, e.g. bronchial artery embolization.

Key steps for safe embolization

- Good-quality preliminary angiography.
- Think carefully about collateral pathways.
- Use the shortest, straightest approach, particularly if coils are involved.
- Always use endhole-only catheters.
- Select the simplest embolic agent that will do the job.

- Test stability of the catheter position with the guidewire if using coils or test injections of contrast if using particulate agents. If the catheter moves during testing, there is little chance of it remaining in place during treatment.
- Use non-heparinized saline to flush catheters and dilute contrast; thrombosis is the aim.
- Use continuous fluoroscopy during embolization. There is no point in a low radiation dose if it results in non-target embolization.
- Monitor the flow. This will be obvious when using particles suspended in contrast. When using coils, perform intermittent runs.
- Adjust your embolic agent delivery as the case progresses. If using particulate or liquid agents, as the territory occludes smaller volumes are needed with each injection. If using coils, remember that as a coil nest enlarges, there is less space for subsequent coils; consider stopping or using smaller, shorter or more tightly packing coils, e.g. microcoils.
- A patient in pain is restless, distressed and often moving; this makes the procedure much more difficult and increases the chances of error. Where the procedure is anticipated to be painful, e.g. fibroid embolization, prescribe premedication and ensure suitable intra- and postoperative pain relief.
- Know when to finish! It is vital to occlude the target lesion; after that has been achieved you are just tempting fate. Remember the maxim: 'The enemy of good is perfect'.

Alarm: Using embolic agents safely

Lethal complications have occurred by inadvertent injections of embolic agents during intervention. Your IR team needs to have a systematic approach to handling embolic agents. This is particularly important for liquid and particulate agents. Always:
- Use a separate trolley to prepare and store particulate or liquid embolic agents.
- Use either different-sized syringes or marked syringes to differentiate the embolic agent from contrast/flush.
- Perform a visual and verbal check with your assistant during preparation and before injection.
- Remember the dead space of the catheter remains loaded with embolic agents. This needs to be carefully flushed through before repositioning for that final glory run.
- If in doubt, chuck it out. Get rid of any 'loaded guns' by discarding any contrast, saline, syringes or catheters, if there is any possibility that they might be contaminated with the embolic agent.

Troubleshooting

Unable to obtain a selective or stable catheter position

Go back to basic principles Make sure that the catheter is the optimal shape for the vessel. Try a more supportive catheter (larger French size or a guide-catheter to support the catheter). There are several possible solutions. Consider an alternative approach, e.g. from the arm rather than the leg. If the optimal position is not obtainable, consider more proximal embolization but remember that the collateral damage will increase.

Problems with coils

The delivery catheter is pushed back during coil deployment Remember that the coil needs some space to form, so a degree of movement is normal when making a dense nest of coils. Movement is worrying when there is little space or when the catheter is recoiling rather than the coil forming. Concentrate on holding the catheter in position. If you find you need three hands, then get assistance from a colleague. A reasonably long coil that has had less than 25% extruded can sometimes be withdrawn along with the catheter. Take great care, as this risks the coil being lost and embolizing elsewhere or even bringing part of the nest back with it. This has to be balanced against the risk of deploying the coil where it is.

 Tip: If only a short amount of coil remains, it can usually be deployed and will often surprise you by shortening back into the target vessel or lying flat against the parent artery wall.

A coil is misplaced This usually occurs when the catheter position is not stable, the coil is incorrectly sized or when deployment is attempted in too short a vessel segment. Only attempt retrieval if the coil is likely to occlude a significant vessel, otherwise you will probably cause more harm than good. Coils can be retrieved using a snare but remember you may fish out more than one! Prevention is better than cure and if you are concerned about the stability of the first coil, a trick is to anchor the first portion in a small branch vessel just beyond the target site. The coil will deploy straight and as the catheter is pushed back will anchor the coil in position.

A coil jams in the delivery catheter This occurs when the coil is the wrong size for the catheter, when there is a tight bend or kink in the catheter or when the catheter has been damaged by previous coils or retains particulate agents. Fluoroscope to determine the position of the coil. First, try to free the coil by flushing with saline; use a 1-mL syringe as this gives the highest pressure. If this fails, try using the stiff end of the guidewire/pusher; unfortunately, this seldom works.

If the coil is in the catheter outside the patient, then cut off the end of the catheter, including the coil. Pass a guidewire through the catheter and exchange it for a new one. If the coil is in the catheter inside the patient, there is no option but to remove the catheter with loss of the position.

 Tip: Do not jeopardize a hard-won position; exchange the delivery catheter before it fails if you feel that there is increasing resistance to coil passage. Consider changing the delivery catheter if using coils after PVA particles.

Problems with particles

The catheter occludes Aggregations of particles form particularly in the catheter hub; this is especially likely if the catheter has not been flushed. First, try to carefully flush with a low-volume syringe (1–2 mL). This generates more pressure, so be careful not to jet the catheter, and emerging embolic material, out of the target vessel. If no success, reach for a guidewire and try to pass it through the catheter. If the catheter is kinked or plugged with a clump of PVA, this will sometimes clear a passage. Kinked catheters will re-kink readily and should be exchanged for a new catheter before continuing. Commonly, neither technique works and it is time to remove the catheter and face getting back into the vessel selectively.

 Tip: Larger particle sizes are more likely to block the catheter; dilute with more contrast to reduce the risk of clumping.

Problems with liquid agents

The difficulty with liquid agents is that, like sale goods, 'when they're gone they're gone'! Very little can be done once you have released the agent into the circulation, so scrupulous technique and attention to detail and prevention are paramount. The only problem that can be remedied is when you are faced with a 'loaded catheter' full of glue or sclerosant and you realize that you have reached your endpoint. At this stage, any further injection will lead to non-target embolization. Stop injecting and DO NOT FLUSH! If you are using glue, then this is the moment to change the catheter. If you are using a sclerosant then try aspirating until flowing blood is obtained. At this stage, there will be minimal agent left in the catheter and you can continue to use it.

The main problem associated with lipiodol is disintegration of the catheter hub and any attached tap – remember not to use polycarbonate! The remedy – as usual remove/replace the catheter.

Complications

Embolotherapy has a high potential for complications and catastrophes. All the standard complications of diagnostic angiography are present. Risks unique to embolization must be discussed pre-procedure with the patient and include:

Post-embolization syndrome Post-embolization syndrome is a consequence rather than a true complication of embolization and occurs as an effect of tissue infarction, with subsequent release of vasoactive substances and other inflammatory mediators. It is most common with solid organ embolization, e.g. the liver, and broadly related to the extent of tissue infarction. After embolization, patients typically develop severe pain within hours, and over the next 24–72 h have fever, nausea and vomiting, myalgia, arthralgia and general debility. Affected patients need support with appropriate analgesia, intravenous fluids and nursing care. Symptoms tend to subside after ~72 h but it can be a worrying time for both the patient and the clinician.

Non-target embolization As we explained earlier, it is usually possible to retrieve a misplaced coil with some skill and determination. Unfortunately, non-target embolization with permanent particulate or liquid agents is irretrievable. The consequences are dependent on the vascular bed affected but may be life-threatening, particularly if the heart or central nervous system is affected. Clearly, great care to avoid this complication is the aim, but for each case you must be aware of the potential innocent bystanders and consent appropriately, prompt recognition and appropriate treatment, surgical or otherwise, may be life-saving.

Abscess formation Ischaemic and infarcted tissue makes a great culture medium and prophylactic antibiotics are essential if a significant volume of tissue is embolized. If patients are persistently pyrexial after embolization, then blood cultures and appropriate imaging are needed. There are circumstances where this is more likely to occur, e.g. open trauma and uterine artery embolization. If possible, warn the patient how to recognize infection and instruct them how this should be managed and to call you if in any doubt.

 Tip: Do not wait if you suspect infection, this is so important that you should always see the patient urgently or arrange for an appropriate colleague to assess them.

Tissue necrosis Necrosis occurs when a tissue has been completely devitalized, usually by occlusion of the capillary bed. This can occur with physical occlusion with very small-particle PVA or with absolute alcohol, which also causes perivascular necrosis. The result will be tissue infarction in solid organs or loss of overlying skin in more peripheral territories. The latter is most common when using sclerosants to manage vascular malformations.

Principles of rendezvous and retrieval procedures

Foreign body retrieval is almost exclusively reserved for iatrogenic problems, most of which will have been of your own making! The techniques and equipment described can also be used for snaring guidewires for pull-through procedures or to reposition misplaced central lines. The majority of foreign body retrieval is within the vascular system, although occasionally these techniques are required in the biliary or urinary system.

The toolkit

See essential equipment: snares (Ch. 17).

There are not many tools at your disposal and, fortunately, most snares are simple to use, so a thorough understanding of the basic principles of how they work and an inventive mind are the keys to success.

Clinical scenarios

Removal of foreign bodies

The key decision is avoid the *'foreign body retrieval reflex'*; consider whether there is a good clinical reason for removing it. This requires an understanding of the likely impact of leaving it in situ; the risks associated with moving or removing it using endovascular techniques; and the risks of alternative strategies. Sometimes, a combined approach is best, e.g. a bullet free in the right atrium has the potential to cause considerable harm in addition to the havoc caused getting there in the first place. It could be removed by cardiothoracic surgery but a better solution may be to capture it with a snare and bring it back to the femoral artery. Clearly, it cannot be extracted safely through a normal sheath but it can be removed by surgical cutdown.

Stents, embolization coils and fragments of catheter and guidewire will probably cause vessel thrombosis. Only if thrombosis is likely to be clinically relevant should retrieval be attempted; if not, leave the foreign body where it is. If something does need to be removed, it is a good idea to heparinize the patient to prevent thrombosis during the procedure.

Catheter and guidewire fragments Guidewire fragments and indeed whole guidewires are sometimes abandoned by inexperienced operators, usually in the context of inserting central lines. These are fairly straightforward to manage.

Key steps in retrieval procedures

- Review the imaging and decide the best approach to the target.

Tip: In practice, this is almost always the common femoral artery or vein or the jugular vein.

- Decide which end of the device you intend to snare. Sometimes, this will be obvious but, as a general rule, choose the end where catheter and snare manipulation are lowest risk and preferably the one which is free in the lumen rather than hard against the wall.
- Choose an appropriately sized sheath: the catheter or wire will almost certainly double back on itself as you pull it into the sheath, so make sure you allow for this (Fig. 36.1). Fortunately, wire fragments are small enough to be withdrawn through a 6Fr sheath even when doubled back. Catheter fragments and bits of central venous catheters are usually easy to capture but will require a substantial sheath. If necessary, experiment with sheath size outside the patient using an identical catheter before starting the procedure.
- Snare the wire/catheter.
- Pull it back into the sheath and out through the haemostatic valve.

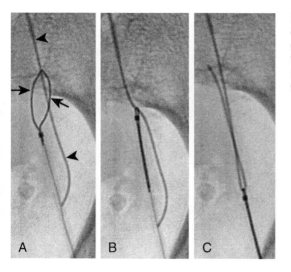

Fig. 36.1 ▦ Snaring a guidewire. (A) The open snare (arrows) is positioned over the guidewire (arrowheads). (B) The snare is tightened to grip the wire. (C) The snare is pulled back into the sheath bringing the guidewire with it.

Tip: If the device jams and will not pull out through the sheath, pull it snugly into the end of the sheath and withdraw the fragment, snare and sheath simultaneously.

Embolization coils The ease of retrieval for coils is critically dependent on the size of the target vessel. If the coil has migrated into a small-calibre vessel, retrieval may require a microsnare. In many situations, vessels of this calibre are not vital and the safest option is to leave the coil alone. Particular care should be taken if the target coil is adjacent to a nest of coils, e.g. when the last coil of an embolization has extruded back into the main trunk. It is very easy to drag several entangled coils back during the retrieval and make the situation much worse.

Stents Partially and even completely deployed stents have been successfully retrieved using snares. It is possible to progressively crimp-down stainless steel stents with a lot of patience but this is not a technique for stents that have undergone minor mispositioning. The stent must be in a site that poses a significant threat to the patient, e.g. embolization to the heart or pulmonary circulation. Unfortunately, the majority of stents will not line-up neatly and require a large sheath or an arteriotomy or venotomy for removal.

The safest option is to consider deploying the stent in a less harmful position, e.g. an iliac vessel. Remember that any of these options is a lot better than a thoracotomy. Self-expanding stents are even more difficult, as only a portion can be compressed and many have 'sharp edges'. They almost always need to be 'parked' safely (Fig. 36.2). This is definitely an area for expert hands only.

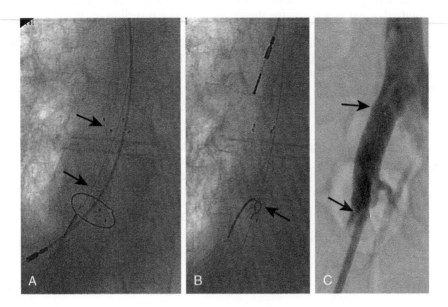

Fig. 36.2 ▧ Retrieving a self-expanding stent from the right atrium. (A) An innominate vein stent (arrows) has been displaced during placement of a pacing wire. A 0.018-inch wire has been passed through the stent and a GooseNeck snare advanced over this. (B) The lower end of the stent is grasped and compressed (arrow); the upper end remains expanded. (C) The stent (arrows) has been pulled back and parked in the common iliac vein.

Bullets and exciting projectiles Intravascular bullets, shot or fragments are occasionally seen in arteries and veins. They are usually brought to a safer place for surgical removal, but a small lead shot can sometimes be safely extracted.

Repositioning central venous lines

The majority of these are subclavian central venous lines that have passed from the subclavian vein into the internal jugular vein (IJV) or from the right subclavian into the left brachiocephalic vein. Either way, non-tunnelled lines can often be readily exchanged by simply pulling them back and using a steerable guidewire to navigate into the superior vena cava (SVC). The line is then removed over the wire and exchanged for a new one. Only in exceptional circumstances is it worth performing more elaborate manoeuvres for a non-tunnelled line. In addition, these lines are relatively stiff, making hooking the line down more difficult.

Tunnelled central lines deserve more effort. The tunnel means that it is much harder to exchange the catheter and therefore more ingenious solutions are required:

1. It is sometimes possible to move the end of the misplaced line into a more favourable position by simply performing a rapid hand injection of saline down the line.

2. If this fails, try passing a stiff Terumo wire through the line. Sometimes attempting to pass the wire around a bend in the line is sufficient to cause it to 'flick down' into the correct position.
3. If this fails, attempt to hook the line down into the target vessel from an alternative access point usually the femoral vein. Negotiate a pigtail catheter to the target line and remove the guidewire allowing the pigtail to form above the catheter. Try to hook the line down by pulling the pigtail back; occasionally, it can be helpful to stiffen the pigtail by passing a guidewire partially round the loop. The same manoeuvre can be performed with a reverse curve catheter, e.g. Sidewinder or SOS Omni catheter (Fig. 36.3).

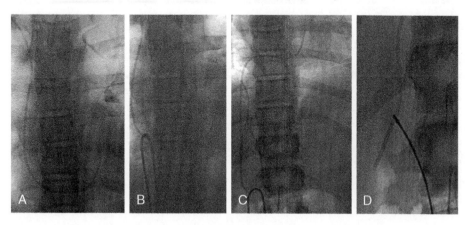

Fig. 36.3 Retrieval of a broken catheter fragment. (A) The catheter tip has migrated into the right ventricle. (B,C) The catheter is hooked with a Sidewinder catheter and pulled down into the inferior vena cava. (D) The catheter is snared prior to being pulled out through the femoral vein sheath.

4. If none of these manoeuvres is successful, then try using a snare. The difficulty with snaring is that the target object has to present a free end to capture. If the end of the misplaced line is in a decent-sized vessel, it is possible to manipulate the snare and the guide-catheter into an appropriate position.
5. If the line is in a small vessel, access with a snare can be difficult. In this case, you need to pass a catheter and wire over the line (step 3. above) and then snare the guidewire. This will require either a large enough sheath to accommodate the original catheter and the sheath catheter or a separate access point for the snare. Once the wire is gripped, simply pull the snare catheter and reverse curve catheter back together; the line will be pulled back with them. If you are feeling brave and have managed to pass enough guidewire over the line, you can remove the catheter leaving the wire in position. The snare is run up alongside it and the wire grabbed and then pulled back.

Rendezvous, pull-through technique or 'body flossing'

This is a special form of guidewire retrieval and refers to putting a guidewire in at one site and bringing it out at another. This gives enormous strength and stability as the wire can be held under tension while catheters are manoeuvred over it. It is typically used when it is simpler to traverse a lesion from one site while the other is the optimal route for intervention, e.g. large stents are best placed via femoral access rather than from the arm.

In the first instance, make sure that you remembered to use a long enough wire; 260 cm is usually required. Getting access to both ends of the wire requires navigating the wire to the target (exit) sheath, then getting it out through the haemostatic valve. The simplest and least expensive option is to steer a hydrophilic guidewire into the target sheath using a shaped catheter. Opacification of the target sheath with contrast will make it much easier to see. This will often succeed but may be quite fiddly. The wire can be manipulated through the valve by passing a smaller sheath inside the larger one (Fig. 36.4); then advancing the wire until through the larger haemostatic valve; remove the smaller sheath and the wire is there. Alternatively, use a snare via the exit sheath to grasp the wire in a convenient location, e.g. iliac artery or the aorta. This is quick but much more expensive. The wire will usually get damaged during snaring, so do not use it again.

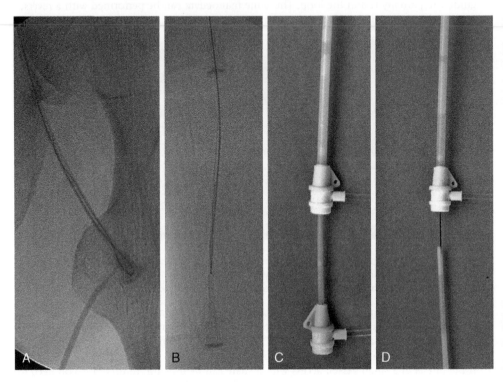

Fig. 36.4 ▦ Bringing a wire out through a sheath. (A) The hydrophilic wire will not pass through the haemostatic valve. (B,C) Sheath in sheath. A smaller sheath has been inserted into the original sheath and the wire has been advanced into it. (D) The smaller sheath is pulled back to reveal the wire.

There are three scenarios where rendezvous is likely to be needed:

1. When the iliac artery has been recanalized from the contralateral approach and a stent cannot be passed over the aortic bifurcation
2. When there is difficulty catheterizing the contralateral limb during aortic stent-grafting. In these circumstances, simply use a small Sidewinder-shaped catheter from the ipsilateral side. This will always pull back into the contralateral limb stump. This allows a guidewire to be passed into the aneurysm sac; do not hesitate to grab a large snare and capture it!
3. When there is difficulty advancing a stent graft through tortuous iliac vessels, despite a Lunderquist wire.

 Alarm: When using through-and-through wires, avoid cheese-wiring the vessels by keeping a catheter over the wire at vulnerable points, e.g. aortic bifurcation when using femoral access.

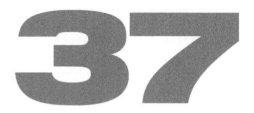

Principles of vascular closure and haematosis

Despite being a great opportunity to talk to your patients, obtaining haemostasis after a diagnostic or therapeutic angiogram is tedious. Hence, the art of staunching the flow is often neglected or delegated to the most junior member of staff in the vicinity. This approach risks haematoma or haemorrhage; make sure you give as much importance to haemostasis as you do to arterial access (Fig. 37.1). In reality, haematoma is a much more common complication of arterial procedures than any other.

Stopping the bleeding is usually straightforward unless:

- The patient is severely hypertensive
- The patient is obese
- The patient is excessively anticoagulated or has a bleeding diathesis
- You did not puncture the artery in the correct place
- You made a bigger hole than normal, i.e. >7Fr
- Or, as is often the case, a full house of the above.

 Tip: If you are anticipating problems, call for help before you remove the sheath. Consider using an arterial closure device. If necessary, leave the sheath in situ, keep the patient heparinized and have it removed surgically. Less than 1% of patients should require transfusion or emergency surgery.

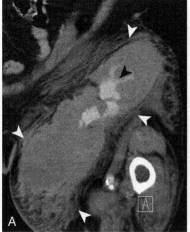

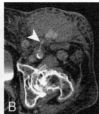

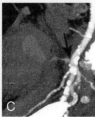

Fig. 37.1 ▨ Fatal haematoma following SFA angioplasty through a 4Fr sheath. The patient was resuscitated following cardiorespiratory arrest and had the artery repaired but succumbed to a CVA. (A) Coronal reformat showing massive haematoma in the left thigh (white arrowheads) with active bleeding (black arrowhead). (B) The point of extravasation is seen anterior to the femoral head. (C) Coronal oblique reformat clearly demonstrating active bleeding from the CFA.

Manual haemostasis: how to prevent haemorrhage and haematoma

If you have only recently given 5000 units of heparin, stop and have a cup of tea before taking out the sheath. When both you and the patient are ready, and have emptied your bladders (do not omit this key step!), you can start.

Remember that the skin entry point is not directly above the arterial puncture site! In antegrade punctures, the skin entry point is above; in retrograde punctures, it will be lower.

Alarm: In 'well-padded' patients, the relationship between the skin entry point and arterial puncture site is complex. Skin entry may be considerably higher if there is a beach ball-shaped abdomen or may be lower if you had to retract a large fold of skin to puncture. Make sure that you can feel the pulse before you pull the sheath.

Key steps in haemostasis

1. Empty all bladders.
2. Attach blood pressure and pulse monitoring and make a baseline recording.
3. Place a finger to either side of the catheter proximal and distal to the hole in the artery. You should be able to feel the pulse. Press firmly down until the pulse reduces; if increasing the pressure abolishes the pulse, you are in control.
4. Look at a clock and check the time.
5. Remove the sheath and continue pressing, feeling the pulse. Watch the puncture site or the patient will develop a haematoma.
6. After 5 min according to the clock, slowly reduce the pressure and check the puncture site.
7. If the bleeding has stopped, get someone else who understands the principles of haemostasis to press for a further 5 min, just to be on the safe side.
8. When the bleeding has completely stopped, the puncture site will remain dry. Place a swab over it, place the patient's hand on the pulse and check that they can feel it. Instruct them to keep pressing until they get back to the ward and to remember to press if they cough, sneeze, etc.
9. Document in the case notes or operation sheet the access site and the required observations.

Special circumstances

Children Most cases will be performed under general anaesthetic. This is great during the procedure but can be problematic for haemostasis. The good news is that most children are thin and the pulse is easy to feel and hence compress for haemostasis. The bad news is that they wake up very quickly and are guaranteed to flex their limbs as soon as they regain consciousness and certainly when the anaesthetist manipulates their airway. It is best to have achieved haemostasis before this! It is always courteous to warn the anaesthetist that the procedure is drawing to a close so that they do not give another dose of muscle relaxant.

Tip: Mention haemostasis in the pre-procedure safety check and politely request the anaesthetist to hold-off waking the patient until you have removed the sheath. Even a couple of extra minutes helps.

Bedrest post-angiography

There is no scientific formula and precious little evidence to tell us what the optimum period of rest is before mobilizing. For uncomplicated 3/4Fr punctures, it is probably reasonable to sit up after 30 min and get out of bed after about 1 h. For larger punctures, a period of 4 h bedrest is probably prudent. Make sure that you advise patients to rest as much as possible for the remainder of the day. Day-case and outpatients should be given clear instructions to rest up and only to exercise the remote control. They and their carer should be shown how to press on the puncture site and told how to contact help if bleeding starts again after discharge.

Troubleshooting

Bleeding has not stopped when you check after 5 min

- Still pulsatile bleeding? Press for at least another 10 min before you check again.
- Gentle ooze? Press for another 5 min before checking.

The bleeding does not stop – there is a range of escalation here

Every time I release, the pressure bleeding starts

- Stay calm and look calm – it reassures the patient.
- If your fingers are numb, ask someone to help you.
- Check pulse, BP and venous access is working.
- Think about the clotting time and consider checking it.
- Make sure you know the vascular surgery phone number.
- If it is still like this after 30–40 min, it is time to make that call.

The groin is okay but the BP is dropping

- Keep pressure on the groin.
- Get help now.
- If the pulse is slow – is this vasovagal? Having someone push on your groin is not pleasant.
- If the pulse is high – then consider retroperitoneal bleeding.
- Check the venous access and start running IV normal saline.
- Check BP and pulse and adjust fluid support accordingly.
- Ultrasound can be useful for a quick assessment, CT is definitive and will show ongoing bleeding.
- It is time to get vascular surgery on speed dial again.
- Send blood for urgent cross-match.

A large haematoma develops

- Stay calm and reassure the patient.
- Make frequent observations of the pulse and blood pressure.
- Try to find the pulse and continue compression. If you cannot do this, ultrasound and colour Doppler are useful. Use the ultrasound probe to direct compression.
- Pressing on a large haematoma will be painful, so give strong analgesics as necessary.
- Inform the vascular surgeon and assess the patient.
- If you achieve control, mark the haematoma margin – this makes it easier for the ward to assess.
- Unless the patient is completely stable, consider CT.

I cannot stop the bleeding no matter how hard I press

- Stay calm and look calm – but it is time to move quickly.
- Get help now – you need at least two other people.
- Try to get the groin pressure on the pulse – often a minor adjustment will get control.
- Check the venous access and get some IV fluids open.
- Check BP and pulse and adjust fluid support accordingly.
- If it comes under control, great – but do not let your helpers disappear for at least 10 min.
- If it does not come under control within a few minutes – it is time to summon the vascular cavalry.

Tip: Remember, if bleeding will not stop you can always tamponade the puncture site by placing an angioplasty balloon from another access point. This will stop the bleeding and allow the patient to be stabilized and everyone else to compose themselves and work out the best solution.

Alarm: If there is any doubt, perform a contrast-enhanced CT scan. This will show the extent of any haematoma, whether there is ongoing bleeding and where it is from (see Fig. 37.1).

Arterial closure devices

Manual haemostasis is effective for punctures up to about 7Fr. Closure devices can seal larger punctures and also allow earlier mobilization than manual haemostasis. Closure devices are not without their own problems and, as with every other intervention, benefits have to outweigh the risks. Obviously we cannot give details or recommendations on every device and, hence, we recommend that you should become familiar with the use and indications for one or two of the devices, ideally with different mechanisms of action. As a general rule, larger holes need more complex devices. Most interventionalists should know a simple device for small punctures (5–8Fr) and some will need a second device for bigger holes.

Devices for helping obtain haemostasis can be divided into passive and active.

Passive devices

These are not directly applied to the arterial puncture. There are a variety of devices which apply external pressure over the puncture site, some of which should be outlawed by the Human Rights Act. Essentially, they are no better than manual compression, but they do have the advantage that they do not tire. It is essential to realize the patient still needs the same level of observation and the device needs to be removed promptly. One device that can be helpful for superficial punctures that continue to gently ooze is the Safeguard (Fig. 37.2). The device is stuck to the patient over the puncture site and the balloon inflated. As the balloon is transparent, the puncture site can be observed while the device is in place. The balloon is deflated periodically to check whether the bleeding has stopped; when it has ceased, the device is simply removed.

Alternatives include materials that promote blood coagulation; these are quite effective when placed directly on a site of bleeding, e.g. a vascular anastomosis. But remember it is just possible that application on the skin does not directly affect the bleeding artery.

Active devices

These are the more commonly used devices and are directly applied to the hole in the artery. The manufacturers are faced with the same problem – closing the arterial defect and some of

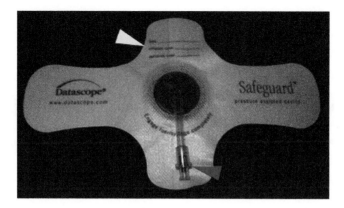

Fig. 37.2 Safeguard external compression device can be used in two ways. (1) Once haemostasis is achieved in the conventional fashion, the device is applied over the puncture site (exactly where you would normally press) and the bladder is inflated with air (red arrowhead). The time and inflation pressure are recorded (yellow arrowhead). (2) The device is positioned and the bulb inflated prior to removal of the arterial sheath. Pressure is applied to the bulb until bleeding stops and the device left in position. In either case the puncture site can be observed through the transparent window. The device is left in position as long as necessary and can be periodically deflated to check for bleeding and skin condition.

the key concepts in the solutions are fairly similar. There are three basic types: suture-mediated, vascular plugs and external clips.

The devices and the techniques for deploying are evolving and improving. The following descriptions are a general overview and are not a substitute for hands-on training. Each system has its own idiosyncrasies and limitations, and these require familiarity and understanding, which should be obtained through specific training.

 Alarm: None of the active devices is infallible and problems most commonly occur when the common femoral artery is diseased.

Suture-mediated closure devices

These devices are typified by the Perclose, Proglide, Prostar (Abbott Laboratories) and the SuperStitch (Sutura). With a suture device, there is immediate haemostasis and the artery may be punctured again immediately afterwards. These devices are capable of closing the largest punctures as the sutures appose the edges of the hole in the vessel, just as they would in surgical repair. Although the mechanisms are different, every device will perform the following four steps:

1. Pass needles through the vessel wall on either side of the puncture
2. Capture the suture material and exteriorize it
3. Tie a locking slip knot on the suture
4. Advance the knot to the vessel and tighten and lock the suture to oppose the arterial defect.

The suture is sited by a process a little like crochet! Fig. 37.3 illustrates the process.

The Perclose is the most commonly use device and is not actually difficult but training is essential; the key steps are outlined below. There are quite a few elements to remember and carry out in the correct order.

Vessel assessment The device needs a minimum of a 5-mm vessel to allow the footplate to open properly. Most manufacturers recommend an angiogram of the puncture site in the

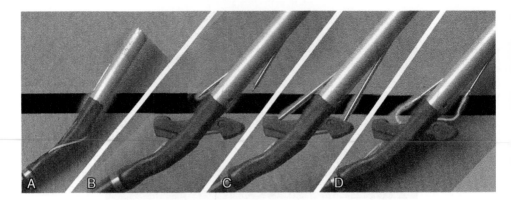

Fig. 37.3 ▦ How the Perclose works. (A) The device is inserted into the artery and held at an angle of 45 degrees. (B) The footplate is opened and the needles advanced. (C) The needles pass through the wall and 'dock' in the footplate. (D) The needles are retracted, bringing the sutures back through the artery wall with them.

oblique plane to be certain that the vessel is a suitable size and the puncture is in the common femoral artery (CFA).

Introducing the catheter The device is introduced over a guidewire, currently available devices are monorail, which means that after the initial portion of the device is inserted the guidewire is removed and the remainder of the device carefully introduced.

Deploying the suture The footplate is deployed in the artery and the device gently pulled back to oppose the footplate to the vessel wall. The needles are then advanced through the vessel wall to the footplate where they 'collect' the suture. The needles are then retracted bringing the suture with them. The sutures are exteriorized and retrieved from the device (see Fig. 37.3).

Tying the knot Take care not to pull the locking suture (for the Perclose the white suture). The locking knot slides down the rail suture assisted by a knot pusher until it is against the arterial wall. If haemostasis has been achieved, the suture is locked and the sutures cut.

Perclose and SuperStitch devices have to be correctly sized to be effective. If the vessel access puncture is too big, the needles will just pass through it rather than puncturing through the adjacent vessel wall. It is possible to get around this problem, using 'pre-closure'. This simply involves deploying the suture after placing a small sheath. The ends of the suture are not tied at this stage and the puncture is up-sized to the larger sheath. When the procedure is finished, the knot is deployed. For really large sheaths, two sutures can be pre-deployed at an angle to each other to give an extra measure of security. Even then, it is prudent not to attempt this unless you are able to control a 20Fr puncture site. In other words, if the suture fails, you will need to be able to control the bleeding and then perform an open repair of the artery.

 Alarm: Pre-closure is sometimes used for truly percutaneous endovascular aneurysm repair. Remember that in these circumstances, it will be difficult to place an occlusion balloon from the contralateral side and separate arm access may be required.

External plugs

These devices deploy material on the surface of the artery to promote thrombosis. There are different variations on the theme, depending on whether there is a temporary intra-arterial balloon that is withdrawn at the time or an absorbable intra-arterial anchor that dissolves over time.

Temporary balloons, e.g. Mynx (AccessClosure) are devices that use a low-profile semi-compliant balloon, which is inserted just into the artery lumen, inflated and then pulled back until it abuts the vessel wall. This 'presses on the inside of the artery' and stops bleeding. With the balloon in place, the procoagulant haemostatic material is deployed outside the vessel. This forms a plug which solidifies. The balloon is deflated and pulled out, leaving the plug in place to seal the hole.

Collagen plug and anchor Typified by the Angioseal (St Jude Medical). The Angioseal comes in 6Fr and 8Fr sizes. This system resembles the plastic tag used to attach price tags to clothing. A collagen footplate is deployed in the artery lumen using a version of a pusher system. The anchor is attached to a thread with collagen 'wadding' on it. The wadding is tamped down the thread with a pusher to form a plug at the puncture site (Fig. 37.4).

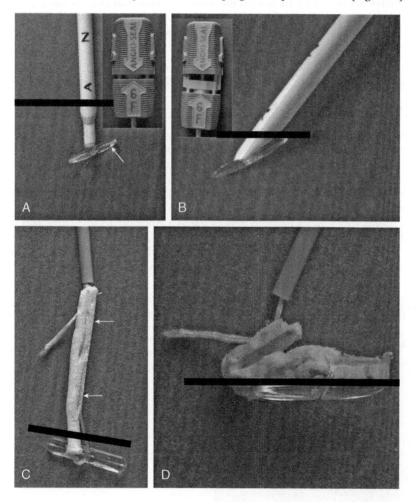

Fig. 37.4 ■ Angioseal: the basics. (A) The footplate (white arrow) is released in the artery. The black line represents the artery wall. The inset shows the delivery mechanism. (B) The footplate is retracted to the end of the delivery catheter (inset shows the delivery mechanism). (C) The catheter is withdrawn to leave the footplate in the artery and the collagen 'wadding' (white arrows) outside the artery. (D) The wadding is tamped down to affect a seal.

Haemostasis is rapid. The collagen footplate dissolves over about 10 weeks and the artery should not be punctured again within 3 months, as there is a risk of dislodging the anchor plate. This subsequently forms an effective embolus.

 Tip: If you do need to access the artery again, the plug can be identified with ultrasound and a puncture made as far away from it as possible.

Nitinol clip

This type of system introduces a permanent circular nitinol clip to oppose the vessel wall and is typified by the StarClose. The key stages are similar to several of the devices above. A special sheath is introduced via a guidewire and the dilator and wire withdrawn. The device is inserted until it clips into the sheath and the footplate is deployed. The device and attached sheath are retracted until they are against the anterior arterial wall and the clip deployed, which also splits the sheath and finally the clip is released and the device removed. The nitinol clip is a permanent feature and should be recorded so that we can try to avoid it at the next arterial puncture.

Complications of manual haemostasis and vascular closure

The risk of complications at the access site varies with a number of factors, including: access site, puncture size, patient body habitus and coagulation. As a guide for interventional procedures, significant haematoma (i.e. delays discharge or requires additional intervention) should happen in <2% of cases. Manual haemostasis remains the gold standard for achieving haemostasis, however vascular closure devices permit earlier mobilization and may reduce complications in high-risk patients. The most common complication for vascular closure devices is failure, which varies between devices but as a guide occurs in 5–10%. Less common but significant complications include vessel occlusion and infection (<1%) (Fig. 37.5). Operator experience is a big factor in reducing these complications and familiarity with both the device and the likely complications and how to minimize risk is essential.

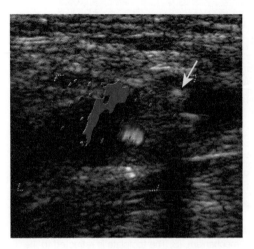

Fig. 37.5 ■ Occlusion of the CFA by Angioseal. Colour flow is seen proximal to the footplate (yellow arrow). At surgery, the footplate caught on plaque in the artery and did not pull back to the deployment catheter tip during phase 3; the collagen plug was partly inside the artery.

Section Four

Intervention

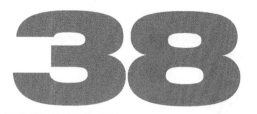

Achieving tissue diagnosis

A combination of increased use of diagnostic imaging and advances in therapeutic interventions means that obtaining tissue to aid diagnosis and cellular typing is now more essential than ever. Most diagnostic and interventional radiologists require core skills in biopsy. The vast majority of lesions can be biopsied with minimal risk. Determining a safe access route and accurate targeting requires a clear understanding of the principles of image guidance for intervention (Ch. 25). The shortest, straightest route is usually the best approach but there are important exceptions to this rule, e.g. peripheral liver lesion. Take time to plan an approach that avoids important structures, e.g. bowel, lung, major vessels and the gallbladder.

To minimize complications, the patient should be fasted for abdominal biopsy and coagulopathy should be excluded. Make sure that the patient has given consent and that all parties are aware of the potential risks (and their consequences) of the procedure.

Pre-procedure

The aim of aspiration or biopsy is to obtain a satisfactory tissue specimen for cytology, biochemistry, microbiology or histology. Make sure that you are clear exactly what is required, any specific requirements for handling and where to send it. Ultrasound is used whenever possible as it allows real-time guidance without exposing you or the patient to ionizing radiation.

The patient

Fine-needle aspiration requires minimal preparation and local anaesthetic is rarely necessary. The vast majority of biopsies are performed under local anaesthesia and patient cooperation is essential. Explain what the procedure entails; in particular, stress the importance of breath-holding during the needle pass. If the patient does not understand or cannot cooperate, then stop now! Most biopsies are not painful; emphasize that analgesia is available if needed. Make sure that the patient is aware that regular post-biopsy observations are normal and do not indicate a problem.

Contraindications

Fine-needle aspiration usually does not require any pre-assessment of coagulation. Biopsy, particularly of vascular solid organs, will usually have a pre-intervention coagulation screen.

- No additional precautions are necessary when the international normalized ratio (INR) is ≤1.5 and the platelet count ≥50,000.

When the clotting is more deranged, consider transfusion of fresh frozen plasma (FFP) ± platelets.

 Alarm: Antiplatelet therapy (e.g. Clopidogrel) will increase the risk of bleeding, seek advice before discontinuing, especially in patients following recent coronary intervention. Always consider the risk–benefit for the individual patient.

Vascular lesion

- Some tumours are highly vascular, e.g. renal cell tumour metastases. Switch on the colour Doppler if there is any doubt. If you need to biopsy a vascular lesion, make sure that the patient is adequately prepared. This may require large-bore IV access and cross-matched blood. Try to avoid the main tumoral vessels and be prepared to plug the biopsy tract and embolize the lesion if necessary.

Obstructed system

- The target for biopsy is likely to be the point of obstruction, e.g. a pancreatic mass, consequently fistula or intra-abdominal leakage can occur. Consider draining the system before biopsy. Attempting drainage after a complication can be very difficult.

Uncooperative patient

- Consider sedation or general anaesthesia.
- Remember that a sedated patient will not be able to breath-hold.

Diagnosis irrelevant to management

- Do not be persuaded to do the biopsy just because it would 'be nice to know'.

Which specimen – cytology or histology

There are two sampling techniques: aspiration cytology and cutting needle biopsy. The local pathology service will guide you on the type of specimen they require. Usually only a few cells are needed to diagnose malignancy but a core of tissue is needed to subtype tumours or assess diffuse liver/renal pathology.

Fine-needle aspiration biopsy

Aspiration cytology, sometimes referred to as fine-needle aspiration cytology (FNAC), is performed with a 21G or 22G needle. The specimen contains only a few cells, but for many conditions, this will establish the diagnosis. The risks involved are very small; FNAC is frequently possible even in hazardous areas.

FNAC is frequently used for neck lesions and nearly always using ultrasound guidance. Ask the laboratory for help if you are uncertain how to handle the specimen, e.g. to make a smear on a slide.

Cutting needle biopsy

Cutting needle biopsy obtains a larger specimen, typically a 1-mm core of 20-mm length for histological analysis.

Tip: Remember that with a fully automatic system, the biopsy is taken from the tissue 10–20 mm in front of the needle tip, depending on the size of the specimen notch.

Biopsy – specific sites

Liver

Liver biopsy is one of the most frequently requested interventional procedures, and it is usually one of the simplest to perform. Biopsies are either targeted to a focal lesion or random cores in diffuse liver disease. Non-targeted biopsies are usually taken from the right lobe. When there are multiple lesions, choose the most accessible.

When taking a biopsy of the right lobe of the liver, a lateral approach is usually chosen. The ribs can interfere with access; choose an approach which allows scanning parallel to the line of the ribs. Sometimes the needle has to be angled up or down to accommodate this.

Tip: To minimize the risk of haemorrhage when taking a biopsy of peripheral lesions, always make a tract that passes through 2–3 cm of normal liver before hitting the target (Fig. 38.1).

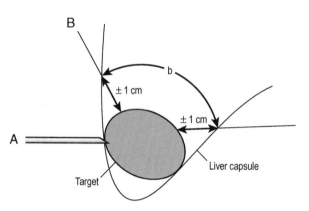

Fig. 38.1 ▨ Direct biopsy of peripheral liver lesions. (A) increases the risk of extracapsular bleeding. Choose an approach (B) that passes through a cuff of normal liver tissue.

Mild shoulder tip pain is not uncommon after liver biopsy and the patient should be warned that this may occur. The risks of biopsy are increased in the presence of biliary obstruction and ascites. Drainage is recommended before biopsy. In the presence of mildly deranged clotting, consider a plugged biopsy.

Plugged liver biopsy

The essence of this procedure is to prevent haemorrhage from the liver capsule by embolizing the needle tract. There are a variety of different materials used for tract embolization, including Gelfoam pledgets, gel foam slurry and coils. If a commercial prepared system is used, then the steps described below for Gelfoam preparation are unnecessary. Using a sheath has the potential advantage of allowing more than one needle to pass through the same tract.

Equipment
- 18G biopsy needle
- 18G sheathed needle
- Gelfoam sheet.

Procedure: Prepare the Gelfoam in advance by cutting the sheet into 1-mm pledgets and soak them in contrast. Discard the needle from the 18G sheathed needle and fit the sheath over the biopsy needle. The needle and sheath are advanced into the liver as a single unit (Fig. 38.2). The biopsy is performed in the conventional fashion. The needle is withdrawn, leaving the sheath in situ and the adequacy of the specimen is confirmed. The tract is now embolized by injecting 1–2 mL of the Gelfoam pledgets as the sheath is withdrawn. Post-biopsy aftercare is the same as for a standard liver biopsy.

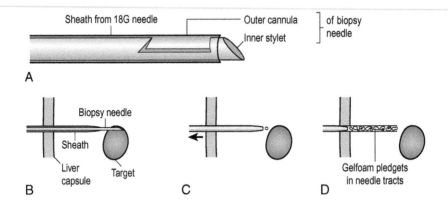

Fig. 38.2 ▨ Plugged liver biopsy technique. (A) The 18G biopsy needle is passed through the sheath of an 18G needle. (B) The needle and sheath are advanced into the liver and the biopsy taken. (C) The biopsy needle is removed and Gelfoam pledgets injected through the sheath as it is withdrawn. (D) The final result is a tract embolized with Gelfoam.

Transjugular liver biopsy

Transjugular liver biopsy (TJB) is a much more complicated and expensive procedure. It is reserved for patients with diffuse liver disease and deranged coagulation or ascites for whom plugged biopsy would still pose significant risk. The rationale for TJB is that there is no puncture of the liver capsule and therefore any bleeding from the needle tract will be contained within the liver or auto-transfuse into the hepatic vein. TJB is not carte blanche to perform liver biopsy in any patient; as always, attempts should be made to correct the underlying coagulopathy before the procedure.

Anatomy: The hepatic veins join the inferior vena cava (IVC) just below the right atrium (see Figs. 38.3 and 49.16). Biopsy is most safely performed from the right hepatic vein 3–4 cm from the junction with the IVC. Angling the sheath anteriorly directs the needle into the maximum volume of parenchyma and minimizes the risk of capsular perforation. Anterior biopsy from the middle hepatic vein should be avoided. Differentiating the right from the middle hepatic vein can be difficult in the AP projection but is easily done from a lateral projection.

Equipment
- Basic angiography set
- 5F sheath
- Cobra II catheter
- Hydrophilic and Amplatz guidewires. A 1-cm floppy tip Amplatz wire is very useful in small livers.

- Transjugular cutting needle liver biopsy set, which contains a 7F long sheath, an angled metallic sheath stiffener, a 5F straight catheter and a long cutting biopsy needle. A metal arrow on the hub of the stiffener indicates the orientation of the curve.

Procedure: The procedure is very similar to the first stages of a transjugular intrahepatic portosystemic shunt (TIPS) procedure.

Access: Ultrasound-guided right IJV puncture.

Catheterization: This is exactly the same as during a TIPS procedure (see TIPS, Ch. 49, p. 358).

Imaging: Hand inject a few millilitres (mL) of contrast to ensure that the catheter is not wedged, then perform a hepatic venogram. The right hepatic vein (RHV) is the target vein and typically has a suitably shallow angle that allows the sheath entry. The angled stiffener within the sheath gives excellent torque control but poor cornering ability and will only negotiate suitably angled veins.

Biopsy: An Amplatz extra-stiff wire is passed into the hepatic vein; take care not to puncture the liver capsule with the guidewire (Fig. 38.3). Exchange the 5F sheath for the reinforced sheath, which is passed 3–4 cm into the hepatic vein. Use the directional indicator on the hub to direct the sheath anteriorly until it abuts the vein wall. The cutting needle is primed and advanced into the sheath until the needle tip is a few millimetres (mm) beyond the end of the sheath in the liver parenchyma. The patient is instructed to breath-hold and the inner stylet is depressed, taking the biopsy.

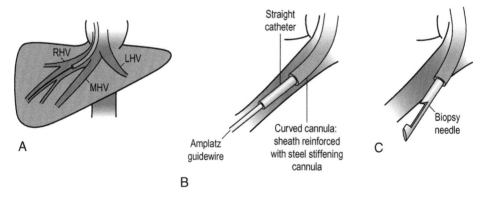

Fig. 38.3 ▥ Transjugular liver biopsy technique. (A) Catheterize the RHV using a Cobra II catheter. Then exchange for an Amplatz super-stiff wire. (B) Advance the curved cannula into the right hepatic vein using a coaxial straight catheter and the Amplatz wire. Remove the catheter and wire to leave the curved cannula in place. (C) Turn the curved cannula anteriorly to abut the vein wall and advance the long biopsy needle into the liver parenchyma to take the biopsy.

Kidney

The kidney is the most vascular organ in the body and biopsy is associated with an increased risk of haemorrhage. Most renal biopsies in native and transplant kidneys are performed to investigate the aetiology of kidney disease. These biopsies should be taken from either the upper or the lower pole of the kidney. Avoid biopsy adjacent to the renal pelvis, as this greatly increases the risks of urinary and vascular complications. There is an increasing trend to biopsy focal renal masses, which reflects advances in immunochemistry and greater use of ablative techniques. Complications occur in about 5% of renal biopsies. Small arteriovenous (AV) fistulae should be treated conservatively as most will close spontaneously. Pain and fall in Hb are indications for CT and transcatheter embolization if bleeding is confirmed.

Adrenal glands

The adrenal glands are usually approached posteriorly in the prone or lateral decubitus position; large lesions can be biopsied anteriorly. In most cases, CT is the best imaging guidance. Always measure vanillylmandelic acid levels in patients who have an adrenal mass with no known primary tumour. When phaeochromocytoma is suspected, α-adrenergic blockade is recommended to minimize the risk of hypertensive crisis.

Pancreas

Pancreatic biopsy is indicated in the investigation of a mass at the head of the pancreas. There is usually associated biliary and pancreatic duct obstruction. If obstructed, the biliary tree should be drained before starting. The pancreatic duct cannot be drained and there is a risk of pancreatitis and pseudocyst formation. Pancreatic biopsy of large masses can usually be performed under ultrasound guidance. Smaller lesions are usually biopsied under endoscopic ultrasound or occasionally CT guidance. The biopsy track may be transgastric but care should be taken to avoid inadvertent biopsy through the transverse colon (Fig. 38.4). Plastic biliary stents are readily seen on ultrasound and can be used to target pancreatic biopsy. As pancreatic biopsy is often painful, sedation and analgesia are recommended.

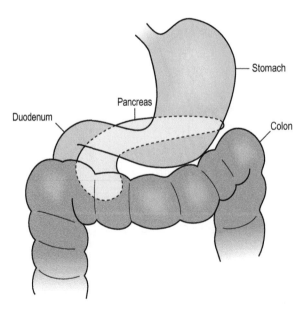

Fig. 38.4 ▦ Relationship between the stomach, pancreas and transverse colon. Transgastric biopsy is acceptable but take great care to avoid the colon.

Retroperitoneum

Most retroperitoneal masses are best biopsied on CT unless they are very large. The retroperitoneum can be approached anteriorly if there is a window without bowel. The posterior approach is particularly useful for paraspinal masses.

Pelvis

The commonest difficulty in pelvic biopsy is identifying a route that does not transgress bowel or bladder. Alternative options include transrectal, transvaginal and transgluteal approaches.

The posterior transgluteal route traverses the sacrosciatic notch and uses CT guidance (see Fig. 39.1). The patient is scanned in the prone position (see Fig. 39.2) and the approach is planned in the conventional fashion. Remember that the sciatic nerve and gluteal vessels pass through the anterior portion of the notch. To avoid them, the tract should pass as close to the sacrum as possible. Burrowing through this much muscle can be difficult and may be uncomfortable for the patient both during and after the procedure.

Ultrasound-guided transrectal and transvaginal biopsy are readily performed and well tolerated. These routes offer a direct approach to posterior collections. Most suitable probes have needle guides. Use sterile covers over the probe and guide.

Transrectal procedures (Fig. 39.3) cause surprisingly little discomfort but this is a 'dirty' route. A cleansing enema is recommended to remove any faecal residue and antibiotic prophylaxis must be given.

The transvaginal approach (Fig. 39.4) is performed with the patient in the lithotomy position. Sedation is recommended as the procedure tends to be uncomfortable and the vaginal wall can be difficult to traverse. The vagina and perineum are cleaned with povidone iodine solution.

Aftercare

There is no fixed regimen for post-biopsy care. The aftercare varies with the site of biopsy, coagulation status and general condition of the patient. Ensure that a written care plan is given to the staff who will care for the patient. If there is no established local protocol, the proforma below can be modified to suit most procedures.

Sample proforma for patient aftercare

Patient name
ID No.
Date
Time
Procedure
Anaesthesia/Sedation
Needle size
No. of cores taken
Uneventful/Complicated (specify)
Specimens – in formalin/saline/dry
Returned with patient/Sent to
Aftercare
Flat bedrest for 2 hours
Pulse and BP
Every 15 minutes for 1 hour
Every 30 minutes for 1 hour
Every 60 minutes for 2 hours
Every 4 hours until discharge
Analgesia as necessary
Other, e.g. fluids only
Information for discharge.

Complications

Fortunately, complications following biopsy are rare and the majority of complications are minor. The risks vary between individual patients and differing sites and are discussed in the relevant sections. The most important complications are:

Bleeding: This may occur even in the best hands, particularly in the presence of a vascular lesion or organ. Ensure that the blood clotting and platelets are optimized before starting.

Alarm: The risk of haemorrhage is highest during:
- Biopsy of vascular organs (liver, spleen and kidneys) in the presence of abnormal clotting
- Biopsy adjacent to major blood vessels
- Biopsy of known vascular tumours, particularly when there is no surrounding normal tissue to tamponade bleeding.
  In high-risk patients it is wise to group and save or even cross-match blood for the procedure.

Perforation of a hollow viscus: Bowel can usually be avoided by using an appropriate approach. If the intestine must be traversed, use a fine needle (22G) rather than a cutting needle.

Pneumothorax: This is common following biopsy of lung or mediastinal masses. Pneumothorax can also occur when the pleural space is traversed during biopsy of upper abdominal lesions. Remember that the pleural space extends much further down posteriorly. This problem can be anticipated and the patient should be warned that it might be necessary to have a chest drain following the procedure.

Fistula: May occur when performing biopsies in the presence of an obstructed system. For this reason, it is advisable to perform drainage before biopsy. This is particularly important in the presence of biliary obstruction.

Infection: This is rare if proper aseptic precautions are taken and the intestine is not traversed. When the bowel is traversed, e.g. transrectal biopsy, then prophylactic antibiotics should be given, e.g. gentamicin (80 mg) and metronidazole (500 mg). If the colon is punctured, seek surgical advice. The patient will usually settle on conservative management, nil by mouth and antibiotics.

Tumour seeding of the biopsy tract: This is rare but can occur with any tumour. The risk can be minimized by passing through a 'normal' section of the target organ or the potential field of resection.

Death: This is usually due to haemorrhage and is very rare in routine biopsies.

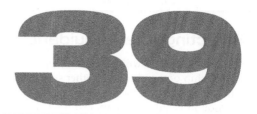

Treating fluid collections and abscesses

Treating fluid collections and abscesses is part of the bread and butter of interventional radiology. The minimally invasive nature of interventional radiology (IR) drainage makes it an obvious choice for many postoperative collections, particularly in the elderly and frail.

Pre-procedure planning

Taking a few minutes to plan the procedure is essential and might mean that you actually plan not to do it!

Selecting collections to drain

The ubiquitous nature of computed tomography (CT) chest/abdo/pelvis scanning in most hospitals means that fluid collections are frequently discovered, particularly in postoperative patients. There are a number of reasons that a fluid collection may be present; haematoma, lymphocele or simple serous fluid for example. Drainage is indicated if there is infection or significant mass effect, e.g. large pleural effusion.

Evidence of an infected collection

- A defined fluid collection with a wall
- Enhancement of the wall
- Gas within the fluid (check it is not a bowel loop!)
- Hounsfield unit (HU) >5 – collections with very low HU are likely to be simple fluid.

Review the CT and look for evidence of infection elsewhere, it is not rare to be asked to drain a small pelvic collection in a patient with a raging pneumonia. A direct discussion with the referring clinician is essential. Draining every collection referred will do patients a disservice as you will almost certainly infect some sterile fluid collections and will certainly have exposed the patients to the risk of drainage without the benefits.

Preparation

Check coagulation and correct coagulopathy. Ensure the patient has received appropriate antibiotic cover, which depends on the site/source of infection – you are likely to make them bacteraemic during the drainage. Abscess drainage can be painful, so get effective local anaesthesia and use parenteral analgesia as required.

Selecting image guidance

Usually, the abscess will have been demonstrated on CT. The CT is invaluable in defining the relationship of the abscess to other structures. Try to plan a route that will allow you to use ultrasound guidance for the actual drainage. That means a route away from bowel, etc. Ultrasound is quicker, allows real-time visualization and does not get you irradiated. If bowel or other tricky obstacles are in the way, then use CT – ideally with CT fluoroscopy.

Diagnostic aspiration

Diagnostic aspiration tends to be used when the nature of the collection is unclear or when there is a small collection that is very difficult to drain. A diagnostic aspirate gives bacterial sensitivity and allegedly reduces the abscess wall tension, which helps antibiotic penetration. Always undertake aspiration under sterile conditions and avoid traversing bowel as there is a real opportunity to inoculate and infect a collection.

In theory, we should tell you to always start with a 20G needle but, in reality, unless the collection is in tiger country, most operators will use an 18G needle – it is easier to steer and you can aspirate thick pus through it. If you use a 20G needle and cannot aspirate then a further puncture is usually needed. If possible, plan the aspiration so that the route is suitable for drainage as if you aspirate pus that is usually the next step.

 Tip: The aspirate is not a fine wine; there is nothing to be gained from sniffing it, gagging and suggesting 'anaerobes'!

Drainage

Drainage is all about getting gravity on your side, so plan the drainage route so that the shortest access is achieved that will result in a drain in a dependent position and preferably with the drain hub below the level of the collection.

Think about the content of the collection. Ultrasound offers the most useful assessment of the viscosity of the collection and the presence of loculi and septa. If the collection is loculated, then target the largest locule first. Look for the following features, which will influence the type and number of drains required:

Anechoic collection – probably clear fluid, e.g. urinoma
Few scattered echoes – turbid fluid, e.g. thin pus
Extensive or swirling echoes – thick fluid, e.g. viscous pus
Diffuse echoes with gas – organized abscess or phlegmon.

 Tip: The ultrasound appearances are not an infallible guide and occasionally will be misleading – always try a diagnostic aspiration.

Equipment

- Coaxial set – if 'danger close'
- 18G sheathed needle
- 0.035 support wire
- Dilators to 1Fr larger than the drain.

Drainage catheter: Use a 6–8Fr catheter for clear fluid, 8–10Fr catheter for thin pus, 10–12Fr catheter for thick pus and a 12–22Fr drain for collections containing debris.

Procedure

The precise technique depends on the type of catheter that has been chosen. Prepare and anaesthetize the skin and the desired puncture site. Make a sufficiently large skin incision to allow passage of the drainage catheter. Pass a needle into the collection, using imaging guidance.

Most operators will use a two-step procedure; fluoroscopy is recommended though the skilled operator can do this under ultrasound alone. Unless it is very tricky, use an 18G needle for the initial puncture as this will allow immediate exchange for a 0.035-inch wire. A supportive guidewire is passed through the puncture needle into the collection. If a 21G needle was used to puncture the collection, either simply re-puncture with an 18G needle or consider using a Neff set to convert to a 0.035-inch wire. The needle is removed over the wire and the track is dilated using fascial dilators to 1–2Fr larger than the drainage catheter. Fix the wire securely to ensure that it does not kink and that you do not lose wire position during catheter exchanges. The catheter stiffener assembly is then passed over the wire into the collection. When you reach either a significant bend or the collection, detach the stiffener, hold the stiffener and the wire fixed in position, and slide the catheter forward over the guidewire (see Fig. 39.1). The stiffener and guidewire are removed and the catheter is allowed to form. Most self-retaining catheters are introduced in this way.

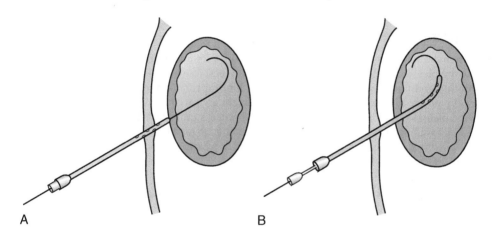

A   B

Fig. 39.1 ▤ Catheter stiffener assembly. (A) The entire assembly is advanced to the edge of the collection. (B) The Luer lock is loosened and the inner stiffener and the wire are held stationary and the drainage catheter pushed forwards.

For a very large and superficial collection, a one-step procedure can be used. The catheter is mounted on a central needle and stylet. A direct puncture technique is used. The central stylet is removed and fluid is aspirated to confirm the tip is within the collection. The needle is held still and the catheter is simply advanced along the needle into the collection. Fluoroscopy is not required. Best attempted after you have a few successful two-step procedures under your belt.

 Tip: Always insert plenty of guidewire as this allows a degree of latitude if you kink the wire.

Whichever technique is used, ensure that there is free drainage and that you have obtained adequate specimens for laboratory analysis. When the collection contains pus, aspirate it as completely as possible. In addition, consider gentle saline irrigation of the cavity as this helps to clear thick pus and other semisolid debris. Make sure that you have a suitable drain bag to attach to the drainage catheter;

 Alarm: Sometimes special adaptors are needed to connect a bag to the drainage catheter. Do not wait until pus is running over your shoes to find this out!

Securely attach the catheter to the patient. There are several ways to do this:
- Suturing the catheter to the skin
- Using adhesive anchor systems
- Using adhesive tape – only secure with waterproof tape.

Make sure that the final position will be practical and as comfortable as possible for the patient.

 Tip: Do not attach a conventional three-way tap to a 12Fr drain – you have just reduced the lumen to 6Fr!

Specific sites

Subphrenic abscess

Subphrenic collections are usually postoperative. They are inconveniently located, as getting below the pleural reflection can be a challenge. The best approach is with a combination of ultrasound and fluoroscopy and it might need a bit of mental triangulation to determine the upward path for the needle. Some centres will accept an intercostal approach on the premise that the pleural surface will be adherent and empyema is unlikely. While this is an option, we would be cautious about this approach for all patients. Remember to add empyema to the potential complications during consent, regardless of whether you deliberately go through the pleural surface or not.

Upper abdominal solid organ abscesses

Liver, renal and splenic abscesses can all be drained percutaneously with reported success rates usually around 90%. Drainage is usually performed under ultrasound guidance and less commonly CT. Peripancreatic abscesses, pseudocysts and phlegmons are common complications of pancreatitis. Infected collections often require drainage. The management of complex pancreatitis is best left to a specialist team but the following guidelines are generally applicable. Collections in the lesser sac can usually be approached anteriorly through the transverse mesocolon between the stomach and transverse colon. Collections in the left paracolic gutter are more difficult and best approached with CT guidance to avoid colonic puncture. Loculated collections may require several drains. As always, frequent review is mandatory. This often entails serial CT scanning. Large pseudocysts, which continue to drain, can be treated by cyst gastrostomy. Increasingly, drainage may be used to provide access for minimally invasive pancreatic necrosectomy – essentially removal of necrotic tissue via endoscopic forceps through a circa 30Fr tract. Planning this access with the pancreatic surgical team is essential. Risks are increased with more vascular organs like the spleen and there is a tendency to use smaller catheters.

Pericolic abscess

These are usually secondary to diverticular disease, periappendiceal or postoperative collections. The aim is often as a bridge to a surgical procedure, however some centres will use this as definitive management – particularly in the elderly and infirm. Imaging guidance is always by CT and care should be taken to avoid puncturing adjacent loops. Further follow-up imaging is usually with CT.

Pelvic collections

The commonest difficulty in pelvic biopsy or drainage is identifying a route that does not transgress bowel or bladder. Gravity causes pus to collect in the prerectal space; this is difficult to access from an anterior approach. Alternative options include transrectal, transvaginal and transgluteal approaches. The commonest approach in most centres is transgluteal drainage.

The posterior transgluteal route traverses the sacrosciatic notch and uses CT guidance (Fig. 39.2). The patient is scanned in the prone position (Fig. 39.3) and the approach is planned in the conventional fashion. Remember that the sciatic nerve and gluteal vessels pass through the anterior portion of the notch. To avoid them, the tract should pass as close to the sacrum as possible. Burrowing through this much muscle can be difficult and may be uncomfortable for the patient both during and after the procedure. Peri-catheter inflammation can cause sciatica even when the catheter is appropriately placed.

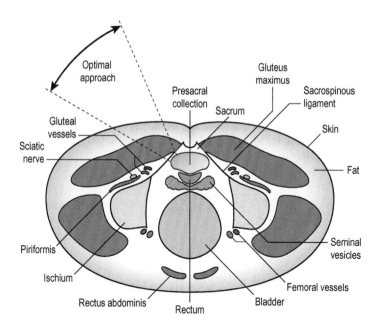

Fig. 39.2 ▇ Approach for transgluteal drainage through the greater sciatic notch. Optimal path is posteromedial to avoid the gluteal vessels and sciatic nerve.

Ultrasound-guided transrectal and transvaginal drainage are readily performed and well tolerated. Although these approaches are unfamiliar, the basic principles of biopsy and drainage apply. These routes offer a direct approach to posterior collections, with the advantage of draining well in the supine position. Most suitable probes have needle guides. Use sterile covers over the probe and guide. The collection is punctured under direct visualization. As always, aspirate some fluid; if it is purulent, formal drainage is performed; if not, the collection is aspirated to dryness. Catheter fixation is difficult and self-retaining catheters are preferred. The catheter can be taped to the patient's thigh and drained into a leg bag.

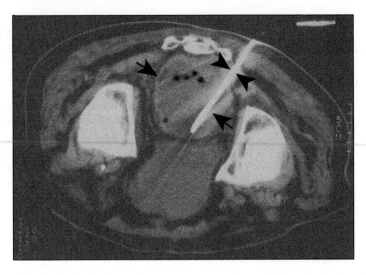

Fig. 39.3 ▨ Transgluteal route for drainage of a presacral abscess (arrows). The catheter (arrowheads) passes close to the sacrum to avoid the sciatic nerve and gluteal vessels that lie anteriorly.

Transrectal procedures cause surprisingly little discomfort but this is a 'dirty' route (Fig. 39.4). A cleansing enema is recommended to remove any faecal residue and antibiotic prophylaxis must be given. Contamination of the collection with faecal organisms is a potential pitfall but is thought not to occur because of the positive intra-abdominal pressure during defaecation. The patient is scanned in the lateral decubitus or lithotomy position. Drains up to 12Fr can be used. Catheter displacement during defaecation is common even with self-retaining catheters.

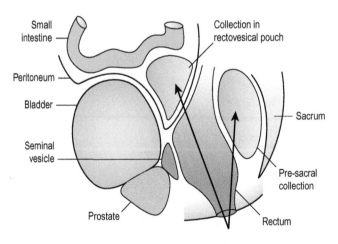

Fig. 39.4 ▨ Sagittal section through male pelvis showing routes for transrectal drainage.

The transvaginal approach is performed with the patient in the lithotomy position (Fig. 39.5). Sedation is recommended as the procedure tends to be uncomfortable and the vaginal wall can be difficult to traverse. The vagina and perineum are cleaned with povidone iodine solution. Catheters up to 12Fr can be used but require employing serial fascial dilators over a stiff guidewire.

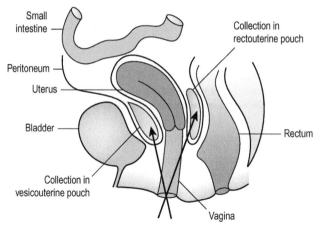

Fig. 39.5 ▨ Sagittal section through the female pelvis to show transvaginal routes for abscess drainage.

Pancreas

Peripancreatic abscesses, pseudocysts and phlegmons are common complications of pancreatitis. Infected collections often require drainage. The management of complex pancreatitis is best left to a specialist team but the following guidelines are generally applicable. Collections in the lesser sac can usually be approached anteriorly through the transverse mesocolon between the stomach and transverse colon. Collections in the left paracolic gutter are more difficult to approach and are best done with CT guidance to avoid colonic puncture. Loculated collections may require several drains. As always, frequent review is mandatory. This often entails serial CT scanning. Large pseudocysts, which continue to drain, can be treated by cyst gastrostomy.

Aftercare

Remember to write in the casenotes if you have inserted a locking pigtail drain, just in case they decide to remove the drain. Give clear instruction to irrigate the catheter with 10 mL of sterile saline three times a day, as this helps maintain catheter patency. In reality, the most effective drainage happens when the interventional radiologist is actively involved in the aftercare – visit the patient on the ward and advise on catheter management.

The volume of fluid drained should be charted. Febrile patients usually settle within 24–48 h if there is adequate drainage. Most simple fluid collections drain quickly, with a steady decrease in the volume of fluid draining. Large inflammatory collections (e.g. pseudocyst, empyema) may take several weeks to resolve.

Thick viscous collections require irrigation and aspiration to ensure effective drainage. It is essential the catheter is aspirated three times a day. Use a 50-mL syringe for maximum suction and then irrigate with 5–10 mL of saline. The drain may need to be repositioned or replaced as the situation evolves.

The drain catheter can be removed when there is minimal drainage (<10 mL/day) and the collection has resolved as documented by CT or ultrasound. Catheters should be promptly removed when they have fulfilled their role, so that they do not become a source of infection in their own right.

Troubleshooting

The drainage catheter will not advance into the collection
- Ensure that the skin incision is large enough.
- Use fluoroscopy to check for wire kinking. If the wire is kinked and there is sufficient wire, pull it until the kink is outside the skin, then insert a dilator and exchange for a stiffer wire.
- Large drains may need to be placed through a peel-away sheath, which is positioned over a stiff guidewire.

The collection is loculated and does not drain freely
- Thin loculi can be disrupted by moving the catheter back and forth within the collection.
- If this is not successful, fibrinous bands can be broken down by instilling streptokinase into the collection. This is particularly useful for loculated empyema.
- Some collections require multiple drainage catheters.

The catheter drains initially but then stops
- Hopefully, the collection is completely drained.
- Re-image the patient to assess the catheter position and the size of the collection.
- The drainage bag has been positioned above the collection, e.g. on the patient's locker. Place the bag in a dependent position.
- The catheter is correctly positioned, but there is a kink in it or the drainage tubing. Kinks are almost always external and are often caused by fiddling with the catheter or dressings. Reattaching it appropriately can often salvage the catheter. If there is any doubt, replace the catheter/drainage tube.
- The catheter may need to be repositioned or replaced if the collection has changed size or shape or if the catheter has been displaced.
- The catheter is blocked. Gentle flushing may clear it. If this fails, try using a guidewire to unblock it. An irreversibly blocked catheter must be exchanged. Catheters which have been in place for a week or more, usually have a well-established tract. The catheter can be removed and a hydrophilic guidewire passed through the tract into the collection. A new drain is then simply positioned over the wire. An alternative option is to cut the hub off the catheter and then pass a sheath over the outside of the catheter. The catheter is removed and a guidewire passed into the collection through the sheath; the sheath is removed and a new catheter positioned over the wire.

Fever does not settle after 48 h
- Failure to improve implies incomplete drainage or another source of sepsis. If this occurs, the patient should be re-imaged. Further drainage is often required. This scenario is common in patients with infected pancreatic pseudocysts.

There is a sudden increase in drainage or a change in the composition of the effluent
- This implies that a fistula has developed; an injection of contrast into the drainage catheter will usually demonstrate the problem. Sometimes it is necessary to perform an alternative study if the fistula tract acts as a one-way valve. A fistula will usually resolve if there is an adequate alternative route of drainage, although prolonged drainage may be necessary. Where there is a connection with an obstructed system, this will also need to be drained if the fistula is to resolve.

Complications

Complications related to drainage are relatively rare but no technique or operator can completely avoid them.

Acute sepsis: Always give appropriate broad-spectrum antibiotics prior to drainage. It is not surprising that sepsis occurs as some bacteraemia during drainage is almost bound to occur. Prompt resuscitation is essential with second-line antibiotics/IV fluids/oxygen and blood cultures. Liaison with the clinical team is essential, as they will need to continue resuscitation and consider moving to a more supportive environment.

Bleeding: If you notice bleeding from the tract during dilatation, the best tactic is to ensure you tamponade the tract by inserting the drain. Most tract bleeding is venous and will settle quickly. Monitor pulse and blood pressure, and if there are any adverse features get a CT to plan further therapy such as arterial embolization.

'Oops I've accidentally kebabed the …': Stay calm and do not be tempted to immediately pull the drain. Depending on the unlucky structure, plan your next move based on ensuring that a safe environment and support are available when you withdraw the tube. Tubes that go through blood vessels need consideration of embolization or stent grafting. Tubes that go through bowel often do not need surgery but a conversation with the surgical team is advised and planned removal with close observation is the usual pathway. If the patient develops signs of peritonitis then surgical intervention is required.

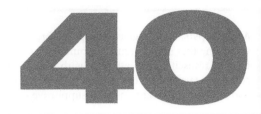

Treating urogenital vascular conditions

There are several conditions which have been grouped together relating to the urogenital tract and which loosely impact on fertility.

Uterine artery embolization

Indications for treatment

The vast majority of uterine artery embolization (UAE) is performed to manage symptomatic fibroid disease and to a much lesser extent, other uterine pathologies associated with menorrhagia. UAE is an alternative to surgery (hysterectomy or myomectomy) for patients in whom medical treatment (e.g. with gonadotrophin-releasing hormone [GnRH] analogues) has failed.

UAE is also important in the management of postpartum haemorrhage (Ch. 46).

The procedure in itself is not particularly technically demanding; however, there is a lot of work in developing and implementing appropriate protocols for assessment, procedural pain relief and post-procedural management. It is essential that the service is delivered in conjunction with a gynaecologist.

Assessment

Patients with menorrhagia and with bulk symptoms are candidates for treatment; they should have both gynaecological and imaging assessment. Ultrasound is principally used to assess the uterus and ovaries, establish the diagnosis of fibroids and assess uterine size. In the majority of centres, dedicated pelvic magnetic resonance (MR) examination is used to assess suitability for UAE and as part of follow-up to gauge the success of treatment.

Suitability for uterine artery embolization

UAE will only succeed if the fibroids are vascular, hence they must show enhancement following contrast on T1-weighted MRI; following treatment evidence of devascularization predicts shrinkage. Pedunculated fibroids may be expelled (or require hysteroscopic removal). If the predominant fibroid is intracavitary then primary removal by hysteroscopy should be considered.

 Tip: Delay embolization for 3 months after treatment with GnRH analogues as the uterine arteries are small and extremely difficult to catheterize during treatment.

Consent issues

Patients should be seen in the interventional radiology (IR) clinic. It is essential that the patient receives both adequate information and an opportunity to discuss the potential complications. Patients undergoing UAE are relatively young, most are hoping to avoid the morbidity associated with hysterectomy. A few will wish to become pregnant, patients wishing to conceive should be assessed for suitability for myomectomy. The risks of UAE are less than those of surgery.

In addition to the usual angiography risks patients should be warned of important side-effects including severe pain and significant complications (Table 40.1).

Table 40.1 Complications of fibroid embolization

	(%)
Risk of recurrence at 5 years	20
Premature menopause	2
Fibroid expulsion	2
Sepsis	1
Hysterectomy	1
Death	<0.01

Equipment

- Hydrophilic 4F catheter
- Hydrophilic wire
- Microcatheter
- Particulate agents: e.g. PVA or microspheres 500–1000 μm.

Procedure

Analgesia: Fibroid embolization is a painful procedure and patients generally have severe cramping pain for 12–24 h, with some milder discomfort lasting for weeks. Analgesia is more effective if given before the onset of pain and at regular intervals. Pre-procedural analgesia usually includes an NSAID given by suppository, an intramuscular opiate and an antiemetic. Intra-procedural analgesia should include an intravenous opiate; midazolam is often also given to alleviate anxiety.

Technique: Bilateral uterine artery embolization is usually required for adequate treatment. The uterine arteries are branches of the anterior division of the internal iliac artery. The internal iliac artery is selectively catheterized with a hydrophilic Cobra catheter. If the uterine artery is suitably large, the Cobra can often be advanced directly into the vessel.

Tip: These vessels are prone to spasm so have a low threshold for using microcatheters.

After selective catheterization has been achieved, embolization with permanent particles is performed, most typically polyvinyl alcohol (PVA). The endpoint of embolization is to-and-fro flow within the uterine artery.

Alarm: The ovaries are very radiation-sensitive. Keep radiation to a minimum. Use pulsed fluoroscopy if possible and avoid performing angiographic runs unless the anatomy cannot be resolved. Hence, there are no illustrations in this chapter!

Aftercare

Work to develop a post-fibroid pain pathway that ensures appropriate access to analgesia – usually opiate. The NSAID should be continued and an antiemetic is required. Most patients can be discharged 24–36 h post-procedure on strong oral analgesia. Make sure to follow the patient with a 3-month follow-up appointment.

Outcomes

UAE is a safe and effective alternative to surgical treatment for uterine fibroids. Fibroid embolization works best for resolution of menorrhagia but is usually effective for bulk symptoms. Expect, on average, a 60% reduction in fibroid volume. About 20% of patients will have recurrent symptoms and may opt for further treatment. As there is a risk of incomplete treatment/recurrence, patients wishing a guaranteed cure may prefer hysterectomy.

Testicular vein embolization

Indications

Testicular vein embolization is an alternative to surgical ligation of the gonadal vein and is used in symptomatic and subfertile patients with varicocele. It is an elective procedure and very straightforward. It is therefore an ideal case on which to learn coil embolization; whether it has any therapeutic benefit for the subfertile is less certain!

Anatomy: Most varicoceles are left-sided; if unilateral then treatment should be unilateral. The left spermatic vein joins the midpoint of the left renal vein. The right spermatic vein joins the anterior IVC just below the right renal vein (Fig. 40.1).

Consent issues

There is no guarantee that varicocele embolization will improve fertility. Technical failure (approximately 10%) is not uncommon, particularly in the right testicular vein. Failure does not preclude subsequent surgical ligation.

Equipment

- Basic angiography set
- Hydrophilic guidewire
- Catheters of choice depending on approach, e.g. hydrophilic Cobra II and Sidewinder II catheters from the groin, Berenstein from jugular vein, microcatheters
- Embolization coils ± sodium tetradecyl sulphate (STS).

Approach: The right common femoral vein (CFV) is often used, but we prefer the right internal jugular vein (IJV). Catheterization is simpler as it is in-line and there is no need for post-procedure bedrest.

Procedure

Catheterize the left renal vein and perform a venogram to demonstrate reflux down the spermatic vein. If reflux is not obvious, gently probe the inferior wall of the vein using a

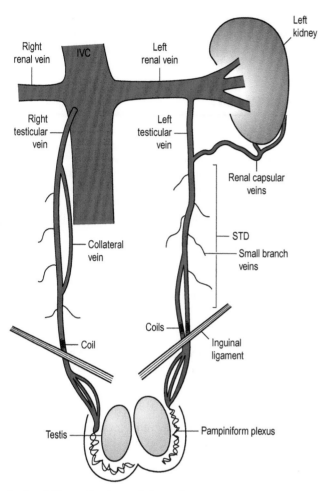

Left
kidney

Right
renal vein

IVC

Left
renal vein

Right
testicular
vein

Left
testicular
vein

Renal capsular
veins

Collateral
vein

STD

Small branch
veins

Coils

Coil

Inguinal
ligament

Testis

Pampiniform plexus

Fig. 40.1 ▦ Varicocele anatomy. Coils are placed in the main veins just above the inguinal ligament. STS may be used to sclerose small branch veins/potential collaterals. IVC, inferior vena cava.

hydrophilic guidewire and the catheter to cannulate the vein. Usually, the gonadal vein arises just lateral to the border of the vertebra. If possible, the catheter should be advanced to the level of the inguinal canal. Occasionally a microcatheter may be necessary to achieve catheterization. Most operators will use 'soft coils', which allow a degree of oversizing and pack down well – a popular choice is the Nestor Coil (Cook Medical). Deploy coils here and confirm blockage of the vein.

Withdraw the catheter to the midpoint of the vein and perform another venogram to look for small collateral veins. These can be treated by further coil deployment, or some practitioners may use a liquid sclerosant, such as STS. Use with caution as the gonadal vein may communicate with important structures.

Alarm: Make sure the coils are appropriately sized and large enough to lodge in the spermatic vein or they will become effective pulmonary emboli.

Troubleshooting

No reflux is seen: You know there is reflux from the ultrasound. Occasionally, there is a competent valve at the top of the spermatic vein and the source of the reflux is a renal capsular vein beyond.

The spermatic vein goes into spasm: Relax! Explain to the patient that this is not uncommon and always self-limiting. Give a small dose of glyceryl trinitrate (100 μg), wait 1 min and then perform a gentle venogram. This is a good time to consider using a microcatheter.

Ovarian vein embolization

Indications

Ovarian vein embolization is the anatomical female equivalent of testicular vein embolization. It is performed in pelvic congestion syndrome and to treat vulval varices when medical treatment (e.g. GNRH analogues) has failed. There are many causes of pelvic pain and it is essential that this patient group has a gynaecological assessment prior to intervention. Prominent ovarian veins on cross-sectional imaging are common and the vast majority will be asymptomatic.

The classical diagnostic features seen at venography are:

- Ovarian venous diameter >10 mm in diameter
- Retrograde ovarian or pelvic venous flow
- Cross-filling across the midline and tortuous collateral pelvic pathways.

Consent issues

In addition to technical failure it is important to explain that symptoms may not be relieved by embolization in up to 20% of patients. Recurrence occurs in approximately 10%.

Procedure

The procedure is similar to varicocele embolization. The anatomy of the ovarian vein tends to be a bit more variable distally and embolization of several branches may be necessary.

Outcomes

Symptomatic relief is rapid and occurs in around 80% of patients with true pelvic congestion syndrome. Recurrence is not uncommon.

41

Treating urological conditions

Nephrostomy

Percutaneous nephrostomy is one of the most frequently performed interventional procedures and is a technique in which every radiologist should feel completely confident. Urgent drainage is required in an infected obstructed system due to the resultant rapid renal loss and septicaemia. Fortunately, nephrostomy is usually an elective procedure, as ureteric obstruction leads to gradual progressive renal loss. Acute renal colic with obstruction and persistent pain or calyceal rupture, while usually not an overnight emergency procedure, does need expedient treatment usually on the next list.

Equipment

- Undilated or minimally dilated system: 21G AccuStick/Neff coaxial access set
- Dilated system: 19G sheathed needle
- Heavy-duty 0.035-inch guidewire (shorter guidewires, usually about 60 cm length make it easier – a short super-stiff Amplatz 4-cm floppy tip is often ideal)
- Fascial dilators to one size greater than the drain size
- 6–8F pigtail nephrostomy drain. Locking pigtails are ideal
- 5F Cobra catheter
- Angled hydrophilic wire
- Give antibiotic cover as advised by local protocol.

Procedure

The performance of a safe nephrostomy requires an understanding of renal anatomy, good ultrasound guidance and basic catheterization skills.

Target zone: The renal arteries and renal veins enter the kidney at the renal hilum and divide into larger anterior and smaller posterior divisions passing around the renal collecting system. The least vascular zone, and therefore the safest area, lies within the arc shown – *aka* Brödel's avascular line (Fig. 41.1). Posterior calyces in the mid and lower pole are the best target and provide the most favourable approach for intervention. Direct puncture of the renal pelvis should be avoided, as this increases the risk of major vascular injury and persistent urine leak. Puncture of the upper pole calyces is only necessary for nephrolithotomy and is associated with a significant risk of pneumothorax (Fig. 41.2). Avoid anterior punctures; in addition to providing the least favourable access and causing renal haemorrhage, you may well traverse the colon, liver or spleen.

Ultrasound-guided puncture: Ultrasound guidance is by far the easiest and safest technique. It is easy to be anxious to get to the needlework, but take time at the start to get the

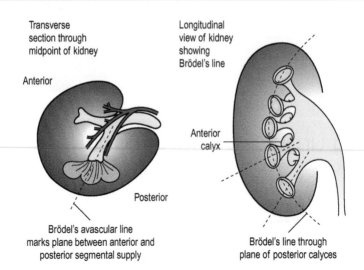

Fig. 41.1 ▨ Optimal approach for nephrostomy – posterior, lower or interpolar calyces along Brödel's avascular line.

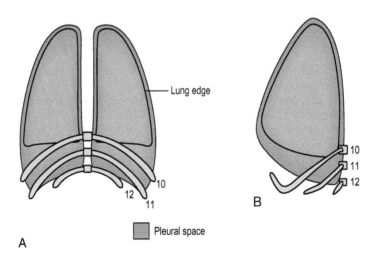

Fig. 41.2 ▨ Surface markings of the pleural spaces and the lungs relative to the lower ribs (10, 11, 12) of (A) the posterior and (B) the lateral chest walls.

ultrasound just right. If you have not read the section on ultrasound-guided punctures (Ch. 26), then read it now, if nothing else!

1. Before all the drapes are applied, scan the patient in either a prone or a prone/oblique position, aiming to find a posterolateral approach to target a posterior interpolar calyx. Mark the potential site of entry on the skin and remember you are aiming at a posterior calyx so the puncture should only traverse the retroperitoneum – that's at the back of the patient! If the puncture is very lateral or even anterior, look for a better window.

2. Drape the patient, infiltrate local anaesthetic along the needle track and make a 5-mm skin nick with a scalpel. Advance the puncture needle under continuous ultrasound guidance. When the needle tip reaches the calyx, advance it 5–10 mm with a darting

motion. There may be a sudden 'give' as the calyx is entered. Apply gentle suction while slowly withdrawing the needle; aspiration of urine indicates entry to the system. Do not completely decompress the system, as it makes subsequent wire and catheter manipulation more difficult.
3. Inject a small amount of contrast to opacify the system and confirm the lie of the land.

Achieving drainage: It seems nothing could be simpler now than to advance the nephrostomy drain into position, but many procedures go wrong at this stage and frustrating hours can then be spent trying to puncture a now undilated system.

1. If you are using a coaxial set (e.g. Neff/AccuStick), initially introduce the 0.018-inch wire, ensuring the soft leading section (the most radio-opaque section on fluoroscopy) is completely within the pelvicalyceal system. The support from the stiffer section of the wire is needed to advance the coaxial dilator system. Exchange the needle for the coaxial dilator system over the guidewire. Remember the metal stiffener does not like corners and unlock the stiffener at the point of entry into the calyx to support advancing the plastic sections.
2. Remove the inner plastic dilator and leave the 0.018 inch wire in place – this is your *safety* wire.
3. Using fluoroscopy, introduce the 0.035-inch guidewire parallel to the 0.018-inch wire, this should advance without resistance. If you are lucky, the wire will pass straight down the ureter but often it will pass into an upper pole calyx or coil in the renal pelvis (see Troubleshooting, below).
4. Advance dilators over the 0.035-inch guidewire to 1F larger than the drain. Leave the dilator in place on the wire to tamponade the track.
5. In an uninfected system, a 6F nephrostomy catheter is adequate, but pus requires at least an 8F drain for satisfactory drainage. Advance the nephrostomy drain until the tip is just within the ureter, then withdraw the wire to form the pigtail.
6. Inject a small amount of contrast to confirm your position.

Alarm: Never over-distend an obviously infected system with contrast. This is a sure way to give the patient septicaemia.

7. If the catheter is a locking pigtail, secure the catheter via the locking mechanism. Some centres also secure the catheter in position with either an adhesive dressing or a suture. Make sure that the catheter is firmly attached or you will be replacing it later!
8. Remove the safety wire once position is confirmed and the drainage catheter is secured.
9. *Finishing off*: remember when documenting the procedure to highlight if you have used a locking pigtail catheter, this is important when removing the drain.

Alarm: Removal without releasing the locking mechanism is painful and can disrupt the pelvicalyceal system or fracture the catheter. Finally, hopefully this catheter will be removed, and in addition to releasing the lock, make sure that the nylon suture does not get left behind when the catheter is withdrawn, as it can act as a nidus for infection or stone formation.

Unless you have performed an immaculate puncture, a formal nephrostogram should be left for 24 h, as blood clot can simulate stones or tumour.
Aspirate the drainage catheter:

- Pus: completely decompress the system
- Blood – rosé-coloured: connect to drainage bag
- Blood – claret-coloured: lavage with normal saline until it clears to rosé.

Troubleshooting

Difficult visualization: Optimize the ultrasound; spend time looking for a good acoustic window before you start.

- Use a suitable probe: 3.5–5 MHz is best for nephrostomy
- Use the best ultrasound machine available.

Aspiration of urine but cannot advance guidewire: The needle/sheath is sitting against the wall of the calyx. Do not use force as the calyx can be perforated. Very gently inject a little contrast to outline the position and carefully retract the needle/sheath and advance the guidewire.

Wire passes into the renal pelvis or an upper pole calyx: Use a Cobra catheter and hydrophilic wire to direct it into the ureter. If there is a proximal ureteric obstruction, allow the wire to coil in the renal pelvis to improve your purchase.

Unable to advance dilators/drainage catheter: Check the skin nick. Have you passed the needle through it? Is it large enough? Enlarge the nick as required.

The guidewire has kinked: The wire most often kinks either at the skin surface or at the renal cortex. If you have inserted enough wire into the ureter or renal pelvis, it will be possible to withdraw the wire until the kink is outside the skin. If there is insufficient wire, advance a 4F dilator into the renal pelvis, this will usually pass over the most kinked wire. Exchange for a new stronger wire and this time do not let the wire ride forward during catheter insertion. Rarely, a stronger wire than the heavy-duty J-wire is needed. Steer a 4F catheter into the ureter, then gently insert an Amplatz wire.

Nephrostomy when the pelvicalyceal system is not dilated: The pelvicalyceal (PC) system may be obstructed but not dilated in two circumstances:

- In a dehydrated septic patient
- When there is a urinary leak from the ureter or PC system usually due to rupture of an obstructed system or following surgery. Fortunately, this is exceptionally unusual for an emergency nephrostomy.

Optimize your chances and use the best ultrasound machine. If the patient is dehydrated consider giving 1 L normal saline and furosemide prior to nephrostomy to try to distend the system slightly.

A coaxial system is best as it is fairly unlikely you will access a suitable calyx first pass. Some operators will use contrast and puncture using fluoroscopic guidance. For the more advanced, inject carbon dioxide after entering the pelvicalyceal system, and, as this floats, it allows targeting of a suitable calyx.

 Tip: Do not try to jump too many French sizes but, as a general rule, go up in steps of two. Remember to dilate the tract to 1F larger than that of the drainage catheter.

Transplant nephrostomy

The good news about transplant nephrostomy is the target is closer and therefore ultrasound guidance easier. As the kidney is in the pelvis you will be aiming for an anterior calyx. It is essential to avoid the temptation to perform a direct puncture of the renal pelvis. Ensure that the path of the nephrostomy catheter passes through parenchyma. Generally, transplant kidneys have a tough outer fibrotic capsule and it will require serial dilators to allow passage of the drainage catheter. Remember to insert plenty of wire; if necessary, use a catheter to steer down into the ureter. Finally, transplant kidneys do tend to be a bit more vascular, so do not be alarmed by bleeding during catheter changes, as the nephrostomy drain will tamponade the tract.

Nephrostomy exchange

Long-term nephrostomy catheters need changed at least every 3–6 months to prevent encrustation and infection. This 'simple' task is usually delegated to the youngest member of the team. If you are really learning and experiencing interventional radiology, then you will know *Robertson's law*: There is no *simple procedure* that cannot become complicated.

- Always opacify the PC system with dilute contrast before you start – it is vital to know where the target is if things start to go wrong.
- Remember to unlock the catheter retention suture – in reality, this usually means cutting off the catheter hub.
- Insert a semi-stiff 0.035-inch guidewire into the catheter – tight J-wires (curve <3 mm) tend to navigate out the catheter side holes, so are best avoided.
- Retract the catheter over the wire to remove.
- Look to see if the retention suture has come out with the catheter. If it is visible in the nephrotomy wound – then gently pull on one end to remove the suture.
- Insert the nephrostomy catheter – dilators are usually not needed.
- Lock, confirm drainage and leave.

Troubleshooting

The wire gets stuck half way down the existing catheter: Fairly common. The catheter is blocked with debris which has been compacted by the wire. Try to clear by flushing with a 1-mL syringe. If this fails, take a stiff Terumo and try to get as far as the first sidehole, as this will allow entry to the PC system. The catheter loop has not been straightened by the wire, so there will be more resistance to removal. Be aware this may be more painful and analgesic may be needed.

The catheter is completely blocked: Ok, this is trickier! Cut the hub off the catheter. Take a suture and pass it through the cut end of the catheter, i.e. puncturing both walls. Thread the suture loop through a suitably sized peel-away sheath. The catheter will serve as the dilator. Use the suture to apply tension and push the sheath over the blocked catheter until it enters the pelvicalyceal system. Take a bow – access preserved.

 Tip: If you do not have a suitable peel-away sheath you can use a conventional sheath or guide catheter to remove the nephrostomy catheter. Remember to introduce a wire into the PC system for the new nephrostomy. Do not deploy it through a conventional sheath!

I've lost access completely (*aka* my assistant lost access completely): Still often recoverable, particularly if the catheter has a mature tract. Use a short forward facing catheter and gently insert it into the tract opening and inject contrast – the tract will often be opacified. It is better to try initially without a wire to gently advance the catheter with occasional injections and navigate up the tract. If the catheter will not go round a curve of the tract, then an angled hydrophilic wire can be useful if used carefully.

Antegrade ureteric stent

Antegrade stenting is performed when long-term ureteric drainage is required. It is more comfortable for the patient than having a nephrostomy and has the obvious advantage of not needing any drainage bag. Ureteric stents can be placed retrogradely or antegradely.

Indications

- Benign or malignant ureteric obstruction; malignant obstruction is by far the commonest indication
- Ureteric injury, often in combination with nephrostomy drainage
- Ureteric calculus undergoing lithotripsy.

Equipment

- Guidewires: 3-mm J, Amplatz super-stiff, stiff hydrophilic
- Catheters: Cobra or Torcon blue
- Peel-away sheath (usually 9Fr)
- Ureteric stent system (pusher/suture or pusher/plug)
- 8F nephrostomy catheter.

Procedure

1. A percutaneous nephrostomy may already be present. Alternatively, perform a nephrostomy aiming for a middle or lower pole calyx.
2. A shaped catheter, either a Cobra or a Torcon blue (Cook Medical, UK) is inserted using a J-guidewire for access.
3. Contrast is introduced via the catheter to outline the ureter and the level of obstruction.
4. A hydrophilic wire (Terumo) is inserted into the catheter and directed down the ureter. The catheter is advanced down the ureter until it is just above the stricture.
5. The hydrophilic wire is gently advanced and rotated and will readily pass through the majority of strictures.
6. The catheter is advanced beyond the stricture and into the bladder.
7. It is useful to distend the bladder at this stage with dilute contrast; this creates space for the pigtail of the stent to form and makes the procedure less uncomfortable for the patient.
8. The guidewire is now exchanged for an appropriately stiff wire, such as an Amplatz super-stiff wire. Try to create a loop of wire within the bladder (Fig. 41.3A), and leave the catheter and wire in situ and prepare/assemble the ureteric stent system.
9. The tract should be dilated to 1F greater than the stent being inserted.
10. The ureteric stent system is inserted over the wire and, holding the wire perfectly still, it is advanced until the distal stent marker lies several centimetres within the bladder (Fig. 41.3B).
11. The proximal end of the stent is positioned within the renal pelvis and the guidewire is withdrawn allowing the distal pigtail to form (Fig. 41.3C).
12. If an inner stiffener catheter is present, carefully withdraw it while keeping forward pressure on the pusher to maintain the stent in position (Fig. 41.3D,E).

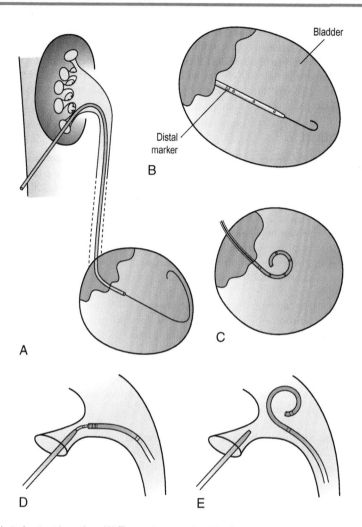

Fig. 41.3 ▨ Ureteric stent insertion. (A) The catheter and guidewire are passed into the bladder. (B) The stent is advanced until the distal marker is in the bladder. (C) The guidewire is withdrawn until a pigtail forms in the bladder. (D) The proximal end of the stent is positioned so that pigtail will form in the renal pelvis. The guidewire is pulled back and final adjustments made to the stent position. (E) The central pusher catheter is withdrawn to release the stent.

13. Usually ureteric stent systems have a variant of one of two methods to allow stent retraction if pushed in too far.
    • Method one is the pusher/suture system: a suture looped through the final sidehole of the stent can be pulled to retract the stent. If the stent is in a satisfactory position, one side of the looped suture is cut close to the skin and the suture carefully removed. This is not foolproof, however. For tips on how to avoid and manage suture-related mayhem, see the Troubleshooting section, below.
    • Method two is the pusher/plug system: this has an inner catheter plugged into the ureteric stent that can be released by pressing a button on the hub that advances a pusher, releasing the stent. Care needs to be taken to ensure that the release button is not accidentally pushed during insertion.

14. If a very avascular procedure has been performed perform a nephrostogram and if you can show drainage then a covering nephrostomy may not be necessary.
15. If it has been a trickier procedure and there is some clot in the system then a guidewire is inserted through the delivery system and a nephrostomy catheter placed in the renal pelvis. The nephrostomy catheter should be capped off and if the stent functions adequately, it can be removed after 24 h.

Troubleshooting

Unable to negotiate the stricture with a guidewire: It is usually possible to negotiate strictures even if no route through can be seen on ureterograms. Use the techniques set out in the principles of crossing stenoses and occlusions but remember it takes skill and patience to negotiate these strictures, not force! Get a ureterogram and advance the catheter so the tip of the catheter is in the apex of the stricture. Use a hydrophilic wire and torque device to gently probe the stricture. This can take some time in the most difficult lesions. If this fails, it is often worth leaving a nephrostomy in and allowing the system to decompress and the ureteric oedema to settle over a few days. If, after several attempts, no route can be found, it may be worth considering extra-anatomical stenting.

Unable to advance the catheter through the stricture: Occasionally, the guidewire can traverse the stricture but the catheter will not follow. Try a 4F or hydrophilic catheter and try to rotate the catheter while advancing through the stricture. If this fails, take a deep breath and withdraw the guidewire and insert a 3-mm J-guidewire down to the level of the stricture before advancing a 9F peel-away sheath into the distal ureter. The increased stability and reduction in friction mean it is now often possible to advance a catheter. Exceptionally, this may fail and it is worth crossing the stricture with a 0.018-inch wire and using a low-profile, small-vessel balloon to dilate the stricture.

Unable to advance the stent through the stricture: Advance a peel-away sheath across a stiff wire into the distal ureter or bladder. The reduction in friction means the stent usually passes readily. Remember to take care not to accidentally pull back the stent when peeling the sheath apart.

The pusher becomes impacted in the stent: With some stent systems, the pusher can become impacted in the stent after the stent has been pushed through. This means when the pusher is withdrawn, the stent comes back with it. Always screen during withdrawal of the pusher and if the stent seems to be coming back with the pusher, rotating the pusher can often separate them.

The retraction sutures are entangled with the stent: In practice, these sutures are often a cause of problems if not handled carefully. Prevention is better than cure and when advancing the stent, always make sure the suture loop is not wrapped round the stent. If, after the loop has been cut, the suture is still pulling back the stent, do not just pull like fury – it is possible to remove the stent, leaving an unsightly exit wound and a failed procedure. An elegant solution is to thread the longest part of the suture loop through a 5F dilator; using this as a buttress against the stent, it is usually possible to withdraw the suture.

Complications of nephrostomy and antegrade ureteric stent

Disruption of the renal pelvis/extravasation of contrast: This will settle, providing the urinary system is adequately drained.

Bleeding: Some degree of haematuria is to be expected, particularly if multiple passes have occurred. Haematuria should clear within 48 h. A blood clot in the pelvicalyceal system will lyse spontaneously because of the endogenous urokinase. Renal angiography ± embolization are occasionally required if there is persistent haematuria.

Inadvertent puncture of adjacent structures: Pneumothorax and colonic, liver and splenic puncture are all possible. These are much less likely to occur under ultrasound guidance.

Percutaneous nephrolithotomy

Percutaneous nephrolithotomy (PCNL) uses percutaneous access to the kidney to dilate a tract that permits stone removal via a nephroscope. Practice varies between centres as regards the roles of the radiologist and the urologist, but more and more urologists are performing this without radiological assistance. The consequence is that you will only be called to assist in complex cases or when something has gone wrong.

As always, reconnaissance is essential and it is vital that you understand the anatomy of the pelvicalyceal system and the stone-bearing calyces, as this will determine the target calyx. Before the procedure, decide with the urologist which calyx is likely to allow the most stone clearance. Remember that more than one puncture may be required to clear a large complex staghorn.

There are a variety of different techniques to achieve PCNL, but, in principle, the case should follow the steps described below.

Accessing the system:
1. The urologist will place a retrograde catheter into the ureter.
2. The patient is turned prone and prepped and draped. Fluoroscopy is used to identify the target calyx and an entry point on the skin; generally, this should be inferior and lateral to the calyx; the exact amount will depend on the size of the patient. If you are targeting an upper pole calyx, the puncture will be more vertical. Remember, with upper-pole punctures, going through the pleura is not good because it will leave a rather large hole probably followed by hydropneumothorax.
3. The urologist can then inject contrast from below to outline the calyx and help distend the system.
4. Usually a 19G sheathed needle is used for access, and this is directed down towards the target calyx. Hitting a stone creates a characteristic feel to the puncture.
5. Now the tricky bit; there will not be much space, as you will have – nine times out of 10 – punctured a stone-bearing calyx. Carefully advance the plastic sheath over the needle until it just enters the PC system. Try to manipulate a stiff hydrophilic wire into the PC system and down into the ureter. If the urologist has put in a retrograde catheter, get them to distend the system a little just prior to puncture, to create some space for your hydrophilic wire.

 Tip: If the calyx is full of stone, try to puncture at the calyceal fornix as there is often a tiny amount of space there (Fig. 41.4).

6. Once you have gained access with the hydrophilic wire, place a catheter into the ureter and exchange for an Amplatz super-stiff wire or similar.

Dilating the tract: Choose between using either balloon dilation (e.g. NephroMax) or serial Amplatz dilators. The serial dilators take more time and involve more X-ray exposure for

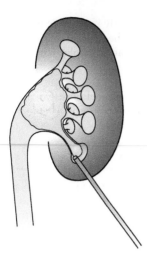

Fig. 41.4 ■ In a stone-bearing calyx, try to aim for the calyceal fornix, as there is potentially more space.

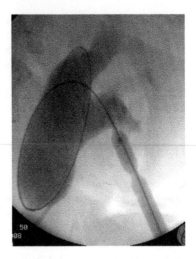

Fig. 41.5 ■ Balloon dilation of the tract. Note careful positioning of the balloon just at the edge of the calyx.

everyone, although they are a bit cheaper – but do not let us influence your choice. A few units use Alken dilators, which are metallic tubes that telescope over each other. The advantages with these are that they are reusable and have a zero tip, so that you can dilate up to the edge of the stone-bearing calyx, without going into the calyx (Fig. 41.5), which might cause calyceal rupture. Either way, take care to think about what the leading edge of the dilation is doing to the kidney – do not push too much into the pelvis as it can completely disrupt the system. If you are using the balloon, remember to pre-load the final sheath onto the balloon shaft. The balloon is then inflated with a pressure device, and fluoroscopy used to confirm that it has completely inflated. With the balloon inflated, the sheath is advanced over the balloon with a twisting motion. This is not for the faint-hearted, as a fair amount of (controlled) force is required to take the sheath into the system. Deflate the balloon and hold your breath – keep the guidewire well down into the ureter.

Removing the stone: It is not unusual for there to be a bit of bleeding at the point of access, particularly from 'cortical vessels' if the sheath has not quite gone in far enough. The urologist usually complains at this point about a variety of aspects of the puncture. This is traditional and resolves once the first stone fragment is visible. If bleeding is genuinely brisk, then simply re-insert the balloon to tamponade the tract.

The stone is then broken up, often by ultrasound and pneumatic drill (Lithoclast) or, less commonly, by laser, and extracted via the tract. This bit can take a while, so get comfortable and make sure they are not pulling out your access wire.

After a while, intermittent fluoroscopy will be used to determine the residual stone burden. It is not always possible to remove all the stone; generally, fragments <4 mm will pass spontaneously.

Which tube to leave behind? There has been a progressive move towards reducing the size of the drainage catheter or even completely doing away with it – tubeless PCNL. This element is likely to vary from centre to centre but, generally, if you are convinced that there is bleeding during the procedure, most operators will leave a larger catheter, e.g. 20 F. An uncomplicated PCNL may well have a smaller 8–10F catheter left in situ.

Complications

The most feared complication is haemorrhage. Immediate management includes clamping the drainage catheter, fluid resuscitation and a low threshold to renal angiography and embolization.

Injury to innocent bystanders during access is a definite risk, and colonic and pleural puncture are the most frequently reported.

42

Treating gastrointestinal conditions

Gastrointestinal interventions fall into two main groups: establishing enteral access for feeding and stenting to treat obstruction secondary to malignancy.

Nasogastric/nasojejunal tubes

Most nasogastric tubes are placed on the ward and most nasojejunal tubes are placed by endoscopists. If a request migrates to interventional radiology for these procedures, it is usually because of problems navigating the nasopharynx. Occasionally, it is an issue with an oesophageal stricture and, in that instance, consider whether oesophageal dilation or stenting would allow the patient to maintain oral intake.

This really should be a simple procedure in the vast majority of cases. Initially, try with the tube that the ward wants to use for feeding. Ask the patient which nostril is best, they usually know, as the ward should have tried several times before coming to you. Anaesthetize the throat with lidocaine spray and lubricate the tube. Some operators will try with the patient sitting up without fluoroscopy for their initial attempt. Usually, the best tactic is to place the patient supine and use lateral screening of the hypopharynx to visualize the action. If they can, ask the patient to swallow as the tube approaches the C6 level. We guarantee that nine times out of 10 the standard tube will go through with a little patience. If this fails, then use a vertebral catheter and hydrophilic wire to navigate the hypopharynx. Most people do not have enough hands to manipulate the catheter and wire and keep the catheter in place at the nose (that's three if you're counting.) Enlist the help of the nurse to hold the catheter at the nose, while you manipulate the catheter. Once the wire is well into the stomach, remove the catheter and place the nasogastric tube over the wire.

If placing a nasojejunal tube you will have to manipulate it round the duodenal loop. The tube may be weighted to help and will often be supplied with an internal wire. Try to get round using the tube; turning the patient onto their right-hand side can be useful. If stuck, a 260-cm Terumo wire and 100-cm vertebral or Headhunter catheter can be used to get round.

 Tip: Nasogastric tubes vary in their internal diameter and endhole configuration – some are blind-ending with sideholes only. Check the tube you plan to place outside the patient. If it is blind-ended, it is usually possible to place the tube by putting the wire through the last sidehole.

Oesophageal stent

Oesophageal stenting is used to palliate dysphagia, particularly in malignant disease. Self-expanding metallic endoprostheses allow durable palliation of dysphagia in a single treatment session, with minimal morbidity and mortality compared to radiotherapy and plastic endoprostheses. Oesophageal stents come in two main types: covered stents and bare stents. Covered stents have lower rates of occlusion secondary to tumour ingrowth but initial designs had a high rate of migration. Improvements in design have reduced the stent migration rate to <10% and most centres will now use covered stents for all patients. A few stents are available that contain a one-way valve to prevent reflux and even have a suture loop to permit repositioning/retrieval. Advances in radiotherapy and chemotherapy mean retrievable stents are an increasingly used option.

Accurate sizing is not important, but using a device that is approximately appropriate in size is required. In reality, few operators measure the true length of the lesion, as the vast majority of these lesions are covered by a single stent. As a guide, the stent length should be at least 2 cm longer than the lesion at either end. Large-diameter stents, i.e. around 30 mm, are best reserved for the dilated oesophagus as they cause considerable pain in a normal-calibre oesophagus.

Equipment

- Oesophageal stent: 18–25-mm diameter
- Hydrophilic guidewire, Amplatz super-stiff guidewire: 260 cm
- Berenstein/vertebral catheter.

Procedure

Review the pre-existing imaging to identify the approximate level of the stricture. The throat is subsequently anaesthetized with lidocaine spray (Xylocaine) and the patient positioned in the prone oblique position. IV sedation is administered and appropriate monitoring commenced.

Using fluoroscopic guidance, the oesophagus is catheterized via the oral route; it is tricky to get an oesophageal stent through the nose later in the procedure! It can take a little time to steer past the epiglottis; use a lateral projection and steer posteriorly. Try to avoid putting a guidewire deep into the trachea as this almost certainly will cause a coughing fit. The catheter is advanced to the approximate level of the lesion and a small amount of non-ionic contrast injected to outline the upper extent of the stricture. The catheter is then used to manipulate the hydrophilic guidewire through the stricture, using the techniques outlined in Chapter 31. If necessary, the catheter can be pulled back while slowly injecting contrast to define the proximal margin. The distal extent of lesions at the gastro-oesophageal junction can usually be outlined by air within the stomach. The position of the stricture can be indicated either by radio-opaque markers placed on the patient or using bony landmarks, but remember these markers are a considerable distance from the oesophagus and even minor patient movement may be significant. The Amplatz guidewire is inserted into the stomach and the stent is then carefully advanced over the Amplatz wire and deployed in position (Fig. 42.1). Deployment mechanisms vary between devices, but most devices are deployed by progressive retraction of a sheath. Most operators do not post-dilate and prefer to wait for the stent to expand itself (Fig. 42.1).

 Tip: If the markers move or there is difficulty being sure of the length and position, use a long angiographic sheath over the wire to depict the proximal and distal extent of the stricture without losing wire position.

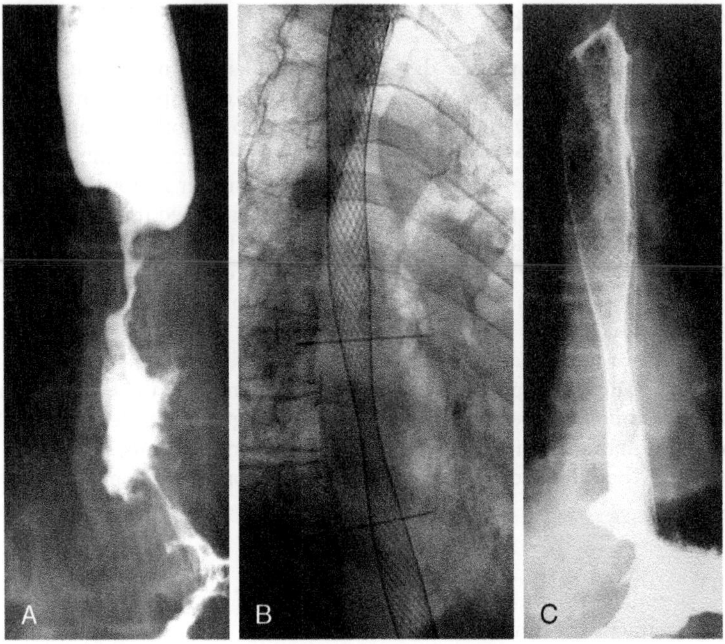

Fig. 42.1 ■ Deployment of an oesophageal stent. (A) Irregular oesophageal stricture. (B) Immediately after deployment the stent was narrow but was not post-dilated. (C) The stent was fully open at 24 h.

Aftercare

Clear fluids are permitted 4 h after the procedure. If this proceeds uneventfully, a light diet may be commenced. It is not essential to perform a routine follow-up oesophageal study. All patients should be advised to cut food into small pieces and encouraged to drink fizzy drinks, particularly cola, as they tend to prevent the stent from progressive sludging with food. If the stent extends over the cardia, the patient should be commenced on a proton-pump inhibitor to alleviate symptomatic oesophageal reflux.

Retrievable stents

Most of the available retrievable stents have a suture loop that will collapse down the stent when pulled taut. This is generally easiest under direct visualization at endoscopy, but it can be undertaken by the skilled interventionalist using a short reverse curve catheter to go through the loop and a long wire, which can be directed retrogradely back up the oesophagus and captured in the mouth. Both ends of the wire are then put through a sheath (12–14F will do) and the sheath gently advanced to just above the stent. The guidewire is pulled tight, and the proximal extent of the stent can just about be withdrawn into the sheath, and the entire ensemble can be withdrawn.

Outcomes

Primary technical success is achieved in 95–100% of patients, with significant relief of dysphagia in most series. Complications consist of migration <10% and haemorrhage.

Troubleshooting

The stent migrates through the cardia: Stent migration is more common with a stent that extends across the cardia and slightly more common with covered stents. If this is partial at the time of insertion, then it may be possible to anchor the stent by inserting an overlapping stent. More often, this occurs some time after the initial insertion and the stent is within the stomach. Most stents are left in situ within the stomach, but if the patient is symptomatic, the stent can be retrieved (but not reused!) at endoscopy, using an overtube.

The stent occludes: An acute occlusion usually indicates food bolus impaction. Perform a contrast study of the oesophagus; if contrast is still percolating through, then try some cola! If this fails, the stent can usually be readily cleared at endoscopy. More insidious onset of dysphagia indicates the stent has become occluded secondary to tumour overgrowth or tumour ingrowth. If tumour overgrowth has occurred, then often a second stent will resolve this. If the problem is tumour ingrowth, then either a covered stent or laser therapy should be considered.

The lesion is high in the oesophagus: The majority of lesions are in the lower-third but high lesions in the upper-third of the oesophagus need particularly critical positioning to avoid stenting open the vocal cords! Endoscopy during stent placement to identify the position of the cricopharyngeus muscle can be very useful. The Ultraflex oesophageal stent comes in a proximal release variant, and this permits more accurate proximal placement. It is generally better to use smaller devices in the upper oesophagus and the Ultraflex stent, which has less radial force, may prove more comfortable for the patient.

The patient develops chest pain post-deployment: This often occurs and is secondary to the expansile force of the stent. The sensation almost always resolves spontaneously.

Oesophageal fistulae and perforations

Covered stents are now usually the first-line intervention in the treatment of oesophageal perforations and fistulae. In particular, malignant fistulae are readily treated by accurate placement of a covered oesophageal stent. Benign perforations are technically fairly straightforward but long-term results may be less favourable due to overgrowth of granulation tissue at the stent margins. In this group of patients, most operators would place a temporary/retrievable covered oesophageal stent.

Percutaneous fluoroscopic gastrostomy

This is a straightforward procedure principally used to provide nutritional support for patients with swallowing disorders. Despite appearing technically fairly simple, it crops up frequently at morbidity and mortality meetings; attention to detail is important.

There are two variants to the radiological technique: the traditional radiologically inserted gastrostomy (RIG, *aka* push) and a new variant, the peroral image-guided gastrostomy (PIG, *aka* pull). The traditional fluoroscopic gastrostomy (RIG) technique places a 12–14F tube, which can be prone to blockage. PIG delivers the gastrostomy tube via the oral route, allowing placement of larger-calibre tubes (14–20F) that are often easier to manage in the long term.

Feeding via a percutaneous gastrostomy is associated with gastro-oesophageal reflux and aspiration in over a third of patients. To prevent this, some practitioners choose to manipulate the tube around the duodenal loop into the jejunum, i.e. percutaneous gastrojejunostomy. The initial technique is similar for both procedures.

Equipment

Commercial kits are available for both the PIG and RIG insertions and in practice, most departments will use a kit. Essentially this contains:

- RIG insertion:
  - 18G Seldinger needle
  - J-guidewire 0.038 inch
  - Fascial dilators to 1F greater than the drain
  - A self-retaining catheter.
- PIG insertion:
  - 18G Seldinger needle
  - J-guidewire 0.038 inch
  - Headhunter catheter
  - Super-stiff wire
  - A 'push' gastrostomy tube and adaptor.

Percutaneous gastrojejunostomy: As above plus:

- Cobra catheter
- Hydrophilic guidewire
- Gastrojejunostomy tube. Some gastrostomy kits have specific extension catheters for gastrojejunostomy.

There is evidence that complications are reduced when suture anchors are used when performing a RIG – they stop the stomach wall being pushed away during dilatation. They may be supplied with the kit or purchased separately.

T-fasteners explained: T-fasteners or anchors can be used to maintain the stomach in apposition with the anterior abdominal wall. Practice is variable, but more practitioners are using T-fasteners/anchors even for a straightforward gastrostomy and certainly in the face of an uncooperative patient, ascites or a post-surgical stomach.

How to use T-fasteners/anchors: T-fasteners, sometimes called suture anchors, are short metal bars attached to a suture/needle, that are delivered through a puncture needle into the stomach (Fig. 42.2). There are a number of designs now available, some of which have a locking mechanism to hold them against the skin of the anterior abdominal wall. In the simplest designs, an introducer needle is preloaded with the suture anchor and directed into the stomach. Contrast is injected to confirm position and a guidewire is then inserted into the needle, which pushes the anchor out into the stomach cavity. The introducer needle may then be removed and traction applied to the suture to bring the stomach into apposition with the anterior abdominal wall. While maintaining tension, the thread is tightened, either by suturing to the skin surface or using the supplied fixation mechanism. The suture is cut after a period of approximately 2 weeks to permit tract formation. We cannot describe the variety of fasteners but make sure you absolutely understand the one on your kit, as inadequate fixation can result in significant complications.

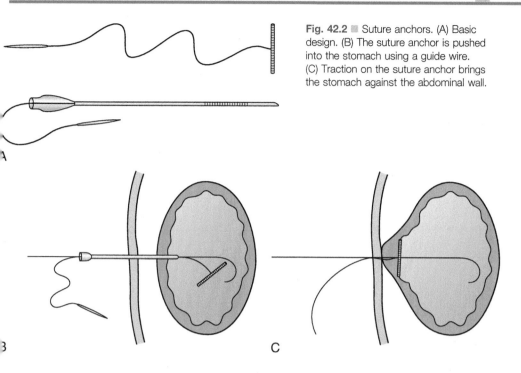

Fig. 42.2 ▨ Suture anchors. (A) Basic design. (B) The suture anchor is pushed into the stomach using a guide wire. (C) Traction on the suture anchor brings the stomach against the abdominal wall.

Push technique

A nasogastric tube is inserted on the ward and any gastric content aspirated. Position the patient supine and before draping; ultrasound the epigastrium to mark L. lobe of liver. The stomach is insufflated with air to bring it into apposition with the anterior abdominal wall; this can be easily confirmed on fluoroscopy. The target is a puncture at the mid/distal body of the stomach, equidistant from the lesser and greater curves to minimize the risk of arterial injury. Avoid puncture through the transverse colon and left lobe of the liver, which are adjacent innocent bystanders (Fig. 42.3).

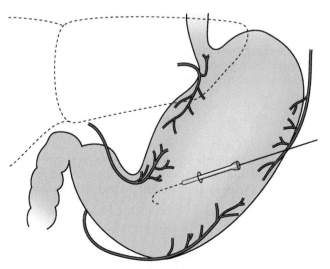

Fig. 42.3 ▨ Puncture site or percutaneous gastrostomy with puncture directed towards the pylorus.

Infiltrate local anaesthesia, go all the way in with the green needle and make a 10-mm scalpel incision. Insert T-fasteners (as above), once the stomach is fixed, puncture vertically down; avoid punctures directed towards the fundus as these will be tricky to convert later to gastrojejunostomy. The final puncture through the gastric wall requires a short stabbing motion. It is usually possible to see the gastric wall tenting away from the needle when it is necessary to make that final thrust (Fig. 42.4). Confirm entry into the stomach by injecting contrast through the needle, then insert the J-guidewire.

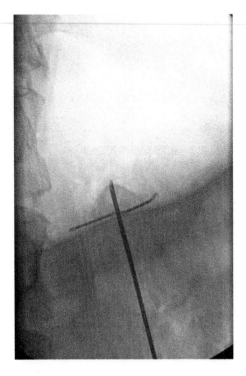

Fig. 42.4 ▦ Characteristic 'tenting' of the stomach wall. Note two suture anchors have been previously deployed.

The next step is tract dilation. You may have a distant memory of anatomy tutorials and the three muscular layers of the stomach. Practically, this means you need to push hard with the serial dilators. Usually, systems then use a peel-away sheath that allows the self-retaining catheter to be advanced into the stomach. There is a variety of different retention methods, including the usual pigtail loop catheters and balloons that tamponade against the gastric wall – remember to pull the balloon up against the anterior wall of the stomach, as this helps reduce air leak. Inject contrast to confirm a satisfactory position, then secure the catheter to the skin.

 Tip: Always keep the guidewire in until the position is confirmed with contrast. If you have somehow not got the catheter all the way in, you have a rescue option through the same gastric puncture.

Percutaneous gastrojejunostomy: If percutaneous gastrojejunostomy is required, the initial steps are identical but a Cobra catheter is used to negotiate around the duodenum; the gastrojejunostomy catheter may then be placed with its distal tip just beyond the ligament of Treitz.

Pull technique

The initial technique for percutaneous access to the stomach is similar, but suture anchors are not required with this technique. The gastrostomy tube for this technique is a completely different design and is pulled down through the oropharynx (Fig. 42.5). This technique can pull down oral flora to the gastrostomy site and therefore a single dose of cefuroxime 750 mg is advised.

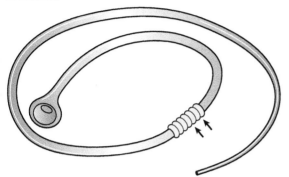

Fig. 42.5 ▥ Peroral gastrostomy tube. Arrows indicate the point of separation of the long dilator from the gastrostomy tube.

A 4F sheath is placed through the gastrostomy tract and the oesophagus is catheterized retrogradely with a Headhunter catheter and hydrophilic wire. This is more difficult than it sounds and can take 10–15 frustrating minutes. The catheter/wire is advanced up the oesophagus and brought out through the mouth. The guidewire is exchanged for a 260-cm stiff wire usually supplied in the kit. Working from the head end, the gastrostomy tube is then advanced over the catheter and wire until the distal end exits the anterior abdominal wall. The 4F sheath will be pushed out by the PIG; this is not a problem and the wire is also pulled out to avoid any risk of 'cheese-wiring'. The gastrostomy tube is now pulled down into the stomach until the external centimetre markings are seen. It is a good idea to prepare the patient at this stage for the sensation of the tube crossing the oropharynx; a reasonably quick passage through the oropharynx is a mercy for the patient. The gastrostomy tube can then be fixed in place with the supplied fixation disc (Fig. 42.6).

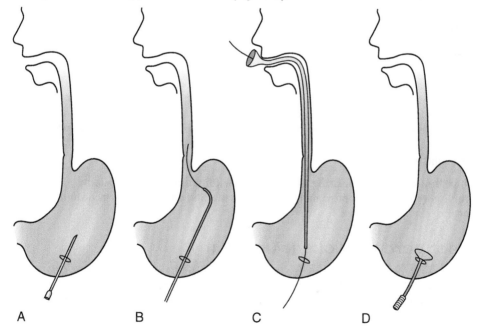

A   B   C   D

Fig. 42.6 ▥ Technique for PIG. (A) Percutaneous access to the stomach. (B) Retrograde catheterization of the oesophagus. (C) Push gastrostomy os advanced over the wire via the peroral route. (D) Gastrostomy tube is pulled down and the internal fixation collar is pulled against the gastric mucosa.

Tip: Remember to watch for the markings on the catheter when you pull through. Most operators are kind and try to pull past the hypopharynx quickly, just don't pull quickly all the way or you can pull the catheter through the abdominal wall.

Aftercare

The patient should fast for 6 h post-procedure, then if they are okay, start water for 6 h.

Troubleshooting

Unable to pass a nasogastric tube: It is often possible to negotiate oesophageal strictures using an angiographic catheter and hydrophilic wire using the techniques described in oesophageal stenting.

Difficult access: If it proves difficult to be certain that you have safe access avoiding other structures, the gastrostomy can often be safely performed under CT guidance.

Difficulty getting the catheter through the gastric wall: A stiff guidewire and a peel-away sheath can be helpful, particularly if trying to negotiate the duodenum for a gastrojejunostomy. Keeping the stomach air distended can also help.

Difficulty accessing the oesophagus retrogradely during a PIG procedure: Pass a wire antegradely down the oesophagus via the nasogastric catheter. It is then usually straightforward to snare the wire using the gastric access.

Access is lost after tract dilation: Unfortunately, it is not usually possible to retrieve this situation. The patient will get a gastric leak from the hole created by the dilation and may have a stormy few days. Inform the ward and give antibiotics and fast and supportive care.

Alarm: All the more reason to make a real effort to maintain access until satisfactory position is achieved with the final catheter. Re-puncture at a later date.

The gastrostomy tube falls out after insertion: If after <7 days, particularly if T-fasteners have not been used, there is unlikely to be a tract. Start again. If >7 days later, a tract is likely to be present, and for long-term gastrostomies this can be maintained by the attending clinical team passing a Foley catheter, until a formal gastrostomy catheter can be replaced.

Complications

Technical success rates are usually in excess of 95% for radiological gastrostomy. Complications occur in approximately 5% of patients and are principally peritonitis or puncture of adjacent viscera.

Direct percutaneous jejunostomy

This is a rare procedure usually reserved for cases in which the stomach is absent or inaccessible. While technically feasible, it is relatively difficult and not a procedure to undertake at the beginning of a career in GI intervention. A nasojejunal tube is helpful to distend the jejunum and the puncture can be made either under fluoroscopy/ultrasound (for the brave) or under CT guidance (for the rest of us). The target jejunal loop needs to be reasonably close to the anterior abdominal wall to allow fixation with a suture anchor. After an appropriate loop has been identified, the loop is distended with saline initially and punctured with the suture anchor needle. The anchor is deployed and a second puncture made to allow careful dilation and insertion of the jejunostomy catheter. Ensure the catheter is inserted a good distance into the jejunum and confirm with contrast injection. The suture loop is usually cut after 10 days.

The most significant risk is leakage/misplacement of the tube and therefore the introduction of feeding needs to be done with care. Some centres will externally drain the catheter for the first 24 h, and introduce saline initially for a test infusion for several hours. If there is any pain the infusion is discontinued and imaging undertaken to determine catheter position.

Alternative techniques for jejunal tube placement are surgical and laparoscopic placement. While these also carry risk they should be considered with the referring team prior to attempting radiological insertion.

Gastric outlet and duodenal stents

Gastric outlet obstruction secondary to either intrinsic or extrinsic tumour involvement can be readily treated by gastrointestinal stent placement; this is usually an endoscopic procedure. Radiological stenting is reserved for failed endoscopy and the technique is essentially the same as for oesophageal placement. Make sure the stomach has been emptied by a nasogastric tube prior to intervention, as an empty stomach is a shorter and easier route. Even with this help, it can be difficult to advance the stent round the greater curve of the stomach and the use of a 90-cm-long sheath can be invaluable. Typically, the stent extends round the duodenal loop and often a 90 × 22 mm diameter Wallstent is used, as it is sufficiently flexible. Remember, this stent will shorten significantly and pay attention to the markers. The Wallstent has three markers, the middle of a marker indicates the expected position of the distal end of a fully expanded stent. In a few patients, it is impossible to advance the stent from an oral route and the procedure can be performed by creating a gastrostomy to allow a much more direct route. It is usual to leave the gastrostomy in situ for a few weeks, rather than removing immediately, as a leak may occur.

Colorectal stent placement

Acute colonic obstruction is a common surgical emergency. Frequently, the patient is dehydrated, frail and has not had sufficient time for accurate staging of malignant disease. Emergency surgery and primary colonic anastomosis are associated with a high surgical morbidity and mortality, and colorectal stenting is an increasingly frequent treatment method for this group of patients.

Equipment

- Vertebral/Berenstein catheter
- Stiff hydrophilic guidewire
- Amplatz super-stiff wire
- Large-calibre sheath: 10–12F, 90 cm long
- Colonic stents: an ever-increasing variety of these devices are available. Most are simple to deploy and we can only suggest that you familiarize yourself with the devices available in your own department. Typically, colorectal stents are between 20 mm and 30 mm diameter and approximately 100 mm long.

Tip: It is easy to find yourself with too short a wire in this procedure, particularly if you 'borrow' an endoscopic stent. Always think about the length of the stent deployment system.

Technique

Rectosigmoid lesions can be negotiated with fluoroscopic guidance alone; however, lesions higher in the colon usually need the company of an endoscopist. The presence of bowel gas and faeces can make fluoroscopy challenging. Place the patient in the left lateral position and administer conscious sedation. Introduce a small amount of water-soluble contrast to outline the stricture. It is often best at this stage to angle the C-arm or turn the patient prone or prone-oblique to profile the stricture. Advance the catheter and guidewire combination and carefully negotiate the stricture. This is often harder than it would appear, as the capacious colon offers little in the way of support for the catheter.

 Tip: Consider using a long sheath to provide additional support.

Once across the stricture, carefully insert the stiff guidewire. If you are using endoscopic assistance make sure that you have a long enough guidewire, this will probably be one from the endoscopy repertoire. The initial challenge is for the endoscopist to hold the endoscope in position whilst you negotiate the stricture. An even greater challenge is keeping the wire in place while the endoscope is removed!

 Tip: Ask the endoscopist to use the shortest scope which will reach the lesion as this will simplify catheter and wire manipulation.

Advance the stent over the wire; this can be difficult if following a tortuous colon and, again, a large-calibre sheath may be invaluable. Centre the stent over the lesion and deploy (Fig. 42.7). Regardless of how tight the stent looks, do not post-dilate. This greatly increases the risks of perforation and misadventure. A successful stent is usually indicated by an escape of gas/faecal fluid, in most cases from the patient!

Finally, arrange for a plain film of the abdomen the next day to assess stent expansion, and check the stent position to make sure it has not migrated.

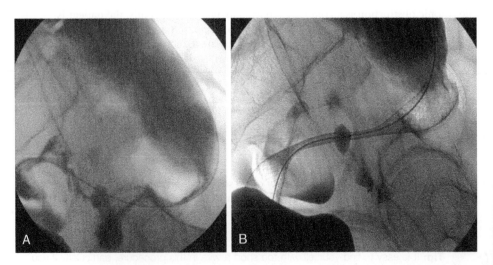

Fig. 42.7 ■ (A) Gastrografin enema showing rectosigmoid tumour. (B) Post-deployment the position is satisfactory, but note that the stent remains narrowed.

Outcomes

Most stents are inserted for malignant obstruction and the overall success rate should be around 90%. Stent placement in the transverse and R colon is more challenging and associated with a higher failure rate. Complications occur in 10% of patients and consist of perforation, migration and sepsis.

Troubleshooting

Cannot negotiate the stricture: Is the colon below the stricture empty? If the colon below the stricture is full of faecal material, then arrange for a bowel washout. Generally, endoscopic assistance helps identify the stricture and the use of a sheath to 'prevent the catheter flopping about' in the colon is helpful.

'Oops, I've perforated the bowel …': Catheter or guidewire perforation is usually without clinical consequence, and it is appropriate to persevere and complete the procedure. Perforation secondary to either balloon dilation or stent expansion is more serious and may lead to surgical intervention.

The stent has migrated: Management depends on the clinical situation. If the stent was placed for temporary relief of acute obstruction, then often there is no need to replace the stent. If a palliative case, the original stent can usually be readily retrieved and another stent placed over the stricture.

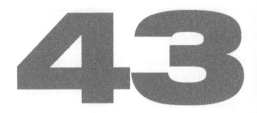

Treating biliary obstruction

Biliary intervention mainly involves biliary drainage and stent insertion. Magnetic resonance cholangiopancreatography (MRCP) and Computed tomography (CT) are the primary tools to investigate stones or other bile duct abnormalities and will usually determine the site and nature of biliary obstruction. Review of CT and MR cholangiography can be invaluable in planning the procedure, particularly for biliary drainage in patients with hilar lesions.

Percutaneous transhepatic cholangiography

Percutaneous transhepatic cholangiography (PTC) is now rarely used as a primary technique to evaluate the biliary tree. In most patients, the role of PTC has been downgraded to a component stage of biliary drainage (PTBD). Before embarking on PTC, remember that patients with jaundice often have deranged liver function and abnormal clotting. Check platelets and coagulation before starting (see Patient preparation, Ch. 1). Correct any underlying coagulation abnormality before proceeding; vitamin K is often all that is required but needs to be given at least a day in advance. In urgent cases, use fresh frozen plasma (FFP). Ensure that the patient is adequately hydrated and that antibiotic prophylaxis has been given prior to the procedure.

Equipment

- Chiba needle or Neff/AccuStick access set
- Connecting tube
- C-arm fluoroscopy and a good ultrasound machine with a suitable probe
- IV access
- Sedatives and analgesics.

Procedure

Planning your approach: Review any cross-sectional imaging before starting to assess the site of the causative lesion, the distribution of duct dilation and to check for ascites. It almost always pays for you to have a quick look with the ultrasound before starting. Look for dilated ducts and consider whether the ducts are uniformly dilated or there appears to be a segmental pattern of obstruction. Hilar lesions should have both lobes drained unless one of the lobes is very atrophic. Ultrasound guidance is always recommended, it is essential for left lobe punctures but is equally valuable to direct right-sided punctures. The patient should be prepared according to the planned approach to the right/left lobe or both. Before starting:

- Take a control film of the right upper quadrant to look for calcification.
- Make sure appropriate intravenous antibiotics have been given to cover Gram-positive and Gram-negative bacteria.

Right-sided punctures

Blind right-sided punctures: This was the preferred technique when PTC was for diagnosis, drainage almost invariably required a second puncture of an opacified duct. A 'blind' puncture is traditionally made from the right flank below the 10th rib. The point of puncture is in the mid-axillary line. Place sponge forceps at the proposed site of puncture, then fluoroscope to ensure it is over the liver and below the pleural reflection.

Tip: Unguided puncture works for uniformly dilated ducts, otherwise use ultrasound to direct operations.

Infiltrate with local anaesthetic down as far as the peritoneum but try to avoid puncturing the liver capsule. The intercostal vessels run along the inferior border of the ribs and therefore it is best to puncture just above a rib. Make the initial pass with the needle, aiming just cranial to the hilum of the liver. Angulate it about 20 degrees cranially and 20 degrees ventrally (Fig. 43.1).

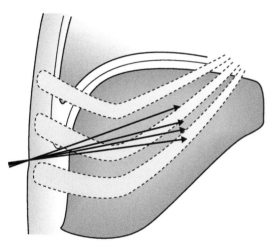

Fig. 43.1 ▪ Pattern of Chiba needle punctures at PTC. Note the pleural reflection extends below the aerated lung.

The needle is advanced into the liver, the central stylet is removed and the connecting tube attached to the needle. Sometimes, bile will drip or can be aspirated from the needle but bile is viscous stuff and you shouldn't bet your life on this happening. Under fluoroscopy, gently inject full-strength contrast as the needle is withdrawn slowly.

Tip: You know you are injecting at the correct rate when the needle tract outlines as a thin line of contrast. Big splurges in the liver parenchyma indicate over-injection.

Clearly, there are lots of tubular structures in the liver other than the bile ducts. When bile ducts fill, contrast tends to flow slowly towards the hilum; in obstructed ducts, the contrast often swirls as it dilutes. Vascular branches are tubular structures that clear the contrast quickly; portal vein and hepatic artery branches flow towards the periphery of the liver, whereas hepatic vein branches flow cranially towards the right atrium. Remember that the biliary radicles course together with portal vein and hepatic arterial branches in the portal triads, so that if you hit one, you are close to the others.

When you hit a bile duct, slowly inject contrast under continuous fluoroscopy. The dependent ducts tend to fill first, so the right posterior duct outlines before the remaining right ducts or the left. The bile ducts have a complex three-dimensional anatomy and anteroposterior and both oblique views are required to analyse them. Take spot radiographs of any abnormal areas. If you are really here only to achieve drainage, then distend only enough to either confirm you are in a suitable duct or where a suitable duct is for your second puncture. Do not over-distend the bile ducts, as this is a sure-fire recipe for cholangitis.

If this is the exceptional case, and you were only in the biliary system for diagnostic purposes, then it is the end of the procedure; pull the needle out and put a plaster over the puncture site. You can press on it if you like but it will not stop the liver from bleeding.

Left-sided punctures

The same principles apply; left-sided punctures are made from a substernal approach with ultrasound guidance (Fig. 43.2). Usually, the target is the segment 3 duct as it is anterior and inferior; try to puncture it as peripherally as possible. This will give you a bit more space, particularly for wire manipulation around the bend of the left main duct towards the hilum.

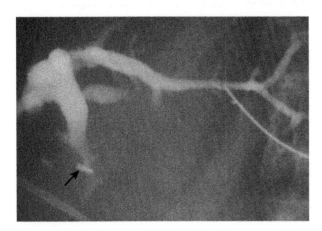

Fig. 43.2 PTC from a left-sided approach showing a surgical clip (arrow) occluding the common bile duct following laparoscopic cholecystectomy.

Interpretation

- **Filling defects** are caused by gallstones, tumour or blood. Gallstones appear as discrete, smooth intraluminal filling defects, sometimes visible on the plain film. Tumour may form mural nodules or strictures. The blood clot appears as extensive serpiginous intraluminal filling defect. Its appearance resembles tramlining, seen in deep vein thrombosis (DVT) (Fig. 43.3).
- **Strictures** are caused by tumour or sclerosing cholangitis. The distribution of strictures should be noted and recorded.
- **Beading** due to sclerosing cholangitis.
- **Dilated ducts** due to downstream blockage.
- **Displaced ducts** due to adjacent mass.
- **Distension of the gallbladder** usually the result of downstream obstruction; this is typically caused by pancreatic carcinoma.

Troubleshooting

Ascites: This increases the risk of bleeding from the liver capsule and makes advancing stiff drainage catheters more difficult as the liver moves away from catheter. If there is extensive ascites, it should be drained before PTC. In the presence of a small amount of fluid, you can proceed if the liver abuts the peritoneum at the proposed puncture site. Many operators would choose to perform an ultrasound-guided left lobe puncture in the presence of small-volume ascites. Make sure that you only make a single puncture of the liver capsule.

You do not hit a bile duct at the first attempt: Do not be surprised, as this is often the case. Angle the needle 5 degrees caudal and dorsal to the initial pass and try again. Do not pull the needle right out of the liver. Stop before you cross the capsule, as fewer punctures = less risk of bleeding. If the patient is not distressed, make up to five attempts and ask the radiographer to alert your boss that you may require assistance.

Contrast extravasate from the bile duct: Unfortunately, you have lost position or were in a small peripheral branch. This nearly always requires re-directing your puncture. If there is residual contrast in the biliary system, you can aim for this.

The left ducts do not fill: The right-sided ducts are dependent and fill preferentially; sometimes the left ducts will only fill if the patient is turned right side up. Be careful not to dislodge the needle as you move the patient.

Extensive intraluminal filling defects are seen: This usually represents haemobilia and is an indication to stop if you are in only for diagnostic purposes. The patient should be closely monitored and resuscitated as necessary. The vast majority of cases of haemobilia will settle with conservative management; however, you should be prepared to perform a CT if bleeding continues (Fig. 43.3).

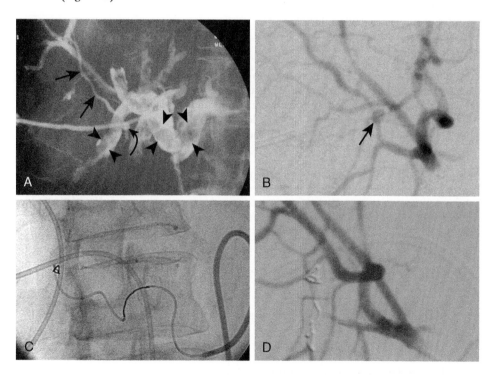

Fig. 43.3 ■ Haemorrhage following percutaneous transhepatic drainage. (A) Cholangiogram shows extensive blood clot (arrowheads) within the bile ducts. Note filling of a branch hepatic artery (arrows) and a false aneurysm (curved arrow) adjacent to the biliary drain. (B) Selective hepatic angiogram confirms the false aneurysm (arrow). (C) Coil embolization via a microcatheter. (D) Completion angiogram showing aneurysm exclusion. Adjacent hepatic artery branches are preserved.

The patient has a rigor on the table: The patient has cholangitis and may rapidly deteriorate. Sepsis is more common in patients with benign strictures than those with neoplastic disease. If the biliary system is obstructed, make sure to place a drain and leave this on free drainage. Contact the referring clinician immediately. Aggressive resuscitation is often required.

Percutaneous biliary drainage

Percutaneous biliary drainage is performed in patients with obstructive jaundice in whom endoscopic drainage is unsuccessful or who have complex hilar lesions. The commonest indications are malignant disease of the bile ducts or pancreas.

Equipment

As for cholangiography, plus:

- Coaxial percutaneous access kit
- Guidewires: curved stiff hydrophilic wire, Amplatz super-stiff wire (long floppy tip)
- Catheters: dilators (at least 4–9F), biliary manipulation catheter
- Drains: there are many alternatives – pigtail, internal external drain, e.g. Ring catheter, Cope loop
- Stents: most people use self-expanding metal stents if permanent drainage is required
- Peel-away sheath (usually 9F)
- Sutures or catheter-retention device.

Procedure

Before starting, review the previous imaging to decide the most promising approach. For distal obstruction, the right-sided approach is usually chosen, as it is technically simpler. For hilar lesions, draining both duct systems will give a more durable result. The left hepatic duct has a longer course before it divides and so a left-sided approach may offer more effective drainage for Klatskin type II and type III tumours (Table 43.1.)

Table 43.1 Number of stents required depending on tumour site

Klatskin type	Site	No. of stents to treat completely
Type I	Common hepatic duct	1
Type II	Confluence of left and right hepatic ducts	2
Type III	Confluence of hepatic ducts and first-order branches	3+

Tip: Sometimes one lobe of the liver has atrophied and it is then too late to salvage function in it; use the other lobe!

Biliary drainage: a step-by-step guide

1. Obtain IV access: give antibiotics, sedation and analgesia – biliary drainage is painful.
2. If performing a 'blind' puncture: use a coaxial set; this allows conversion to a 0.035-inch wire if you hit a suitable duct. Frequently, in an unguided puncture, the initial duct entered on the right is not appropriate for drainage of hilar lesions, usually

as it is too near the hilum. Use the first puncture to opacify the biliary system and fluoroscopically target a more suitable duct with a second Chiba needle.

3. If performing an ultrasound-guided puncture; use a coaxial set and choose a duct away from the hilum of the liver. Once in the duct, opacify with contrast to ensure a suitable position.

4. Puncture the duct: aim for a point where the duct is large enough to accommodate the catheters and drains that you plan to use, but remember that there are fewer complications the more peripherally you puncture. In fluoroscopically guided puncture, rotate the C-arm or the patient to demonstrate the position of the needle relative to the duct. When you are close to the duct, it will move as the needle is moved back and forwards. When you reach the duct, it will indent as the needle tip contacts it. There is usually 'a give' when the duct is entered.

 Tip: While targeting a duct, it is important to know whether the needle is anterior or posterior to the target. Swing the C-arm; if the duct moves in the same direction as the needle it's behind the duct, if the duct moves in the opposite direction it's anterior. Simple?

5. Confirm intraduct position: free backflow of bile indicates that you are in the duct. If this is not forthcoming, either inject a small amount of contrast or try to see if the guidewire will pass along the duct; make sure you put a decent length of the 0.018-inch wire into the duct (certainly all the opaque floppy section).

6. Exchange the 0.018-inch wire for the 0.035-inch J wire: using the coaxial set.

7. Dilate a tract into the duct: this is usually uncomfortable, so remember to give the patient adequate analgesia/sedation. Use 5F or 6F dilators, depending on the size of catheter you intend to use.

8. Introduce the catheter you hope to use to cross the stricture; most operators use either a Cobra or a biliary manipulation catheter.

9. Take a sample of bile: for microbiology ± cytology.

10. Cross the stricture: this is often harder than it sounds. We usually start with the curved hydrophilic wire. The process is similar to crossing a stricture or occlusion in a blood vessel (see Ch. 31).

11. Confirm intraluminal position: always ensure that you are either in the distal bile duct or through to the duodenum.

12. Exchange for the Amplatz super-stiff wire: aim to have the wire into the 3rd part of the duodenum.

13. Position the drain catheter/stent: internal/external drains must have sideholes on each side of the obstruction but not into the liver parenchyma. Stents must completely cover the lesion.

14. Confirm free drainage: make sure you do this before you attach the catheter!

15. Fix the drain catheter to the skin: there are many options for this; none is foolproof, so either use a suture or a proprietary skin fixation device.

Which drainage catheter

The choice depends on the anatomy.

Straight drain: Only used as a last resort as a temporary measure when it is not possible to negotiate through a stricture into a large enough duct to form a pigtail. Straight catheters are easy to remove, often unintentionally. They should not be trusted and should be exchanged for a 'proper drain' as soon as possible.

Pigtail drain: Use these when you cannot cross the obstruction but can access a sufficiently central duct. Even pigtail catheters can be inadvertently dislodged, so a self-retaining device, e.g. a locking pigtail loop, is preferable. Pigtail catheters are usually used with a sense of shame as a temporary measure until a definitive drainage procedure is performed.

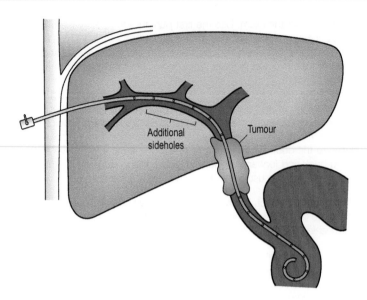

Fig. 43.4 ■ Internal/external biliary drainage catheter. Note that additional sideholes are often required to drain the proximal biliary tree.

Internal/external drain: These drains are more secure than straight catheters or pigtails. They have multiple sideholes over a long length of the catheter (Fig. 43.4). When they are placed across the stricture, bile can be drained externally to a bag, or internally to the duodenum. Additional sideholes may be punched along the proximal catheter to permit drainage from the intrahepatic biliary tree. Take care that no sideholes extend proximal to the liver parenchyma as bile may then drain into the peritoneal cavity, particularly in patients with ascites. The position of the most proximal sidehole can be determined by this simple test: before inserting the drain, put a green needle into the most proximal sidehole, then advance a guidewire into the drain. The guidewire will stop at the needle. Bend the guidewire at the hub of the drain. Insert the drain into the patient. Final positioning can be determined by using the previously bent wire to indicate the most proximal sidehole. Note the position and then advance or pull back the drain as necessary.

Rarely, internal/external drains may be used for long-term drainage. In this case, they should be allowed to drain externally for about a week before converting to internal drainage. The advantages of internal/external drainage are:

- Bile salts are not lost.
- It allows the patient to be ambulant without a bag.
- Skin excoriation is less common.
- The drain can be readily replaced over the wire if required.

Troubleshooting

Guidewire or catheter reluctant to advance: Bile is an effective lubricant and passage of guide wires and catheters is usually easy. If you experience difficulty, this usually indicates a problem, e.g. you are not in the duct any more. Stop and confirm intraluminal position by aspiration ± contrast injection.

Initial cholangiogram fades: Either inject more contrast through the initial puncture needle or through the catheter if you used the PTC tract to access the biliary tree.

Unable to cross the lesion with the guidewire: Do not be despondent; it is often very difficult to cross an occlusion in a very dilated system. Put in a pigtail drain (preferably self-retaining) and leave the catheter on free drainage for 2–3 days. When you try again, the system will be less capacious and less oedematous; frequently, it is now much simpler.

Unable to cross the lesion with the catheter: Try a 4F hydrophilic catheter or a tapered van Andel catheter. If this is not successful, try to pre-dilate the lesion with a low-profile angioplasty balloon. If the balloon will not cross the entire lesion, try to dilate it incrementally. It is sometimes necessary to sacrifice the guide wire position and re-cross the lesion with a 0.018-inch guidewire to allow use of a low-profile angioplasty balloon. These rarely fail to cross the lesion.

Unable to cross the lesion with the drain or stent: Consider balloon dilatation. If this fails, make sure that you have a stiff guidewire across the lesion and then insert a peel-away sheath. Cross the lesion with this if you can; if not, position it close to the obstruction and try again.

Biliary bleeding: Stop and put in a drain. Resuscitate the patient as necessary and monitor closely. Try again in 48 h.

Drainage stops: Review the patient yourself. Often, there is a benign cause, such as kinking of the drain tube. If this is not the cause, try flushing the drain with saline as this may salvage a blocked catheter. If none of the above is successful, bring the patient down and fluoroscope to assess the drain position. If this looks ok, perform a cholangiogram through the drain to determine the problem. If the drain has come completely out of the liver you will need to start again.

Biliary stenting

Plastic and metal stents are available. Metal stents have a longer patency but cannot be removed; they are generally avoided in benign disease or when the patient has a long life-expectancy. Stents can be placed endoscopically, percutaneously or as part of a combined procedure with initial radiological biliary drainage and subsequent endoscopic placement of the plastic drain.

Plastic stents

These stents are cheap but are more likely to occlude than metal stents. Endoscopic stent placement is the first choice in most centres, with the other techniques reserved for those patients in whom endoscopic access has failed. The combined procedure, as its name suggests, involves percutaneous and endoscopic techniques. The radiologist performs a percutaneous drainage and passes a catheter and long guidewire (4.5 m!) into the duodenum. The endoscope is now positioned alongside the catheter and the guidewire is snared. The wire is pulled out through the endoscope and then used to deliver the stent. The radiologist's job is to keep tension on the guidewire and to abut the percutaneous catheter against the stent. The stent and catheter can then be pulled through the stenosis. Plastic stents can be placed percutaneously but require at least a 10F tract compared with the 6/7F tract required for a metal stent, and are therefore rarely used percutaneously now.

Metal stents

Many units now deploy metal stents for malignant biliary obstruction. This is associated with extra capital costs, but these are offset by:

- Better patency, reducing the cost of re-intervention as they will frequently stay patent for the remainder of the patient's lifetime
- Ability to treat the patient in a single session in radiology because of the smaller tract size (usually 6F or 7F)
- The patient is spared the inconvenience of an external tube
- Smaller tracts are required through the liver.

A variety of self-expanding metallic stent types are used in the biliary system. In practice, 10-mm diameter stents are used in a variety of lengths *circa* 90 mm. The Wallstent has been extensively used to palliate jaundice. It is flexible and comes in sufficiently long lengths to allow most lesions to be treated. The alternative is to use a Nitinol-type self-expanding stent. While there is perhaps less experience with this stent type in the biliary system, it does have the advantage of very predictable shortening and placement. More recently, partially and completely covered self-expanding stents have become available for common duct lesions. Covered stents, particularly fully covered, do seem to migrate more readily, however they may potentially offer longer patency at least in some trials.

Percutaneous gallbladder drainage

Indicated to drain an infected gallbladder in a critically ill patient, particularly in intensive care patients. The widespread use of CT in patients with sepsis means that a lot of gallbladders now get scanned and start to worry clinicians. Increasingly, the difficulty is determining whether the gallbladder really is the source of sepsis; even after CT there are often several possibilities. Try to guard against reflexly draining slightly thickened gallbladders in patients with elevated inflammatory markers. The technique also provides an alternative option for imaging the biliary tree in patients in whom endoscopic retrograde cholangiopancreatography (ERCP) and PTC have failed.

Equipment

- Coaxial set (Neff/AccuStick)
- Short Amplatz super-stiff guidewire
- Dilators to 1F larger than the drain
- 8F locking pigtail drain.

Procedure

There are two potential approaches: transperitoneal or transhepatic. For transabdominal drainage, the acutely inflamed gallbladder will be thick-walled and adherent to the anterior peritoneum and can be drained from an anterior transperitoneal approach. Gallbladders that are not in contact with the anterior abdominal wall are better punctured transhepatically. In this way, any bile leakage will not cause peritoneal irritation. An additional advantage of transhepatic puncture is that the gallbladder shrinks towards the drainage catheter, whereas with transabdominal puncture, the catheter may be displaced when the gallbladder decompresses.

Use ultrasound to guide gallbladder puncture and take particular care to maintain access and insert a self-retaining catheter. Put plenty of drainage catheter into the gallbladder as the gallbladder will shrink rapidly on drainage and can retract away from the drain. Take a bile specimen and send it for culture – antibiotic sensitivity is helpful in sepsis. Vasovagal reactions are not infrequent and atropine should be readily available. Drainage is usually performed for at least 2 weeks to allow a mature tract to form. Cholangiography should be performed to confirm cystic duct patency before the tube is removed. If there is obstruction, infection will recur or a biliary fistula will form. Clamp the tube for 48 h prior to removal, to confirm satisfactory internal drainage.

Roux loop access

Many patients with benign biliary strictures will have choledochoenterostomy, usually to a proximal jejunal loop. Benign strictures tend to recur and therefore an access loop of bowel is sometimes apposed to the anterior abdominal wall. Roux loop access is preferable to percutaneous transhepatic access to the bile ducts when repeated intervention is required

Equipment

As for percutaneous drainage.

Procedure

Access: The Roux loop is punctured percutaneously. This sounds straightforward, but the bowel loop in question looks just like any other. Kind surgeons fix the Roux loop to the anterior abdominal wall and place radio-opaque marker clips to identify it, which greatly simplifies the procedure. However, it is more likely that there will be no markers, so either:

- Perform a limited abdominal CT to identify and mark the position of the loop that is anastomosed to the bile duct (see Ch. 26, p. 113) *or*
- Perform a percutaneous cholangiogram using a Chiba needle and then aim for the correct loop – usually much harder.

Catheterization: Puncture the bowel loop with a Neff set. Inject contrast to confirm intraluminal position, then introduce the guidewire. Dilate the tract and then place a heavy duty J-wire well into the lumen. You can now place a shaped catheter into the loop, a biliary manipulation catheter is often used, and use this to negotiate through the loop to the anastomosis. The anastomosis can be difficult to find, clips are often visible, and try to watch for the catheter engaging. The bowel loop is much wider than the target, which means that the catheter flicks out easily; gentleness, patience and care are required (some interventionalists find these attributes in short supply). Once identified, it is usually fairly easy to cross the stricture with the ubiquitous hydrophilic wire and perform dilatation.

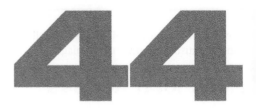

Treating cancer

Treating tumours

Understanding ablative techniques

The objectives of tumour ablation are to increase patient survival and sometimes to palliate local symptoms and painful tumours. There are several techniques which cause either tissue heating (radiofrequency [RF], microwave, laser, focused ultrasound) or freezing (cryotherapy). Advantages over surgical tumour resection are due to the minimally invasive nature of these therapies, which allows a wider spectrum of patients to be treated and reduces morbidity and mortality. Some treatments are performed on an outpatient/day-case basis, with potential to decrease costs.

Imaging guidance for ablation

Fluoroscopy, ultrasound, computed tomography (CT) and magnetic resonance imaging (MRI) are the modalities used, with ultrasound and CT being the most useful and practical.
    Imaging has five distinct purposes:

- **Planning:** ultrasound, CT, MRI and more recently, positron emission tomography (PET) are used for planning/assessing suitability.
- **Targeting:** ideal qualities of a targeting technique include clear delineation of the tumour(s), treatment electrodes and the surrounding anatomy, coupled with real-time imaging and multiplanar and interactive capabilities (Fig. 44.1).
- **Monitoring:** important aspects of monitoring include how well the tumour and/or target is being covered by the ablation zone and whether any adjacent normal structures are being affected at the same time.
- **Controlling:** MRI is currently the only modality with real-time temperature monitoring. When using cryotherapy, CT clearly delineates formation of the iceball.
- **Assessing treatment response:** post-procedural imaging.

Size of lesion: Increase in size is normal during the first 1–4 weeks due to reactive changes after ablation. At 3 months, the lesion should be equal to or smaller than the pre-procedural size. Considerable involution is expected by 6 months and thereafter.

Contrast enhancement: A lack of enhancement suggests adequate tumour ablation.
    Another important follow-up tool is tumour markers – elevation in organ-specific tumour markers points to recurrence or new lesions.

 Tip: If using ultrasound guidance, start with the deeper portions of the tumour to prevent microbubbles produced during ablation of the superficial parts blocking your view!

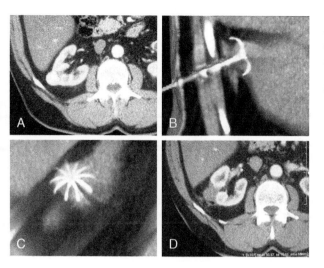

Fig. 44.1 ▦ (A) Exophytic renal tumour. (B) Tined electrode opened within tumour. (C) Confirmation of electrode coverage in different planes. (D) Post-procedure image showing satisfactory ablation.

When using CT, utilize the multiplanar images and reconstructions for better evaluation of probe and electrode tips – this is especially important when using expandable multi-tined probes.

Radiofrequency ablation

RF ablation (RFA) is the most widely used minimally invasive image-guided tumour ablation technique and is used for treating a wide variety of focal primary or secondary tumours in many organs, particularly the liver, lung, bone and kidneys.

General principles of RFA

- Tumour size should be <4 cm if a complete cure is the aim, regardless of the site of origin.
- Curative tumour ablation treatment must include an 0.5–1-cm margin of healthy tissue around the target lesion in order to treat any microscopic satellite foci and avoid early local recurrence.
- Multiple overlapping spheres (Fig. 44.2) or cylinders of necrosis may be needed to achieve adequate ablation of tumour, and systems that are based on coaxial guidance can be advantageous for larger lesions.

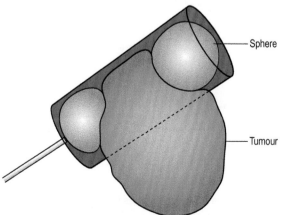

Fig. 44.2 ▦ Multiple spheres may be needed for complete tumour ablation.

Sphere

Tumour

- For tumours >5 cm, the main role of RFA is to debulk the lesion prior to chemotherapy or for pain relief.

There is a variety of different systems available for RFA, but the core principles and science behind RFA remain the same. In essence, RFA applicators are introduced percutaneously into the target tumour using CT or ultrasound guidance. The applicators have straight or expandable electrodes (Figs. 44.1 b and c, 44.3). A high-frequency alternating current (460–500 kHz) is delivered through the lesion, which causes agitation of ionic molecules producing localized frictional heating within the tissue. The electrical current exits the body through grounding pads attached to the thighs (Fig. 44.4). Local tissue temperatures between 60°C and 100°C produce protein denaturation, immediate cell death and coagulative necrosis of the tumour.

 Tip: The endpoint of ablation is assessed either by a change in electrical impedance or by measurement of the temperature at the electrode tip. Check that you are familiar with the parameters of the equipment you are using.

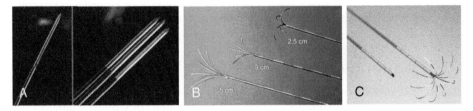

Fig. 44.3 ▧ (A–C) Common electrode types.

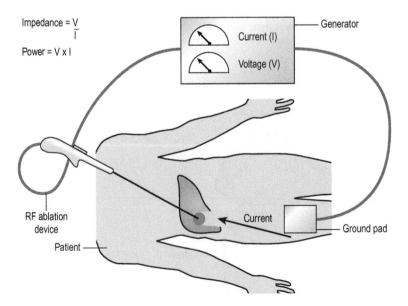

Fig. 44.4 ▧ Patient with generator and grounding pads. The RFA probe acts as the cathode of an electrical circuit that is closed by the application of dispersing pads on the patient's thighs.

Contemporary systems vary in power, size of needles, electrical parameters, and, most importantly, the electrode technique to maximize treatment volumes. Temperature and impedance changes during RFA reflect tissue cooking or overcooking. Although temperature and impedance are measured in several of the systems, each one uses one parameter to maximize treatment diameter. There are system-specific treatment algorithms which require varying degrees of operator input. Temperature information at the periphery of the thermal lesion (from thermocouples on the RFA probes or external thermocouples) may help to assess skip areas next to vessels from the heat sink.

Microwave ablation

Microwave ablation relies on agitation of water molecules around the probe to heat the surrounding tissue. The technique can be used percutaneously, laparoscopically or with open surgery. Optimal tumour size for treatment is <3 cm. Microwave typically produces higher intra-lesional temperatures than RFA and is less prone to heat sink effect.

There are several different device modifications available. Many needles need active cooling with saline to reduce the risk of heating non-target tissue proximal to the antenna tip. Several devices types allow placement of multiple antenna to permit treatment of a larger volume of tissue. Active monitoring of treatment is possible with placement of intra-tumoral thermocouples.

Cryotherapy

Cryotherapy uses related freeze/thaw cycles to cause cell death. The nature of the effect is complex and depends on the temperature reached, the speed of cooling, the rate of thawing and the number of freeze/thaw cycles. In simple terms, at temperatures from 0 to −20°C extracellular ice crystal formation causes cell death by osmotic dehydration (solution effect injury). At lower temperatures, e.g. −20° to −40°C, intracellular ice crystal formation leads directly to cell death. In addition, damage to capillary endothelium leads to coagulation and tissue hypoxia.

The cryoprobe is inserted into the tumour under image guidance and rapid expansion of argon induces cooling (Joule Kelvin effect) with subsequent helium flushing controlling the thaw cycle (Fig. 44.5). The technique can be used percutaneously, laparoscopically or at open surgery. The best results are achieved in tumours <4 cm, however in patients unsuitable for other treatment modalities using multiple probes, it is possible to treat much larger tumours

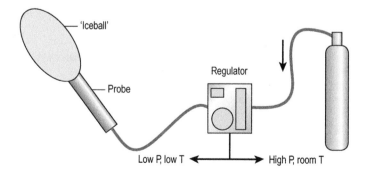

Fig. 44.5 ■ Argon gas stored at high pressure is supplied to the probe via a regulator. The sudden drop in pressure results in a temperature drop. This is transmitted to the tissues surrounding the uninsulated portion of the probe, resulting in an 'iceball' visible under US, MRI or CT imaging. P, pressure; T, temperature.

with cryotherapy. The main advantage of cryotherapy is that the iceball produced is readily visualized on CT, MR or ultrasound (US) scanning with immediate demonstration of target tumour destruction. Cryotherapy is not for the faint-hearted; multiple probes are required but it is very controllable as a technique. The control of the iceball makes cryo particularly suitable for central renal lesions. Typically cryotherapy treatment sessions take 1.5–2 h and usually it is kinder to have the patient under general anaesthesia.

Alarm: Patients with cirrhosis and liver tumours can develop 'cryoshock', which has a poor prognosis and, although technically tempting, the pendulum is swinging away from treating this group with cryotherapy.

There are limited numbers of cryotherapy systems available but all use the same technology. Multiple probes are required, typically 4–6 probes will be used to treat a lesion that is 5 cm. Argon and helium are relatively expensive and coordinating delivery of gases can be a hassle.

Irreversible electroporation

Irreversible electropolation (IRE) is a relatively new form of ablation that utilizes microsecond pulses of direct current to induce cell membrane damage and cell death by apoptosis. Unlike other ablation techniques based on thermal techniques, IRE offers a degree of tissue selectivity; structures formed predominately of protein are not affected by IRE and therefore collagen-based structures such as vessels and ductal systems can be preserved. The transition zone between ablated and non-ablated tissue is narrow, in theory, only a few cell layers, and complex treatment fields can be configured by placement of multiple electrodes. Finally, IRE is not sensitive to thermal sink effects and allows effective treatment closer to vascular structures. It may sound as though IRE is the perfect ablation technique but it does have its own complexities; strong muscle contractions mandate deep muscle relaxation, ECG synchronization of pulses is required to minimize the risk of cardiac arrhythmia and differences in local electrical conductivity can impair treatment volumes. Although experience is limited, this technique has particular promise in treatment of tumours that are challenging to thermal techniques due to vascular proximity such as pancreatic lesions.

Procedure

Ablation: key procedural steps

The key to complete and successful ablation is the precise placement of the electrode relative to the tumour.
- Review all pertinent cross-sectional images, including MPR.
- Note the size and number of tumours, and the anatomical relationship of the tumour to vital structures.
- Plan the point of entry, a safe trajectory, and the end position of the needle; understanding image guidance is essential. (See Chapter 26 for intervention for useful tips.)
- If using RFA, ensure ground pads are secure and be familiar with the electrode/ generator and regimen for heating.
- Ensure adequate analgesia and sedation for during and after the procedure; some treatments will require general anaesthesia.
- Inject local anaesthetic from the skin to the surface of the target organ (except for lung lesions).
- Advance the electrode towards the tumour along anaesthetized tract and deploy.
- At the end of the procedure, perform scan to check for any immediate complications.

Adjunctive techniques

These are used to increase the safety and applicability of RFA and other ablation techniques and have resulted in some ingenious solutions.

Minimizing collateral damage: Protecting adjacent viscera from thermal injury is an important consideration. Other organs and viscera can be displaced away from the intended ablation zone. Several techniques are described.

- **Fluid displacement (hydrodissection):** sterile isotonic solution (e.g. dextrose if RFA is being used) is used to separate the tumour and the organ deemed at risk by injection through a fine needle inserted between them.
- **Balloon displacement:** the use of fluid-filled balloons positioned between the kidney and adjacent viscera has also been described.
- **Gas displacement:** instillation of carbon dioxide or air to form an insulating thermal cushion is another successful technique.
- **Retrograde** or **percutaneous antegrade** infusion of chilled water during RFA of the kidney protects the adjacent collecting system from thermal injury during ablation of central tumours (Fig. 44.6).

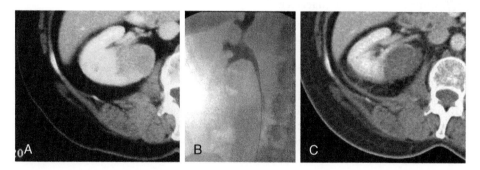

Fig. 44.6 ▦ (A) CT scan of central renal tumour. RFA of this was likely to cause ureteric heat injury. (B) Internal ureteric cooling with cold irrigation via catheter to reduce heat injury. (C) Post-ablation scan demonstrated no hydronephrosis and no ureteric stricture.

Improving access: An improved window can sometimes be created to improve the path to the tumour.

Intentional pneumothorax: An iatrogenic pneumothorax is created by instilling air into the pleural surface without producing injury to the lung surface. This can be performed for the treatment of upper-pole renal cell carcinoma with RFA or for central lung tumours.

Pitfalls and limitations

- **Tissue vaporization/charring:** temperatures above 100 °C vaporize water and carbonize the tissue adjacent to the electrode, both of which degrade the electrical conductance and result in suboptimal treatment effect. Vigilant intralesional temperature monitoring helps avoid this scenario.
- **Heat sink phenomenon:** if the target lesion abuts a blood vessel 3 mm or larger, the flowing blood carries heat away from the adjacent tumour, reducing effectiveness. Heat sink effect can be minimized by reducing blood flow using an occlusion balloon (Fig. 44.7), embolization or pharmacological modulation of blood flow.
- **Size of lesion:** see discussion above.

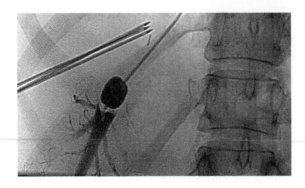

Fig. 44.7 ▦ Occlusion balloon within hepatic vein to reduce heat sink effect.

Complications

New techniques bring new complications and essentially the potential complications can be divided into three categories.

Complications of electrode placement

- **Bleeding:** depends on tumour location and character of the underlying parenchyma.
- **Infection:** strict sterility; risk factors are diabetes and biliary enteric communication (for liver RFA).
- **Tumour seeding:** commoner in superficially located, poorly differentiated hepatocellular carcinoma. Meticulous technique is required for initial placement of the electrode, with care taken to ensure optimal positioning on the first pass. Use coaxial needle, with the advancement of the inner electrode only through the tumour. 'Hot withdrawal' technique to coagulate tract site may reduce tumour seeding and also reduce bleeding rate.
- **Pneumothorax:** similar to lung biopsy; traversing fissures or long transpleural tracts increases the risk.

Complications of thermal therapy

- **Post-ablation syndrome:** this presents with constitutional symptoms such as fever (low-grade) and arthralgia. Seen more commonly when large tumour volume is treated. Supportive treatment with pain medication and rest is all that is required. Strict adherence to aseptic technique and eradication of pre-existing infection prior to the procedure help avoid post-ablation syndrome.

 Alarm: Persistent fever after 2–3 weeks should raise suspicion for infection.

- **Non-target damage:** bile duct strictures, cholecystitis and perforated bowel have all been recorded. Colon is at higher risk than small bowel (more mobile) or stomach (thicker wall and fewer adhesions).
- **Grounding pad burns:** The grounding pads heat up during RFA; if you are in any doubt if you feel the leading edge of the pad during treatment. Grounding pad burns are well recognized and largely avoidable by checking of the pads prior to use for blemishes and periprocedural checks to monitor any temperature increases.

Organ-specific complications

- These are covered in the sections on specific applications.

Implants

Electronic devices: Cardiac pacemakers may require temporary deactivation during RFA due to potential interference with pacemaker function. In patients with an automatic implantable cardioverter-defibrillator the ventricular arrhythmia sensor should be deactivated.

Small implants, such as cochlear implants, represent an unknown risk.

Metal implants

- Metal jewellery and cosmetic body piercing should be checked for and removed.
- Large implants (hips, knees) are safe.

Liver tumours

Primary hepatocellular tumours

Primary hepatic tumours are increasing in incidence. Transplantation offers the best chance of a cure. Patients unsuitable for surgery are considered for ablation, chemo or radio embolization or chemotherapy with sorafenib. The choice between these agents is dependent upon number of tumours, volume of disease, location of disease and background liver function. For patients with suitable disease, ablation offers the best chance of local control and in patients with tumours <5 cm in size delivers comparable results with hepatic resection but with better preservation of hepatic function.

Hepatic metastases

The optimum treatment remains hepatic resection for secondary liver tumours. Small-volume (<4 cm in diameter) colorectal metastases have been treated with ablation but, as there are likely to be micrometastases, recurrence rates are higher than for hepatocellular carcinoma. Chemoembolization has generally produced disappointing results for colorectal metastases however radioembolization has shown some promising results in patients who have previously had chemotherapy. At present, radioembolization remains a complex treatment and its use is restricted to specialist centres and a small patient cohort.

Bland embolization

Embolization with standard particulate agents is used to treat carcinoid tumours to provide symptomatic relief. In hepatoma, particulate agents and coils can be useful in the treatment of acute bleeding but anti-tumoral effects are better with trans-arterial chemoembolization (TACE) and radioembolization.

Transarterial chemoembolization

TACE is a treatment used for irresectable hepatoma. The treatment delivers high doses of chemotherapy directly to the tumour and combines this effect with hypoxia to induce tumour regression. Selection criteria will vary between units but generally TACE is considered for patients with a single tumour >5 cm (tumours below this are usually suitable for resection or ablation) or multifocal disease.

TACE is possible due to the dual blood supply to the liver from the hepatic artery and portal vein. Occlusion of a segmental hepatic artery produces tissue hypoxia but the residual portal vein supply prevents hepatic infarction. Hence, determination of portal vein patency is a key component of pre-intervention assessment. Patients with segmental portal vein occlusion can be treated but the risk of complications increases significantly. Inevitably, there is a loss of hepatic function with TACE and patients with severely impaired hepatic function (e.g. Child's C, bilirubin >50 mmol) are at a high risk of hepatic failure. Finally, there is risk of hepatic abscess post-treatment, which increases markedly if there is a biliary enteric fistula (25%).

Equipment

- Standard vascular catheters and microcatheters
- Embolic agent: usually, either
  - DC Bead: These are microspheres which are loaded with doxorubicin, beads come in a range of sizes to allow predictable tumour embolization. Dosage varies between centres and should be reduced in patients with impaired hepatic function

  or
  - Lipiodol + cisplatin or doxorubicin: emulsified mixture of iodized oil and chemotherapeutic agent. This is cheaper than DC Bead but not as stable a mixture.

Procedure

Plan the procedure from the CT/MRI; look for tumour/s location, arterial variants and segmental supply, portal vein patency, gallbladder (if present try to avoid the cystic artery) and the quality of the access vessels. Give appropriate antibiotic cover. The usual access point is the groin and selective catheterization of the feeding vessels performed and access to the segmental feeding vessel achieved usually with a microcatheter. The embolic agent is delivered via the microcatheter until the flow slows. In large tumours, it is possible to run out of embolic agent (particularly with DC Bead). It is usually better to come back another day rather than continuing with bland embolization, as the patient will have had a big enough hit for the day.

Aftercare

Patients are usually in hospital for 24–48 h post-TACE. It is not unusual for the patient to have postoperative right upper quadrant pain, nausea and vomiting, though these usually subside quickly and prophylactic analgesia and antiemetics should be given. Liver function tests and renal function are checked – transient disturbance is to be expected.

Complications

Post-embolization syndrome (5%); hepatic failure (2%); liver abscess (1%); cholecystitis (1%); death within 30 days (1%). Plus the usual complications of selective catheterization.

Follow-up

The vast majority of patients require a course of treatment. Usually, the response is determined by a CT scan 4 weeks after the intervention and further treatment targeted at residual disease.

Radioembolization

Radioembolization with Yttrium 90 (Y90) is a promising technique but requires more work during assessment and delivery and is more expensive than TACE. It is indicated for both primary and secondary liver tumours that are unsuitable for surgical resection or conventional intravenous chemotherapy.

There are variations in technique, depending on whether glass (higher dose per sphere/less embolic burden) or resin (lower dose per sphere) is used. Determining the exact arterial anatomy and the presence of shunting is essential for radioembolization for both sphere types. Pre-intervention angiography delineates the arterial vessels and delivers a dose of Tc-99 macroaggregated albumin into the hepatic artery at the anticipated site of treatment and subsequent radioisotope scan of the chest and abdomen used to determine the shunt fraction (the proportion which stays where it is intended in the liver) and identify non-target uptake. If resin spheres are being used, then selective embolization of non-target vessels is commonly required before radioembolization in order to prevent necrosis outside the liver, e.g. R gastric/cystic artery, etc. Strict protocols and precautions must be followed to avoid exposing the staff to excess radiation, and participation of nuclear medicine experts and physicists is mandatory. The angiography suite is prepared to minimize the risk of radioactive spill and a specialized delivery system is used to deliver the Y90. The Y90 is not opacified and the delivery is undertaken after test injections at the preferred delivery site.

Y90 radioembolization shares similar potential side-effects to TACE though post-embolization syndrome is usually less severe. In the short term after treatment, the patient needs to take precautions to avoid close contact with pregnant women and children due to radioactivity.

Portal vein embolization

Portal vein embolization (PVE) is used to induce hypertrophy of the future liver remnant prior to resection. It is usually necessary when the remaining liver volume is estimated to be <30%, though this will vary depending on the baseline liver status. Patients with established cirrhosis will tolerate hepatectomy less well and require a future liver remnant volume of around 40%. PVE is typically required to hypertrophy the left lobe of the liver when a right or extended right hepatectomy is being performed.

Equipment

- Coaxial puncture set, e.g. Neff/AccuStick
- 5F access sheath
- Catheters to access portal branches
- Liquid/particulate embolization material + coils (a large variety of agents have been used PVA, Gelfoam, glue to name but a few).

Procedure

Review available cross-sectional anatomy for venous anatomy, residual liver volume and tumour/s location. Transhepatic access is obtained via one of the liver segments to be embolized. Once the portal vein is punctured a 5F sheath is inserted. The adjacent peripheral portal vein branches are catheterized; this can be harder than you think from the ipsilateral approach, and embolization with liquid/particulate agents is undertaken.

 Tip: Consider forming a small reverse curve catheter in the main portal vein to help access segmental branches.

A variety of liquid and particulate agents has been used. Bear in mind that the peripheral portal venous branches need to be occluded distally and this takes a significant volume of embolic agents. The proximal segmental portal vein branches are then embolized with coils and tract embolization with coils or Gelfoam performed.

Aftercare

Complications include haemobilia, haemoperitoneum, portal vein thrombosis. Post-embolization syndrome is seen though not as frequently as one would expect.

Follow-up

Serial CT scanning is performed to assess hypertrophy of the residual liver segments.

Hepatic ablation

Liver ablation with RFA or microwave is a relatively common procedure due to the high incidence of primary and secondary hepatic malignancies that are unsuitable for surgical resection due to either tumour size, position, number of tumours or coexisting medical conditions. Ablation may frequently be used in combination with TACE or chemotherapy.

Central (near the hilum) lesions should be avoided because of the risk of central bile duct and vascular injury. Consider the use of coaxial access needles to allow for easy repositioning of probes in larger lesions, as image guidance may become obscured as treatment progresses; this is particularly common with ultrasound. Tract ablation is advisable in the liver to reduce tumour tract seeding and bleeding particularly in hepatocellular carcinoma.

Large tumours and those in difficult sites, such as near the dome of diaphragm or pericardium are best treated using CT guidance under general anaesthesia for respiratory control and accurate needle positioning. Caution should be used when treating patients with significant liver impairment, e.g. Child's grade C, as they are more likely to have coagulation disorders or liver failure post-treatment. Similarly, bleeding complications are more common with concurrent systemic chemotherapy. Liver abscess is common in patients with low-grade biliary sepsis or biliary enteric communication, which should be regarded as a relative contraindication.

Bleeding is an infrequent complication following either RFA or microwave ablation and bleeding adjacent to an ablated lesion usually stops by itself. Follow-up CT is essential in patients who have had intra-procedural bleeding or significant ongoing pain.

Renal tumours

The detection of small renal cell carcinomas has increased markedly as we continue on a quest to CT every part of every patient attending hospital. The natural history of these tumours is unknown and they are frequently detected in elderly patients with limited renal reserve and life expectancy. Renal ablation has been shown to offer a minimally invasive method of achieving local control with 3-year disease-free survival rates exceeding 90%. When intervention is warranted, the choice between nephrectomy/laparoscopic partial nephrectomy and ablation will depend on individual patient circumstances and unit expertise, but ablation plays an increasing role.

Renal embolization

The most frequent indication for embolization in renal cancer is in the control of post-biopsy bleeding. The increasing role of ablation has increased the frequency of renal tumour biopsy and, with that, the number of post-biopsy bleeds. In the majority of instances, these are readily treated with micro-coil embolization, which allows preservation of the maximum volume of renal parenchyma.

Renal cell carcinoma: Preoperative renal embolization to reduce intra-operative blood loss is infrequently performed, as there is limited evidence of effectiveness, certainly in terms of survival. Selected individual patients with locally advanced tumours may benefit but need detailed discussion. Advanced irresectable renal tumours, which present with persistent haematuria may be helped by embolization. As always, examining the CT is valuable to assess the arterial supply and distribution of disease. It is rare to confidently identify the culprit vessel in this group and far more common to treat the most likely area. Vessels are usually embolized using a combination of particulates (often polyvinyl alcohol [PVA]) and coils. Judgement is required to estimate the volume of tissue to embolize to stop/reduce bleeding versus infarct the renal volume – remember it is possible to go back for a second procedure, so a degree of caution can be employed.

Renal angiomyolipoma (AML): AML is a benign tumour with hamartomatous features, which can present as a sporadic isolated lesion or in association with tuberose sclerosis when bilateral tumours are most frequently present. Angiomyolipoma can present acutely with rupture, renal angle pain and retroperitoneal haematoma, though more commonly they are detected by cross-sectional imaging and are asymptomatic. Multiple lesions are associated with poor renal function. Asymptomatic lesions with a significant vascular component are treated when they are >4 cm; lesions <4 cm are followed up by US or CT. At angiography, AML display arterial hypertrophy, irregularity and intralesional aneurysms. Embolization can be performed with a variety of agents but probably the safest approach is subselective embolization with PVA. Coil embolization is often added in patients presenting with acute haemorrhage. Preserving renal function is important, particularly in bilateral disease, and care should be taken to perform as selective a treatment as possible.

Renal ablation

Indications for renal ablation have expanded over recent years and it is no longer the last port of call for patients unsuitable for other nephron-sparing treatments. Patients may frequently opt for percutaneous ablation as a first choice as long-term follow-up now suggests similar results to partial nephrectomy with less morbidity. Small (<4 cm) and exophytic tumours are best suited for treatment with ablation, however patients with larger or central tumours may be successfully treated particularly if unsuitable for conventional treatment. Similarly, patients with inherited renal cancer syndromes, such as Von Hippel-Lindau, may benefit from intermittent repeated ablation rather than surgery.

Treatment of central lesions will increase the risk of complications and tumour recurrence over peripheral exophytic lesions. A variety of scoring systems is available to quantify the risk, e.g. the renal nephrometry score. Thermal damage to the psoas muscle or nearby nerves may cause transient intercostal, groin or leg numbness or hip flexion weakness.

 Tip: Anterior lesions on the right kidney frequently will lie close to the duodenum and may be unsuitable for percutaneous approach. Work-up imaging in various patient positions (prone, oblique and lateral) may save time during the procedure.

Thoracic system

Until recently, interventional oncology in the thorax has been largely restricted to palliation of disease either by superior vena cava (SVC) stenting or bronchial stenting. Lung ablation is becoming increasingly established and can offer a curative intervention for patient groups that are unfit or otherwise unsuitable for surgical resection.

Bronchial stent

Tracheobronchial stenting is a useful and simple technique for the palliation of stridor secondary to airways compression and invasion by tumours within the upper mediastinum.

In specialist centres, tracheobronchial stenting has been used in the treatment of benign disease such as post-intubation tracheal stenosis. The technique is usually restricted to the trachea and main bronchi and best reserved for tumours that do not have bulky intraluminal disease. Occasionally, patients will receive treatment, such as laser, to reduce intraluminal disease with subsequent airway stent. Generally, self-expanding stents are used, and covered and uncovered stents are available. Some of the stents are designed to have retrieval loops for easier removal.

Preparation

These patients are usually breathless, with reduced oxygen saturations, and appropriate monitoring by skilled personnel is essential. With luck, the patient will have recently had a CT to assess the mediastinum and it is usually possible to measure the size of the affected airway from this examination. As a rough guide, 10–12-mm self-expanding stents are suitable for the main bronchi and 14 mm upwards for the trachea.

Technique

It is possible to perform this technique without the aid of a bronchoscopist, but why make life hard for yourself? The bronchoscopist will navigate the vocal cords and may even be able to get beyond the tumour. In addition, they will anaesthetize the airway more thoroughly than a radiologist can, and this may mean that you are not trying to deploy a stent during a coughing fit. The throat should be thoroughly anaesthetized with lidocaine spray and conscious sedation may be required. The bronchoscopist can usually identify the area of compression, and external radio-opaque markers can be used to mark the target area. Get the markers correct as opacifying the bronchi with contrast is not a great option. Pass a suitably long wire (260 cm) through the instrument channel of the scope. Take care manipulating the wire in the bronchi, as it is still possible to start a paroxysm of coughing. Carefully remove the bronchoscope. If you are already through the tumour and confident that you know the site of the stenosis, now is the time to load on the stent. Occasionally, it is necessary to inject contrast to outline the stenosis. It is nearly impossible to see non-ionic contrast, as it is coughed up so quickly; it is better to use 10 mL of the more viscous Lipiodol. Once you have markers applied to the target lesion, it is usually straightforward to deploy the stent over the target. The only potential difficulty is the cough. Be patient and wait for it to subside before deployment. The bronchoscopist can then go back down (carefully) and directly visualize the stent to admire your work – try to discourage them from going into the stent 'to have a look' – stent displacement is a real risk. Often it is obvious from the oxygen saturation monitor that you have done the patient some good.

Complications

Covered and non-covered stents are available and frequency of complications varies between designs. All complications are commoner with use in benign disease and this is an area for expert consideration. Overall complication rate is about 15% with stent ingrowth, migration and fragmentation all described.

Superior vena cava obstruction

Superior vena cava obstruction (SVCO) causes distressing symptoms, including facial and upper limb oedema, headache and drowsiness. The majority of cases are secondary to intrathoracic malignancy, particularly central bronchogenic carcinoma (Fig. 44.8). Patients with malignant SVCO usually have a poor life expectancy and the aim of therapy is palliation of symptoms. SVCO can also occur in patients with benign conditions, particularly following repeated central line placement, e.g. dialysis catheters. Unless SVCO is treated promptly, extensive venous thrombosis can develop and greatly increases the complexity of intervention.

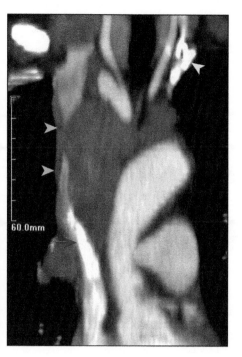

Fig. 44.8 ■ CT reformat showing SVCO (turquoise arrowheads) due to a large mediastinal mass. Note collateral veins in the left side of the neck (yellow arrowhead) and dense contrast in the lower SVC (red arrow) due to filling from the azygous vein.

Alarm: The greater use of CT means that patients are sometimes referred based on the CT scan rather than their symptoms. SVC stenting is invaluable in symptomatic patients but does not benefit the asymptomatic (though it does expose them to significant risk).

SVCO is one of the most gratifying conditions for the interventional radiologist to treat. Patients often feel marked improvement immediately the stent is deployed.

Assessing SVCO

The aim of investigation is to delineate the extent of the venous obstruction and thrombosis and to plan the subsequent intervention. This is now invariably chest contrast-enhanced CT (CECT) and coronal reformats will usually serve to delineate the cause and extent of the problem. It will also demonstrate complicating factors such as tumour invasion or thrombosis (Fig. 44.9).

Alarm: Stenting SVCO is a palliative treatment; there is a procedure-related mortality rate of approximately 2–4% related to pulmonary embolism and venous tears resulting in haemopericardium.

Treatment of SVCO

There are two very different clinical scenarios.

Uncomplicated stenosis or occlusion: This is quick and easy to treat. Benign strictures may respond to angioplasty alone but the majority of neoplastic lesions will be treated by primary stenting (Fig. 44.10).

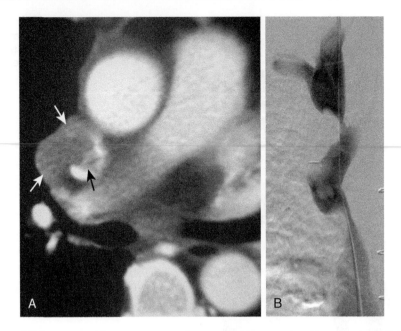

Fig. 44.9 ▓ SVCO. (A) Initial CT shows tumour adjacent to (white arrows) and invading the SVC (black arrow). (B) The venogram performed via a sheath in the right IJV confirms the findings.

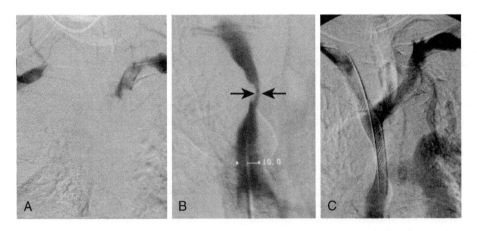

Fig. 44.10 ▓ SVCO. (A) Peripheral injection does not demonstrate the central veins. (B) Injection through a catheter in the innominate vein demonstrates a simple stenosis (arrows). Note measurement of the SVC diameter. (C) Following deployment of a single Wallstent, excellent bilateral drainage is restored.

SVCO complicated by thrombosis: The aim of treatment is to re-establish flow without causing pulmonary embolism. There are two distinct strategies: primary stenting or stenting following thrombolysis and thrombectomy. The former is quick but may require additional stents. The thrombus is often organized and difficult to clear, making thrombolysis and thrombectomy a more complicated and time-consuming option.

Equipment

- Basic angiography set
- Guidewires: curved hydrophilic wire, Amplatz super-stiff wire 180 and 260 cm

- Catheters: 4F straight, Cobra II, Berenstein, 80 cm, 8-, 10-, 12- and 15-mm angioplasty balloons
- Sheaths: start with a small sheath to cross the lesion and then escalate to the size needed for the balloon/stent
- Stents: 8–16+ mm diameter. The venous Wallstent is the most frequently used device.

Procedure

Access: Femoral and jugular access are the commonest routes.

The shortest, most stable route is via the right internal jugular vein, however neck access can be difficult in an oedematous, breathless patient.

Catheterization: Cross stenoses in a standard fashion using a shaped catheter and a hydrophilic wire. Exchange for an Amplatz wire before angioplasty/stenting. If necessary, cross the lesion from the arm and then exchange for a 260-cm guidewire, which can be snared and brought out of a femoral sheath (see Ch. 36).

Runs: Perform venography to delineate the obstruction and demonstrate the major collateral channels. Assess the extent and distribution of any thrombus.

Technique

As a general rule, use angioplasty for benign disease and stents for malignant disease. Organized thrombus can be stented over directly. When there is extensive fresh thrombus, an attempt can be made to debulk it by mechanical thrombectomy or thrombolysis using a low-dose infusion. Before starting thrombolysis, it is essential to exclude cerebral metastases and other potential bleeding sites such as the primary tumour. Thrombectomy will not clear all the venous thrombus but rather will create a central channel that will allow stenting. The majority of operators will use a bare self-expanding stent. Covered stents are sometimes used when faced with tumour invasion/ingrowth but caution is required, as there is an increased risk of migration and venous collaterals are occluded. Choose a stent which will completely cover the lesion and be firmly anchored in the stricture and adjacent vein; in practice, 12–16 mm. Most operators try to leave at least 60% of the stent above the lesion to reduce the risk of migration. Do not leave the end of the stent low in the right atrium, as it may cause emboli or even perforation. The stent can be dilated with a balloon to an appropriate diameter. Following deployment, perform a venogram to demonstrate patency.

 Alarm: In the presence of thrombosis, there is a risk of pulmonary embolus during stent placement, especially if the stent is placed from the femoral approach, as the stent opens from the jugular end towards the SVC and may 'toothpaste' the thrombus.

Complications

Major complications occur in approximately 4% of patients including SVC rupture, pericardial tamponade, pulmonary embolism, stent migration and cardiac failure/arrhythmias. The mortality rate for SVC stenting is between 2–4%. Minor complications include access haematoma, chest pain and re-stenosis.

Outcomes

Technical success rates are 95–100% with appropriate patient selection. The presence of SVC thrombus or tumour invasion increases the risk of re-thrombosis. Re-intervention is possible but not commonly required as this patient group often has a short life expectancy due to the overall burden of disease.

Troubleshooting

Poor flow or extensive collateral filling: Perform further angioplasty/stent deployment.

Both brachiocephalic veins are involved: When there is bilateral obstruction, it is usually only necessary to treat one side to relieve symptoms.

There is a large discrepancy in size between the venous segments to be stented: This is an indication to use a Wallstent, which will taper to fit the narrower vessel. This will significantly increase its final length; make sure that you allow for this.

The patient becomes hypoxic or hypotensive: *This is an emergency!* Call the cardiothoracic surgery and arrest teams as things can deteriorate rapidly. Resuscitate them promptly and consider the possibility of pulmonary embolism, SVC perforation and cardiac tamponade.
    Perform a venogram and include images of the central pulmonary arteries:

- If there is evidence of a leak, then a covered stent should be deployed.
- If there is a large central pulmonary embolism, consider macerating it with a catheter.
- If these are negative quickly perform a cardiac ultrasound looking for pericardial fluid. SVC perforation can lead to rapid cardiac tamponade and death.

Inferior vena cava obstruction

Inferior vena cava obstruction (IVCO) is considerably less common than SVCO but again mainly secondary to advanced tumour. Affected patients often have gross leg and lower body oedema. The basic principles are identical to SVCO, but particular care should be taken to avoid stenting over the renal or hepatic veins. The IVC has a large calibre and there is significant potential for stent migration, so choose a suitable stent diameter carefully (Figs 44.8–44.10).

Percutaneous lung tumour ablation

This is now one of several treatment modalities available to treat primary or secondary lung tumours and can be thought of as an alternative to stereotactic radiotherapy or metastasectomy. Cryotherapy is effective in treatment of rib pain from metastatic bone disease.
    Lung tumour ablation is best performed using CT under general anaesthesia. Suspended respiration or high-frequency oscillating ventilation is useful to limit lesion movement. Access should allow the shortest and safest route avoiding fissures or bullae. RFA, microwave and cryoablation are suitable for lung ablation, however the bulk of literature focuses on RFA and microwave. Imaging during/following procedure will show evidence of a halo of ground-glass shadowing surrounding the lesion suggesting adequacy of treatment. Follow-up with CECT and PETCT is suggested, although enhancement or activity of the lesion may persist initially despite adequate treatment.

Bone tumours

Painful osteolytic secondary bone tumours are common and are often treated with radiotherapy. Persistent pain after radiotherapy can be difficult to treat and extremely limiting for the patient. Cementoplasty and vertebroplasty can be invaluable in the treatment of this patient group.

Cementoplasty

Cementoplasty is the injection of bone cement into osteolytic lesions to achieve mechanical support in areas of weakened bone. Lesions that are predominately osteoblastic are unsuitable for treatment as they do not permit sufficient diffusion of cement. The most common indication is painful metastatic bone disease though benign pathologies such as sacral insufficiency fractures may be treated. Typical sites are within the pelvis and vertebrae, although long bone and peripheral lesions have also been treated. Initial imaging with MR ± CT is undertaken to delineate the extent of the disease and plan approach.

Equipment

- Specific bone biopsy needles
- Bone cement.

Procedure

In the treatment of metastatic disease, the procedure may sometimes be combined with thermal ablation to achieve initial destruction of tumour cells prior to stabilization. Ideally the procedure is performed under general anaesthesia though it is possible under deep sedation, this will require anaesthetic support. Simple lesions may be targeted under fluoroscopy but more complex lesions will require CT guidance. Specific bone needles are required to penetrate the cortex. Position is confirmed before slow injection of bone cement. A number of injection systems have been developed for use in vertebroplasty and these are usually also used for cementoplasty.

Complications

Cement leakage into either the venous plexus or adjacent soft tissue. This risk is higher when previous imaging has shown cortical breach by tumour. The risk is reduced by using an appropriate from of bone cement and injection system.

Outcomes

Approximately 80% of patients will experience a significant reduction in pain. The effect is usually within 1–3 days, which offers an advantage over other treatments such as radiotherapy.

Vertebroplasty

Vertebroplasty is the percutaneous injection of bone cement to stabilize vertebral fractures. Pain secondary to vertebral compression fractures (VCFs), which is refractory to medical therapy, is the primary indication. Other indications include the treatment of vertebral metastatic disease and myeloma and much less commonly painful vertebral haemangiomata.

Procedure

Patients should have an MR scan prior to intervention. Vertebra which have lost >75% of their height or have no marrow oedema are unsuitable for intervention. Vertebroplasty for VCF is usually offered if initial conservative management had failed for a period of 1–2 months providing there is persistent marrow oedema on the MR scan.

The procedure is performed under conscious sedation, a small number of patients require general anaesthesia (GA) either because they fail to tolerate an attempt under conscious sedation or because the intent is to treat multiple lesions. The commonest form of imaging guidance is bi-plane fluoroscopy via a transpedicular route. CT can be used and is particularly valuable for difficult cases. The bevelled needle is introduced along the pedicle aiming to puncture within the oval ring of the pedicle and aiming to stop with the tip in the anterior half of the vertebral body. The needle bevel is then rotated to the midline to allow dispersal of cement across the vertebral body. Specialized radiopaque bone cement is used via an appropriate injection system. Injection is made under continuous fluoroscopy looking carefully for evidence of cement leaks. If it is not possible to adequately fill the vertebral body, then a puncture of the contralateral pedicle may be necessary. After optimal filling of the vertebral body the needle stylet is replaced and the needle removed.

Complications

Complications are commoner in malignant disease. Cement leakage is the complication of most concern. Leakage into the spinal canal or exit foramina can cause radiculopathy or spinal cord compression and paraplegia. Cord compression requires urgent neurosurgical opinion for consideration of decompression. Cement can leak into the perivertebral venous plexus and therefore enter the venous system with risk of pulmonary embolism. Fortunately, in the majority of patents, such leaks are asymptomatic. Finally, leakage into the paravertebral soft tissue can occur, this is rarely of consequence. Other complications have been described including infection, pneumothorax and collapse of adjacent vertebral bodies.

Outcomes

Success rates are based on relief of pain and rates of 80–95% are quoted for vertebral compression fractures. Pain relief is a little lower in malignant disease but still a creditable 70–90%.

Embolization of bone tumours

Embolization is mostly used before internal fixation of vascular tumours, the aim is to reduce perioperative blood loss. Embolization is occasionally used as a means of pain control or as primary therapy in the treatment of some benign tumours. CT/MR provide valuable information about tumour extent and proximal arterial anatomy, but DSA remains invaluable for defining the true extent and nature of the arterial supply for bone tumours.

Malignant disease: Renal and thyroid bone metastases are the commonest indications.

Benign disease: Aneurysmal bone cysts and giant cell tumours are locally aggressive highly vascularized bone tumours. Management is usually surgical but this can be complex, particularly for large pelvic lesions. Embolization alone may induce ossification of aneurysmal bone cysts.

Equipment

- Basic angiography set
- Embolic material: typically PVA and Gelfoam
- Microcatheters.

Procedure

Lesions in the pelvis and proximal femora are often best approached from a contralateral approach; catheterization is easier and it keeps you out of the radiation. Initial angiography is invaluable in understanding the various sources of supply and making a plan for intervention. Microcatheters may be necessary for selective catheterization of the predominant feeding vessels. Look carefully for arteriovenous shunting before proceeding with embolization. A wide variety of agents can be used but the commonest and probably safest is PVA 300–500 μm (increase size if there is AV shunting present). In very vascular lesions, it may not be possible to occlude all the arterial supply to the lesion but it is almost always possible to make a substantial difference. The interval between embolization and surgery should ideally be <48 h. Longer periods mean that infarction and oedema can make surgery more difficult.

Complications

Complications are related to the site of the lesion and include all the usual risks with the addition of non-target embolization dependent upon the adjacent structures; in the pelvis this may include bladder, uterus and rectum.

Outcomes

There are no large trials but small case series experience supports the utility of embolization in both benign and malignant tumours.

45

Achieving angiographic diagnosis

Having a high-quality route map of the target vascular bed and, if necessary, the access to it are the keys to successful vascular intervention. They determine the choice of approach, the best equipment to use and the suitability for intervention. A preliminary diagnostic angiogram is seldom now required and non-invasive diagnostic imaging using ultrasound (US), magnetic resonance angiography (MRA) and computed tomography angiography (CTA) is the norm. Therapeutic decisions and approach are planned on this basis.

The skills necessary to perform high-quality angiography are still mandatory as digital subtraction angiography (DSA) is required in the following contexts:

- Intervention
- When small-vessel detail is required
- Where non-invasive imaging has failed or cannot be tolerated
- To arbitrate when non-invasive imaging is not conclusive and a definitive answer is needed.

Diagnostic digital subtraction angiography

Obtaining good-quality diagnostic angiograms is central to any successful endovascular intervention, remember to apply the basic principles of angiography (Ch. 29) and catheterization (Ch. 30).

This chapter details the indications, equipment, procedural details and views for all the common sites. If a pump injection is recommended, then we have assumed 300 mg/mL-strength iodine will be used. When hand injections are recommended, 300 mg/mL is too viscous for rapid injection and we would suggest dilution with saline to approximately 200 mg/mL.

Lower limb arterial diagnosis

Imaging the lower limb arteries is most frequently requested to investigate chronic ischaemia (intermittent claudication, rest pain and ulceration) or acute ischaemia (Fig. 45.1). Less common reasons are trauma, vascular malformation and tumour. The choice of imaging modality and the study should be tailored to obtain the information necessary for the clinical scenario (Table 45.1). A standard peripheral angiogram covers from the infrarenal abdominal aorta to the ankle (Table 45.2). Lateral foot views are mandatory if distal intervention for critical limb ischaemia is being considered.

Equipment

- Basic angiography set

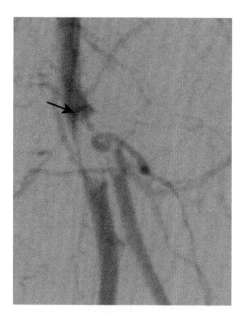

Fig. 45.1 Typical appearance of an embolus (black arrow) involving the bifurcation of the common femoral artery. The filling defect has a convex meniscus and is sited at a bifurcation. The underlying artery is normal and there are no collaterals.

Table 45.1 Lower limb arterial imaging depends on the clinical scenario

Scenario	Modality
Elective	
Intermittent claudication	MRA > CTA > Ultrasound[a] > DSA
Chronic critical limb ischaemia	MRA > CTA > DSA
Assessment of bypass graft	Ultrasound diagnosis then DSA for intervention
Popliteal aneurysm	Ultrasound for diagnosis and size, MRA for inflow/outflow
Popliteal entrapment	Ultrasound initial diagnosis, MR/MRA for delineation of type
Tumour/vascular malformation	Ultrasound for flow (high or low), MRI for extent, angiography for intervention
Acute	
Acute limb ischaemia	CTA/MRA, DSA depending on availability and expertise
Trauma	CECT for vascular and nonvascular injury, DSA for intervention

[a]Ultrasound can be used to perform a basic screen of the femoropopliteal segment but this does not answer issues regarding inflow and outflow, hence MRA is the preferred tool due to speed and increased coverage.

- Catheter: pigtail or straight, 3F 30-cm length, 4F 60-cm, 90-cm or 120-cm (femoral, brachial and radial approach, respectively). Always use the femoral route unless contraindicated.

Procedure

Access: Tailor to the planned intervention. Diagnostic angiography for peripheral vascular disease is traditionally performed from the symptomatic leg unless the femoral pulse is absent

Table 45.2 Typical parameters for a lower limb angiogram

View	Contrast volume (mL)	Injection rate (mL/s)	Frame rate (FPS)	Field size (cm)	Inject delay (s)	X-ray delay (s)
AP aorto-iliac	15	8	2	40	1.5	0
Oblique aorto-iliac	15	8	2	28	1.5	0
AP proximal thigh	10	5	2	40	0	0
AP distal thigh	10–15	5	1	40	0	Increase as necessary
AP calf vessels	10–20	5	1	40	0	Increase as necessary
Lateral foot	10–20	5	1	28	0	Increase as necessary

AP, anteroposterior; FPS, frames per second.

or very weak. This ensures optimal images of the affected side. Straight catheters can be pulled back into the external iliac artery for single-leg views. There is no risk to the asymptomatic limb.

Catheterization: Position the catheter below the renal arteries.

Runs: Tailor the examination to the individual patient.

Supplemental views: Additional views are frequently required pre- and post-intervention or in the presence of prosthetic joints; the answer is almost always an alternative projection, either an oblique view or a lateral. Adjunctive manoeuvres, such as flexion of the contralateral leg in a patient with a knee joint prosthesis, will help achieve an unimpeded lateral view (Fig. 45.2).

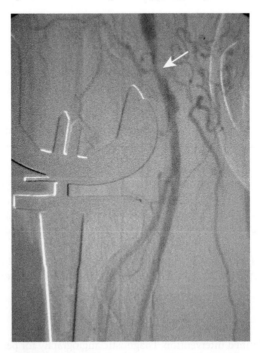

Fig. 45.2 High-grade stenosis behind a knee prosthesis (white arrow) seen on the lateral knee view. This was not seen on AP or shallower obliques.

Tip: Remember the diagnostic maxim: one view is one view too few. We are trying to visualize 3D structures. If in doubt, try another run at 90 degrees to the original.

Iliac obliques The iliac vessels are tortuous and oblique views are essential to allow full assessment before and after intervention and also to demonstrate the origins of the internal iliac arteries in profile.

Tip: Remember to use the contralateral oblique view, e.g. LAO for the right iliac system.

Profunda oblique To see the origins of the profunda femoris artery (PFA), superficial femoral artery (SFA) and femoropopliteal/distal grafts, i.e. right anterior oblique (RAO) 30–50 degrees for the right PFA.

Focal stenoses Any stenosis can be more accurately assessed if an additional oblique view is taken. Experiment with 30 degree obliques in either direction to try to profile the lesion.

Lateral foot views Both feet – the 'Charlie Chaplin' – place both heels together, turn toes out, 40-cm field.

Single foot – externally rotate the foot and rotate C-arm the opposite way to obtain lateral projection, 28-cm field.

Troubleshooting

Poor views of the distal run-off, this is usually the result of slow flow, contrast dilution and movement:

- Increase the volume and strength of contrast delivered
- Collimate to a single limb
- In the ipsilateral limb, pull back a straight, multi-sidehole catheter into the external iliac artery (EIA) to direct all of the contrast to the area of interest
- In the contralateral limb, use a shaped catheter (e.g. Cobra II or RDC) to catheterize the contralateral EIA
- Use a vasodilator such as tolazoline or glyceryl trinitrate (GTN) to increase flow.

Tip: Use iso-osmolar contrast in patients with critical ischaemia. This reduces the pain/heat associated with contrast injection. Everyone is happy, the patient stays still, you save time and improve your images!

Arterial bypass graft imaging

Imaging aims to demonstrate mechanical problems:

- Anastomotic stenoses caused by neointimal hyperplasia. Usually within the first year
- Intragraft stenosis, particularly at valve cusps and in composite vein grafts
- Progression of disease in the arterial inflow or outflow. Usually after the first year
- Graft kinking during knee flexion. This should always be excluded following thrombolysis if no other abnormality is found (Fig. 45.3). The graft usually kinks a few centimetres above the knee joint; this is best appreciated in the lateral projection.

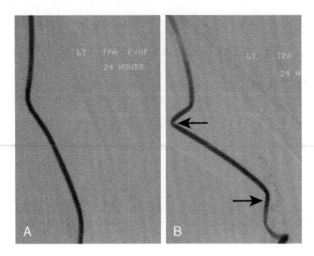

Fig. 45.3 ■ Following thrombolysis, lateral views with the knee straight (A) and flexed (B) reveal kinking (arrows) as the underlying problem.

Arterial bypass graft DSA

Graft angiography can be difficult due to scarring over the femoral arteries and limited access. Success is much more likely if you spend time ascertaining the graft anatomy, material and the results of the Duplex ultrasound before you start. Give prophylactic antibiotics when puncturing synthetic grafts, e.g. cefuroxime 750 mg IV.

Equipment

• Basic angiography set.

Procedure

Access: Use ultrasound guidance to target puncture, use Table 45.3 as a guideline for choosing the point of access.

Table 45.3 Access sites for graft angiography

Graft configuration	Angiography approach	Intervention approach	Tips
Axillofemoral	Radial or brachial	Brachial for proximal lesions graft or CFA for distal problems	
Aortofemoral	CFA or brachial	CFA or brachial	
Iliofemoral crossover	Donor side CFA	Either CFA	Steep angulation at origin, establish access with Amplatz wire, then introduce long sheath or guide-catheter for support
Femoro-femoral crossover	Donor CFA	Either CFA or graft	
Femoro-popliteal/distal	Antegrade CFA	Antegrade CFA for distal problem, retrograde for inflow	Cobra or RDC useful to access graft origin

Catheterization: The majority of at-risk grafts will be infra-inguinal, and antegrade puncture is usually required. Most grafts come off the common femoral artery (CFA) anteriorly and steep ipsilateral anterior oblique views are useful to profile their origins and to guide selective catheterization (Fig. 45.4).

Runs: A satisfactory angiogram must show the graft inflow and run-off and include views of the proximal and distal anastomoses in profile (Figs. 45.4 and 45.5). Magnified oblique views should be used to demonstrate stenoses. When imaging vein grafts, demonstration of contrast jetting as a result of valve cusps requires runs at 6 frames per second (FPS). These should be viewed with a wide contrast window (Fig. 45.6).

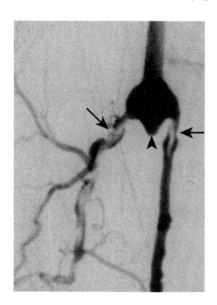

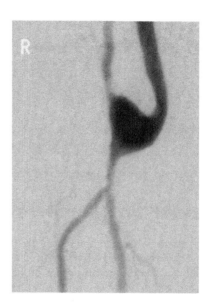

Fig. 45.4 ▪ Oblique view showing non-occlusive thrombus in the profunda femoris artery (black arrows) and origin of the femoropopliteal vein graft. The stump of the native SFA (arrowhead) lies in between.

Fig. 45.5 ▪ Profile view of the distal cuff of a below-knee femoropopliteal vein graft. The popliteal artery is diffusely narrowed below the graft.

Tip: The Doppler is right! If the lesion cannot be identified at angiography, wheel in an ultrasound machine and re-scan to mark the lesion.

Troubleshooting

Difficulty inserting the sheath: Review the basic principles of vascular access.

Difficulty catheterizing the graft origin Once you have chosen the optimal projection, use roadmap or fluoroscopy fade for guidance. A shaped catheter, usually a Berenstein, Cobra or RDC, can be directed towards the graft origin.

Difficulty visualizing the graft origin Contrast in the CFA patch, the stump of the SFA or in the PFA may obscure the graft origin. Position the catheter with its tip in the proximal graft; contrast can then be refluxed to show the graft origin. A frame rate of ≥2 FPS is necessary. Laterally running grafts are best shown with the ipsilateral posterior oblique view.

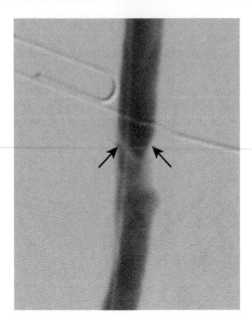

Fig. 45.6 ▨ A valve cusp (arrows) that was causing significant stenosis in a vein graft.

Upper limb arterial diagnosis

Upper limb ischaemia represents only 4% of peripheral vascular disease and is not as frequently associated with generalized atherosclerosis as lower limb ischaemia. Disease is usually focal, affecting the origins of the great vessels. In thoracic outlet syndrome (TOS), vascular compression by bone or ligament is associated with distal embolization, Raynaud's syndrome and subclavian aneurysm. Imaging depends on the clinical scenario (Table 45.4).

Table 45.4 Upper limb arterial imaging depends on the clinical scenario

Scenario	Modality
Elective	
Chronic upper limb ischaemia	MRA[a] > CTA > ultrasound; DSA for intervention. Vasodilator may be required to differentiate spasm from fixed lesions in digital arteries. MRA can be combined with oral vasodilator and DSA with intra-arterial vasodilator
Thoracic outlet syndrome	Ultrasound with postural manoeuvres as initial screen. MRA using blood pool agent and postural manoeuvres subsequently
Acute	
Acute limb ischaemia	CTA, MRA, DSA depending on availability and expertise
Trauma/dissection	CTA for vascular and non-vascular injury, DSA for intervention

Ultrasound does not demonstrate origins of the great vessels.
[a]Dedicated MRA is needed for the hand vessels.

 Alarm: Arch aortography and selective catheterization of the great vessels carry a risk of stroke, so particular care must be taken during catheter and wire manipulation and catheter flushing. Never flush a blocked catheter in the aortic arch.

Equipment

- Basic angiography set
- Catheters: 90-cm 4F pigtail, Berenstein, Headhunter, Sidewinder
- Guidewires: angled hydrophilic guidewire
- GTN or other vasodilator.

Procedure

Access: Diagnostic angiography is usually performed from the femoral approach. Therapeutic intervention is often easier from the brachial artery or with combined femoral and brachial access.

Catheterization: Use a pigtail catheter for arch aortography. A Berenstein catheter will engage the vast majority of arch vessels if used properly.

Runs: Begin with an arch aortogram to show the origins of the great vessels. Additional views may be needed to show the proximal subclavian arteries, particularly when they are tortuous. In suspected TOS, perform runs with the arms raised above the head and also in the Roos position (elbow flexed 90 degrees, shoulder abducted 90 degrees and dorsiflexed). It is possible to see as far as the elbow from an arch injection; a selective catheter should be advanced peripherally to image the distal arm vessels. Use iso-osmolar contrast when imaging the digital arteries. Remember that the radial and ulnar arteries often arise from the axillary or brachial arteries; failure to recognize this will lead to misinterpretation.

 Tip: To obtain high-quality images of the digital arteries, invert the C-arm and place the hand on the image intensifier, immobilizing it with a sandbag. Use a vasodilator to increase flow and discriminate fixed lesions from spasm (Fig. 45.7).

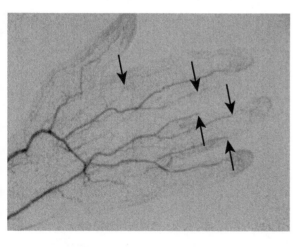

Fig. 45.7 ■ 'Blue digit syndrome'. Hand arteriogram following intra-arterial GTN. There are multiple digital artery occlusions (arrows) secondary to microemboli from a subclavian stenosis. The middle finger is particularly ischaemic.

Interpretation

Vascular compression during postural manoeuvres also occurs in about 30% of normal subjects; subclavian artery irregularity or aneurysm is a more valuable sign of TOS (Fig. 45.8). Diffuse atheroma affecting the subclavian and axillary arteries is most commonly caused by radiotherapy. A proximal high-grade stenosis or occlusion may cause a subclavian steal; this is usually asymptomatic. You should expect reversed flow in the vertebral artery from the duplex; if not, it will only be seen on late images from the arch aortogram.

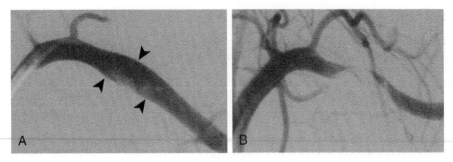

Fig. 45.8 ▨ Thoracic outlet stenosis presenting with distal embolization. (A) There is a subclavian aneurysm containing thrombus (arrowheads). (B) Arm abduction results in marked compression of the subclavian artery.

Troubleshooting

Unable to catheterize an arch vessel
- Remember the basic rules; identify the target vessel on an overview.
- If the arch is unfolded, the Berenstein catheter may be difficult to control; try using a Headhunter 1 catheter, which has a wider primary curve.
- If the target vessel is angulated backwards, then a reverse curve catheter, such as a Sidewinder may be helpful.

Poor visualization of the distal vessels
- Use a vasodilator to increase flow and also to discriminate spasm from irreversible fibrosis.
- Use iso-osmolar contrast and try increased contrast strength.
- Selectively catheterize and advance the catheter into a peripheral position.

Aortic arch arterial diagnosis

CTA and MRA have almost completely replaced DSA in the investigation of patients with aortic syndromes, penetrating ulcer, dissection, intramural haematoma and traumatic injury.

Aortic arch DSA. Paradoxically, arch angiography has become more frequent in the context of thoracic aortic stent grafting and carotid artery intervention (Fig. 45.9).

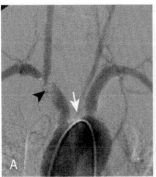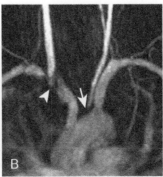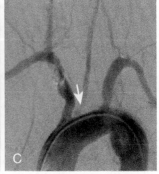

Fig. 45.9 ▨ (A,B) AP projections from arch aortogram and MRA showing calcified plaque causing innominate (arrowhead) and left CCA (arrows) stenosis. (C) LAO 30 degree projection gives a better view of the final line arch morphology and the left CCA (arrow) but obscures the innominate.

Equipment

- Basic angiography set
- Catheter: 90-cm 4F or 5F pigtail.

Procedure

Catheterization: Position the pigtail catheter in the ascending aorta just above the aortic valve.

Runs: A 30 degree LAO to show aortic arch and origin of the great vessels (centre on the aortic arch); a 60 degree LAO may be helpful during stent grafting and in trauma cases (Table 45.5).

Table 45.5 Suggested runs for arch aortography

View	Contrast volume (mL)	Injection rate (mL/s)	Frame rate (FPS)	Field size (cm)
LAO 30 degrees, LAO 60 degrees AP	40	18–25	2–4	28–40

Interpretation

Look for irregularity in the lumen in the region of the ligamentum arteriosum as this is the usual site of injury (Fig. 45.10). A ductus bump appears as a smooth bulge only on the inner curvature.

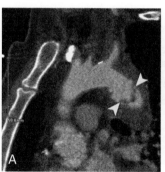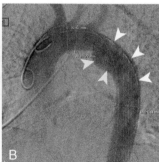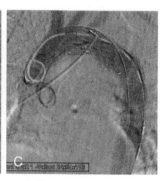

Fig. 45.10 Aortic trauma: the chest X-ray showed mediastinal widening. (A) CT reformat showing intimal/medial tear (yellow arrowheads) and adjacent haematoma. (B) Arch angiography with calibrated catheter (white arrowheads) shows false aneurysm (yellow arrowheads) distal to the left subclavian artery. (C) Following stent-graft repair.

Renal arterial imaging

Renal arterial imaging is needed in four groups of patients:

- Those with renal vascular pathology
- Those with renal transplants
- Potential live renal donors
- Patients with renal tumours requiring embolization.

Magnetic resonance and CT angiography have largely replaced diagnostic renal angiography. DSA remains the 'gold standard' and is still required in case of doubt or to demonstrate distal disease such as fibromuscular dysplasia (FMD) (Fig. 45.11). Renal arterial imaging is most frequently requested to investigate renal artery stenosis (RAS), even though the benefit of renal revascularization is questionable except in renal transplants. The remainder of referrals are for trauma, tumour, pre-transplantation assessment or, rarely, arteritis (Table 45.6).

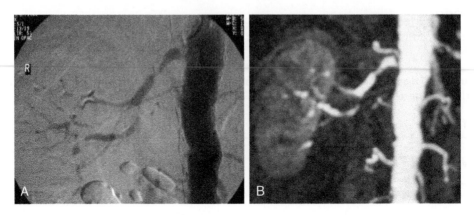

Fig. 45.11 ▧ Multifocal renal artery stenosis. (A) DSA; (B) MRA. Note that the MRA does not demonstrate the calcification in the aorta and renal arteries.

Table 45.6 Renal arterial imaging depends on the clinical scenario

Scenario	Modality
Elective	
Renal artery stenosis	MRA[a], DSA for intervention and for detail of small vessels
Live renal donor assessment	MRA, CTA, including venous and ureteric phases. DSA if any doubt. Note: radiation dose issue with CTA in a healthy patient
Renal tumour embolization	Check the contralateral kidney and plan approach on CT/MRA
Renal artery aneurysm	CTA or MRA for roadmap and assessment
Acute	
Trauma/bleeding	CTA for vascular and nonvascular injury, DSA for intervention

[a]*MRA is unable to exclude subtle lesions of FMD.*

Renal artery DSA

Equipment

- Basic angiography set
- Flush aortogram: 4F pigtail catheter
- Selective angiography: Cobra II, RDC, Sidewinder II.

Procedure

Access: The right CFA is usual for diagnostic angiography; the contralateral CFA often provides better access for selective angiography and intervention as the catheters tend to deflect towards the contralateral side of the aorta.

Catheterization: Plan the procedure based on the cross-sectional imaging. Position the catheter at L1 and start with a flush arteriogram in the optimal oblique projection (commonly LAO 15)! This is good, safe practice; an aortic injection will answer most questions.

Runs: See Table 45.7.

Table 45.7 Typical parameters for renal angiography

Run	Field size (cm)	Catheter position	Contrast volume (mL)	Injection rate (mL/s)	Frame rate (FPS)
AP aortogram	40	L1 adjust as needed	15–20	15–20	2
15 degree oblique	28	As needed	15–20	15–20	2
Selective	28–20	Proximal renal	10	5	2

Flush aortogram Aim to show the origins of the renal arteries in profile (Fig. 45.12). The renal arteries arise at L1/2. Multiple projections may be necessary in the diseased or aneurysmal aorta. In these cases, rotational angiography is helpful if it is available.

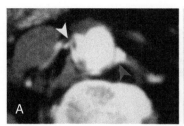 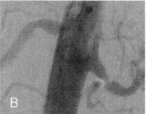 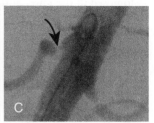

Fig. 45.12 (A) Axial CT in a patient with bilateral renal artery stenosis showing typical position of the origins of the renal arteries, right (yellow arrowhead), left (red arrowhead). (B) The right renal artery appears normal on first run (RAO) but the origin is not seen. (C) The LAO view reveals a high-grade stenosis of the right renal artery (arrow). It is essential to obtain views of both renal artery ostia in profile. The same applies to MRA images.

Selective angiography: Is used to resolve detailed intrarenal anatomy or in rare instances when the renal artery origin cannot be seen in profile. A Cobra II or RDC catheter is the first-choice catheter. Occasionally, a Sidewinder or arm approach will be necessary to deal with an acutely angled artery. Hand injection of 10 mL of contrast is usually satisfactory.

Troubleshooting

Only one kidney seen: time to check how many were present on the non-invasive imaging? Only one – relax; however, if there were two:

- Ensure the catheter is high enough
- Fluoroscope to check for nephrogram, e.g. ectopic kidney
- Check late-phase angiogram for renal perfusion via collaterals.

Contrast in the superior mesenteric artery (SMA) obscures the right renal artery.

If the catheter is too high, contrast fills the SMA. For subsequent runs, pull back the catheter and try alternative oblique tube positions.

Unable to profile the renal artery ostia: If all else fails, catheterize selectively but take care in the presence of stenosis.

Imaging potential live renal donors: The objective is to select the appropriate kidney for donation. The left kidney is usually chosen as it has the longer renal vein. The transplant surgeon needs to know:

- The number and position of renal arteries
- The presence of any disease in the renal vessels
- The number and position of the renal veins
- The ureteric anatomy.

Renal transplant artery imaging

In established transplants, chronic deterioration in function or hypertension may indicate renal artery stenosis (RAS). In a recent transplant, acute dysfunction occurs secondary to rejection, thrombosis of the artery or vein, or less commonly, a poorly fashioned anastomosis or transplant artery kinking. Most transplant arteries are anastomosed to the anterior external iliac artery. Cadaveric transplants arise from a Carrel patch (Fig. 45.13), this is simply a patch of donor aorta incorporating the transplant artery. Arteries from live donors do not have a patch and normally have an end-to-side anastomosis to the external iliac artery, or, occasionally, end-to-end anastomosis to an internal iliac artery. In children, the graft may be anastomosed to the lower aorta.

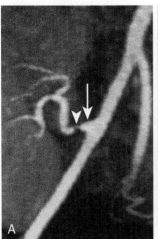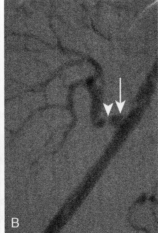

Fig. 45.13 ▦ (A) MRA and (B) CO_2 angiogram of a cadaveric renal transplant showing typical appearance of the Carrel patch (arrows) and stenosis (arrowheads) distal to this.

Renal transplant artery DSA

Catheter angiography follows an abnormal MRA or duplex either for intervention or in case of doubt regarding the diagnosis.

Equipment

- Basic angiography set
- Catheters: 4F straight, RDC for selective angiography
- Wires: 3-mm J, Terumo.

Procedure

Access: Ipsilateral CFA for diagnosis; the contralateral CFA is often better for intervention.

Catheterization: Contrast in the internal iliac artery or the contralateral iliac artery often obscures the transplant renal artery. To minimize this, use a hand injection run to establish the position of the catheter just cranial to the transplant artery.

Runs: A hand injection is mandatory for selective catheterization (Table 45.8).

Table 45.8 Suggested runs for renal transplant angiography

Position	View	Contrast volume (mL)	Inject rate (mL/s)	Field size (cm)	Centring
Above renal artery	AP, multiple obliques or rotational angiography	10–15	5	28–20	Over renal artery and kidney

Interpretation

RAS occurs at the anastomosis, and focal smooth stenoses distal to this are often clamp injuries. In transplant rejection, there is pruning of the intrarenal vessels. If there is early venous filling, look hard for a post-biopsy arteriovenous fistula.

Tip: Look at the operative notes to see the site and type of anastomosis and the number of renal arteries.

Troubleshooting

The transplant artery is tortuous or overlapped by other vessels:

• Craniocaudal tilt and rotational angiography may be necessary.
• If satisfactory views cannot be obtained, try selective catheterization. Contrast can be refluxed to show the anastomosis.
• Try a higher frame rate.

Hepatic artery imaging

Diagnostic hepatic angiography has been superseded by CT, MRI and ultrasound. Angiography is requested only when intervention is an option and is essential when considering patients for liver tumour embolization and selective intra-arterial radiotherapy (SIRT) (Table 45.9).

Table 45.9 Hepatic arterial imaging depends on the clinical scenario

Scenario	Modality
Elective	
Liver tumour embolization	MR/MRA; check the portal vein is patent, DSA prior to SIRT and for intervention
Liver transplant artery stenosis	Ultrasound/CTA diagnosis, DSA for intervention
Acute	
Trauma	CECT for vascular and nonvascular injury, DSA for intervention
Haemobilia	CECT unless secondary to percutaneous transhepatic procedure

Anatomical variants of the hepatic arterial supply are common (Fig. 45.14). In most patients, the hepatic artery is a branch of the coeliac axis, this arises anteriorly from the aorta at T12/L1. Transplant vascular anatomy may be surprising; the transplant hepatic artery may be anastomosed to the recipient hepatic artery or via a conduit to the aorta or iliac artery. Check the operative notes before starting!

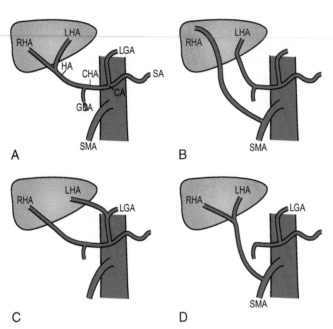

Fig. 45.14 ▒ Common variants of hepatic arterial supply. (A) Conventional anatomy – 55%. (B) Replaced right hepatic artery (RHA) arises from the superior mesenteric artery (SMA) – 16%. (C) Replaced left hepatic artery (LHA) arises from the left gastric artery (LGA) – ~20%. (D) Replaced common hepatic artery (CHA) arising from the SMA – ~2%. CA, coeliac artery; GDA, gastroduodenal artery; HA, hepatic artery; SA, splenic artery.

Hepatic artery DSA

Equipment

- Basic angiography set
- Catheters: Cobra II, Sidewinder II (hydrophilic Cobra catheter, microcatheter)
- Guidewires: 3-mm J, angled Terumo.

Procedure

Access: Usually the right CFA, but sometimes the arm approach will be necessary due to the angulation of the coeliac axis.

Catheterization: A Cobra catheter will be successful in most cases; if it will not engage the coeliac axis or remain stable, a Sidewinder is the next choice. Selective catheterization of the common hepatic artery and its branches may be required, particularly when assessing tumours or embolizing.

Tip: Catheters often pass preferentially into the splenic artery, which comes more anteriorly off the coeliac axis. A Terumo wire can usually be negotiated into the hepatic artery and the catheter will follow it. If this fails, the Sidewinder tip can be shaped with a bend to the right.

Runs: Runs should be centred to include all of the liver, including the right hemidiaphragm and chest wall. Less contrast is required for distal selective angiograms. Magnified oblique views of the liver hilum are often required (Table 45.10). SIRT requires specific highly detailed demonstration of the hepatic arterial anatomy including its branches and anastomoses.

Table 45.10 Typical parameters for hepatic angiography

Catheter position	Contrast volume (mL)	Injection rate (mL/s)	Frame rate (FPS)	Field size (cm)	Projection	Run length (s)
Coeliac axis	32	8	2–1	40	AP	To portal vein ≈20
Selective Hepatic artery	5–15	Hand	2	20–28	AP and RAO 20 degrees	≈5
Splenic artery	20	5	2–1	40	AP	To portal vein

Vascular tumours (e.g. hepatoma and carcinoid) show neovascularity and an abnormal parenchymal stain (Fig. 45.15). Arterial injury following percutaneous transhepatic cholangiography (PTC) usually manifests as a small pseudoaneurysm, which can almost always be selectively embolized.

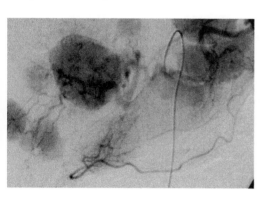

Fig. 45.15 ▥ Carcinoid syndrome. Late arterial phase image from a coeliac axis injection showing multiple hypervascular liver metastases.

Tip: The hepatic artery is prone to spasm when catheterized. Have a low threshold for prophylactic antispasmodic agents. Take care not to misdiagnose spasm as encasement.

Troubleshooting

Unable to pass a guidewire into the hepatic artery:

- Check that the catheter tip is not in the splenic artery by gently injecting contrast and avoiding reflux.
- If the Cobra catheter is pushed out by the wire, try a reverse curve catheter.

Consider a using a guide catheter.

Unable to selectively catheterize the hepatic artery:

- Put plenty of guidewire into a peripheral hepatic branch or the gastroduodenal artery.
- Keep the wire under tension while gently rocking the catheter from side to side; only apply gentle forward pressure, and let the catheter find its own way in.

- Try a softer catheter, e.g. a hydrophilic Cobra.
- Try from the arm; the caudal angulation of the mesenteric vessels lends itself to this approach.

Spasm in the hepatic artery

- This is very common and minimized by administering prophylactic GTN and using microcatheters.

Mesenteric arterial imaging

Three categories of condition will require your input:

- Gastrointestinal bleeding: covered in the section on treating haemorrhage (Ch. 49).
- Mesenteric ischaemia
- Mesenteric aneurysm.

Non-invasive imaging is the default, not least because the production of satisfactory mesenteric angiograms is challenging, particularly in patients with acute gastrointestinal bleeding (Table 45.11).

Table 45.11 Mesenteric arterial imaging depends on the clinical scenario

Scenario	Modality
Elective	
Chronic mesenteric ischaemia	US as rapid screen for proximal disease; MRA, CTA
Mesenteric aneurysm	Usually incidental finding on CT, further assessment with dedicated CTA, DSA for intervention
Chronic gastrointestinal bleeding	Conventional and capsule endoscopy have almost completely replaced DSA
Acute	
Upper gastrointestinal bleeding	Endoscopy[a] is first choice for diagnosis and therapy. CECT if negative endoscopy or if postoperative. DSA if endoscopy positive and embolization needed
Lower gastrointestinal bleeding[b]	Bleeding rectal varices should be excluded first. Apart from this, endoscopy is rarely helpful due to lumen full of blood. Three-phase CECT will demonstrate active bleeding and site and allows targeted angiography
Acute mesenteric ischaemia	CECT – don't forget to look at the intestine as well as the vessels as there is no point in revascularizing a 'black pudding'

[a]Ask the endoscopist to place radiopaque clips at site of bleeding.
[b]More philosophical musings on lower gastrointestinal bleeding later!

Mesenteric DSA

Equipment

Personal preference is important here:

- Basic angiography kit
- 5F sheath
- Catheters: 60-cm Pigtail, Cobra II, RDC, Sidewinder, SOS Omni for selective catheterization. Hydrophilic catheter or microcatheter for distal catheterization
- Hydrophilic guidewire.

Procedure

Access: Right CFA unless difficulty catheterizing the mesenteric vessels, in which case consider an arm approach.

Catheterization: Head straight to the vessel of interest. Perform an overview of each target arterial territory before proceeding to more selective angiography. For LGIB starting with the SMA will be a winner in many cases. The visceral arteries arise anteriorly from the aorta and selective catheterization can be frustrating for even the most experienced angiographer. If you are struggling start with a lateral flush aortogram. Contrast layers posteriorly in the aorta, so it is sometimes necessary to use a larger, faster contrast bolus (20–30 mL at 15–20 mL/s). Centre on L2/3 just anterior to the spine and use filters to eliminate flare caused by bowel gas.

Start with the right tool: The mesenteric arteries

- A Cobra II will often engage the coeliac axis (Fig. 45.16). If this fails, try a Sidewinder II catheter.

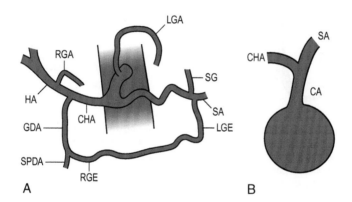

Fig. 45.16 ■ The coeliac artery (CA). (A) Principal arterial branches. (B) Cross-section showing why catheters and wires preferentially enter the splenic artery (SA). CHA, common hepatic artery; GDA, gastroduodenal artery; HA, hepatic artery; LGA, left gastric artery; LGE, left gastroepiploic artery; RGA, right gastric artery; RGE, right gastroepiploic artery; SG, short gastric artery; SPDA, superior pancreaticoduodenal artery.

- The SMA can usually be catheterized with a Cobra II. It can be advanced distally over a hydrophilic wire for super-selective views of the ileocolic and right colic arteries, which are the most common sites of bleeding (Fig. 45.17).
- The IMA arises acutely from the anterolateral aspect of the distal aorta (Fig. 45.18). Perform a steep RAO angiogram of the distal aorta to show its origin; there is often a 'sentinel plaque' adjacent to the origin. Catheterization is easiest with a short reverse curve catheter such as the SOS Omni or Sidewinder I.

Runs: See Table 45.12.

- Paralyse the intestine. If you cannot abolish peristalsis with Buscopan or glucagon, there is little hope of success!
- Use breath-hold if the patient's condition permits. If not, wake the radiographer and try multimasking.

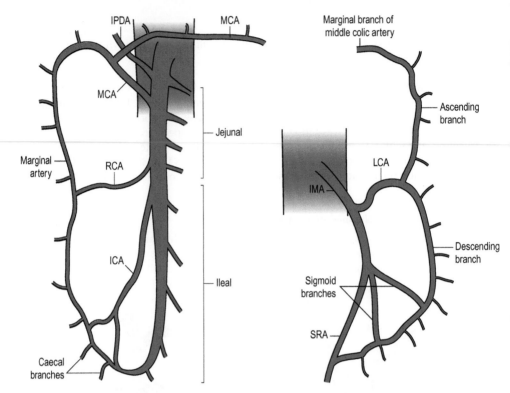

Fig. 45.17 ▨ The principal branches of the superior mesenteric artery. The origin of the ICA marks the transition between jejunal and ileal branches. ICA, ileocolic artery; IPDA, inferior pancreaticoduodenal artery; MCA, middle colic artery; RCA, right colic artery.

Fig. 45.18 ▨ The inferior mesenteric artery (IMA). LCA, left colic artery; SRA, superior rectal artery.

Table 45.12 Suggested runs for mesenteric angiography

Run	Field size (cm)	Centring	Contrast volume (mL)	Injection rate (mL/s)	Frame rate (FPS)
Lateral flush aortogram	40	Mid abdomen	30	20	2
SMA AP	40	Mid-abdomen	30	6	2–1
IMA AP	28	Rectosigmoid	10	Hand	2–1
IMA RAO 25 degrees	28	Rectosigmoid	10	Hand	2–1
IMA LAO 30 degrees	28	Ascending colon and splenic flexure	10	Hand	2–1
Coeliac axis	40	Epigastrium	30	6	2–1
Gastro-duodenal artery	28	Epigastrium	15	Hand	2
LGA	28	Epigastrium	8–10	Hand	2

Gastrointestinal bleeding

See Chapter 49.

Mesenteric ischaemia

This is an important but often overlooked diagnosis. The classic presentation is post-prandial pain ('mesenteric angina') leading ultimately to food avoidance and weight loss. In many cases significant stenoses of one of the mesenteric arteries will be asymptomatic due to collateral supply. Symptomatic mesenteric ischaemia is uncommon unless at least two of the visceral arteries are significantly diseased, the SMA and coeliac axis are almost always both involved.

Mesenteric ischaemia imaging: MRA and CTA are the first-choice investigations and will demonstrate the site and extent of disease and allow planning of surgical and radiological intervention. Visceral angiography is virtually confined to treatment.

Tip: Mesenteric vascular stenosis should be suspected when a large marginal artery of Drummond is seen during peripheral angiography (Fig. 45.19). Similarly, large pancreaticoduodenal arteries suggest stenosis of the coeliac axis or SMA (Fig. 45.20).

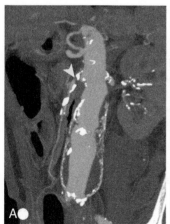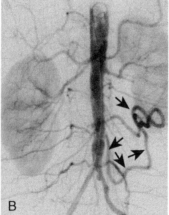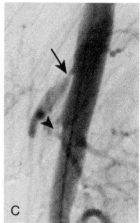

Fig. 45.19 ▦ Images from patients with 'intestinal angina'. (A) Reformat from CTA showing high-grade stenosis (yellow arrowhead) of the superior mesenteric artery (SMA), which is heavily calcified. (B) AP DSA in a different patient shows hypertrophy of the inferior mesenteric artery (IMA) (arrows). Branches of the SMA are filling via the IMA. Lateral flush aortogram (C) showing high-grade stenosis of the coeliac axis (arrow) and occlusion of the SMA (arrowhead).

Mesenteric ischaemia DSA

Approach: Consider the arm approach for intervention.

Catheterization: Begin with lateral flush aortogram with a pigtail catheter above the coeliac axis (T11/12) to delineate the arterial origins before selective catheterization.

Troubleshooting

A vessel is seen on the anteroposterior (AP) arteriogram but cannot be identified on the lateral aortogram: This is usually due to proximal occlusion with reconstitution via collaterals (Fig. 45.20). The coeliac axis and SMA often communicate via a hypertrophied pancreaticoduodenal arcade.

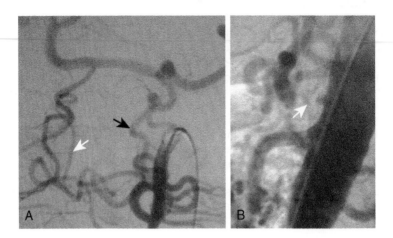

Fig. 45.20 ■ (A) SMA injection showing filling of the coeliac axis via hypertrophied pancreaticoduodenal (white arrow) and pancreatic collaterals (black arrow). (B) Lateral flush aortogram showing occlusion of the coeliac axis (white arrow).

A smooth impression is seen on the superior aspect of the coeliac axis: This is the result of extrinsic compression by the median arcuate ligament of the diaphragm. The diagnosis is confirmed by showing a normal appearance on a lateral flush aortogram with the patient in the right lateral decubitus position. This finding is seen in 20% of asymptomatic patients. A few patients have severe compression of both coeliac axis and SMA and are candidates for surgery.

Tip: Selective catheterization is only required when distal disease is suspected on the flush angiogram. Do not attempt to cross a tight stenosis unless you are prepared to treat it!

Mesenteric aneurysm: False aneurysms following surgery, trauma or infection/pancreatitis are the most common and important as the risk of major haemorrhage is very high. True aneurysms are uncommon and often diagnosed incidentally on CT performed for other indications. Less is known about them than renal artery aneurysm. High-flow aneurysms can be associated with stenosis of the coeliac axis or SMA. When identified, it is usual to perform a CTA to delineate the anatomy. DSA is usually only necessary during intervention (embolization or stent grafting).

The equipment and runs are the same as for other selective mesenteric angiography.

Pulmonary vascular imaging

The bronchial and pulmonary arteries have a distinct set of pathologies, which are best considered in terms of the clinical problems for each circulation (Table 45.13).

Table 45.13 Bronchial and pulmonary imaging depends on the clinical scenario

Scenario	Modality
Elective	
Recurrent haemoptysis	CECT and bronchoscopy to evaluate lungs. Bronchial artery embolization (BAE) if underlying pathology. Pulmonary angiography if suspected tuberculosis. Rasmussen aneurysm
Pulmonary arteriovenous malformation (PAVM)	Non-contrast CT for diagnosis. Pulmonary embolization for treatment
Acute	
Suspected pulmonary embolism	CECT, DSA only for insertion of IVC filter and mechanical thrombectomy
Active haemoptysis	Bronchoscopy, CECT for vascular and non-vascular injury, DSA for bronchial artery embolization

Bronchial artery imaging

The only reason to image the bronchial arteries is as part of the investigation of massive haemoptysis. CECT will demonstrate the bronchial artery anatomy and may be able to demonstrate important collateral supply. Before setting forth, it is crucial to appreciate that the bronchial circulation is complex tiger country. A little knowledge will help you and the patient survive.

Bronchial artery anatomy: Like the liver, the lung has a dual blood supply from the pulmonary and bronchial arteries. Normal bronchial arteries are 1–2 mm in diameter but they hypertrophy in chronic inflammatory pulmonary conditions such as bronchiectasis and become the source of massive haemoptysis. Fortunately, most patients can survive without their bronchial arteries, hence these are sometimes embolized to manage massive haemoptysis. The majority of bronchial arteries arise at the T5/6 level but variations are common, including multiple and conjoined bronchial arteries and common bronchointercostal arteries. In common with other visceral arteries, the bronchial arteries arise anteriorly. Combined bronchointercostal arteries arise posteriorly.

Bronchial artery anastomoses: Bronchial arteries also supply oesophagus, mediastinum, and pulmonary arteries and often have anastomoses with the anterior spinal artery. The latter is essential to recognize if embolizing! The bronchial arteries can also anastomose with arteries that supply tissue in contact with the pleura, this includes the subclavian arteries and their branches, internal mammary arteries, intercostal arteries, phrenic arteries and even coronary arteries. These variant anatomies are particularly relevant if embolization has been performed.

 Tip: The majority of bronchial arteries are found within the air lucency of the left main bronchus, i.e. where you can see the left main bronchus when screening.

Bronchial artery DSA

Equipment

- 5F sheath
- 3-mm J-guidewire

- 5F 90–100-cm-long pigtail catheter
- Terumo wire
- A variety of selective catheters – multipurpose and reverse curve shapes can be effective but the variable anatomy of the bronchial arteries makes prediction of the correct tools something of a lottery!

Procedure

Use the CECT to plan the procedure as far as possible.

Access: The right femoral is normal but consider any approach that simplifies selective catheterization.

Catheterization: No holds barred here, be prepared to try a variety of catheters until you find one that fits. Microcatheters are essential for embolization.

Runs: Start with a flush aortogram (40 mL at 20 mL/s) with the catheter just beyond the left subclavian artery centred on T6. Then play it by ear.

What to look for: Conventional bronchial arteries branch away from hilum and are not normally seen beyond the medial half of the lung. Abnormal bronchial arteries are hypertrophied and may reach further into the parenchyma (Fig. 45.21). Anterior spinal branches arise close to the midline and have a characteristic course, initially running cranially and medially, then bending suddenly downwards to pursue a midline vertical course.

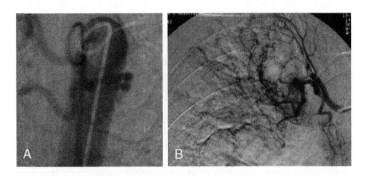

Fig. 45.21 ▨ Bronchial angiography. (A) Flush aortogram showing origins of a right bronchial artery and a combined trunk. (B) Selective catheterization of the right upper bronchial artery prior to embolization.

Troubleshooting

Unable to see bronchial arteries:

- Check you have included the aorta from the left subclavian onwards.
- Try another run in a magnified oblique projection.
- If this fails, then try 'systematically trawling' the aorta around T5/6, injecting contrast as you do. Start at 12 o'clock and work your way round the clockface, paying particular attention to the area of the air shadow of the left main bronchus. Feel for the catheter engaging and look for filling of the bronchial arteries.
- If still no success, then it is time to search for aberrant arterial supply from one of the vessels above.

Unable to catheterize the bronchial arteries:

- Go back to basic principles and ensure that you have a catheter pointing in the correct direction.
- It might be that they are tiny – check the previous CT to try to identify them.
- Try a reverse curve catheter such a SOS Omni.

 Alarm: Be careful not to wedge the catheter; with your luck, it will be a vessel feeding the anterior spinal artery. If you think the catheter might be tight in the vessel then place the hub of the catheter in a bowl of saline before removing the guidewire. If the catheter is wedged in the vessel, saline rather than air is sucked in, preventing an air embolus.

Pulmonary artery imaging

Pulmonary angiography is very rarely required as a diagnostic modality but indicated in pulmonary thrombectomy for massive pulmonary embolism or occluding symptomatic PAVM.

Pulmonary artery DSA

Equipment

- 5F sheath
- 3-mm J-guidewire
- 5F 90–100-cm-long pigtail catheter
- Terumo wire
- ECG monitoring and pressure kit required.

Procedure

Access can either be from the femoral vein or from the basilic or jugular vein. Most practitioners use femoral venous access. In patients with pulmonary embolism (PE) the IVC should have been assessed for the presence of thrombus, make sure you review the cross-sectional imaging before starting.

 Alarm: It should go without saying: do not puncture a grossly swollen leg. Embolization of the underlying ileofemoral thrombus may cause embarrassment to both the patient and you. Stop and consider alternative access points, such as other groin, jugular vein or basilic vein.

 Pulmonary angiography: step-by-step guide

1. In patients with PE: if the IVC has not been assessed, obtain an IV cavogram. Use a hand injection of 20 mL non-ionic contrast via the side-arm of the sheath. Use Buscopan or glucagon to paralyse the gut. If there are filling defects within the IVC, consider an alternative access point from above.
2. Advance the 5F pigtail catheter over the J-wire until the loop of the pigtail lies just below the right atrium.
3. Insert the Terumo wire into the pigtail catheter and advance (Fig. 45.22). The wire will progressively unfurl the pigtail until the wire points to about 1 o'clock, almost invariably straight at the pulmonary trunk. Carefully advance the wire across the tricuspid valve – get your assistant to watch the ECG – and the wire almost always goes into the left main pulmonary artery. Advance the catheter until it is in the left main pulmonary artery.

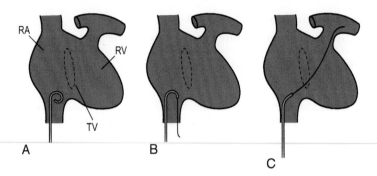

Fig. 45.22 ▓ Technique for pulmonary artery catheterization. (A) Pigtail and hydrophilic wire at the upper inferior vena cava. (B) Advance the guidewire which opens the pigtail loop. (C) The wire usually goes through the tricuspid valve into the pulmonary artery. RA, right atrium; RV, right ventricle; TV, tricuspid valve.

4. Measure the pulmonary artery pressures:
   a. Systolic pulmonary artery pressure <50 mmHg, then angiography is safe
   b. Systolic pulmonary artery pressure >50 mmHg, then pull the catheter back into the right ventricle
   c. Measure the right ventricular pressures – if the right ventricular end diastolic pressure (RVEDP) is >20 mmHg, non-selective pulmonary angiography is dangerous.
5. If this is your first pulmonary angiogram, now is a good time to shout very loudly for help. If you remain determined, selective pulmonary angiography with hand injections of contrast into areas identified by the CT/V/Q scan may be very useful.
6. Give a test injection with 10 mL of contrast, and make sure the end of the pigtail catheter is not in a small pulmonary artery branch. Connect the catheter to a pump injector. Set the pump for 40 mL at 20 mL/s.
7. Assuming you are using DSA, ask for 6 FPS – the faster frame rate will help overcome misregistration secondary to cardiac motion. Start with an AP view.
8. Look carefully through the first run. If you have definitely identified an embolus, then you have finished the examination and may proceed to item 12.
9. Proceed to perform further runs in RAO 30 degrees and LAO 30 degrees.
10. Pulling the pigtail catheter back into the pulmonary trunk, then gently advancing, the Terumo guidewire enters the right pulmonary artery. The guidewire often loops into the right pulmonary artery; by gently manipulating the wire, a right lower lobe pulmonary artery can be entered with the wire. Make sure you advance the catheter well into the right main pulmonary artery at least as far as the hilum, as the catheter always tends to come back slightly when the wire is withdrawn.
11. Repeat the AP, LAO and RAO projections for the right lung.
12. Look through the standard projections. If there are any questionable areas, consider a repeat run, possibly magnified or in a different projection.
13. Before withdrawing the catheter, straighten out the pigtail with the Terumo wire. This prevents an unnecessary thoracotomy to retrieve a catheter firmly entangled in the chordae tendinae of the tricuspid valve.

Troubleshooting

Failure to catheterize the pulmonary artery:

- Bad luck! Did you really use the rules in Chapter 30? Enlarged right ventricles can cause difficulty with the wire repeatedly entering the apex of the right ventricle.
- Carefully use a Headhunter or Berenstein catheter with a Terumo wire to manipulate into the pulmonary artery.

Pulsatile injection with poor peripheral pulmonary artery filling despite 40 mL at 20 mL/s:

- Check the psi rate on the pump – fast injections require higher psi. The catheter packaging will tell you the maximum rate for that catheter. Rarely, 50 mL at 25 mL/s is required.

Breathless patient and poor DSA images:

- Ask the radiographer to get more mask images at the beginning of the run. It may be better to do a run at 2 FPS with the patient breathing or consider selective angiography of relevant territories.

Complications

- Pulmonary angiography is a relatively safe procedure. Overall mortality rate is 0.2%.
- Cardiopulmonary collapse is the main cause of death. It usually occurs in patients with severe pulmonary hypertension and right ventricular end diastolic pressure >20 mmHg or right ventricular strain diagnosed echocardiographically.
- Right ventricle perforation 1% – usually no sequelae.
- Symptomatic persistent arrhythmia.

Carotid and vertebral arterial imaging

Advances in CT, MRI and ultrasound have virtually eliminated the indications for diagnostic carotid angiography. Carotid artery stenoses should be measured accurately using calipers and analysed according to the NASCET study criteria, which form the basis for treatment (Fig. 45.23). Dissection of the carotid artery causes string-like narrowing (Fig. 45.24).

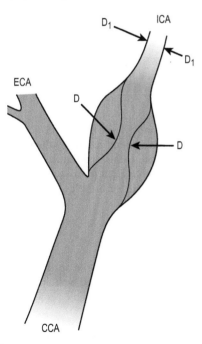

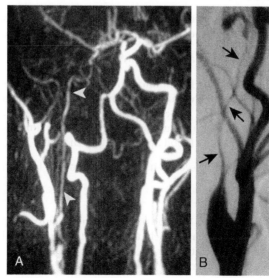

Fig. 45.23 ▓ NASCET criteria. NASCET % stenosis = $[1 - (D/D_1)] \times 100\%$. CCA, common carotid artery; ECA, external carotid artery; ICA, internal carotid artery.

Fig. 45.24 ▓ Typical 'string-like' appearance of carotid dissection. (A) MRA: the right internal carotid artery (ICA) is dissected (arrowheads). (B) Lateral view from a selective carotid angiogram showing IAC dissection (arrows). (Image (B) courtesy of Dr P Turner.)

In most centres, carotid angiography is now the domain of neuroradiologists as part of cerebral angiography for the investigation and treatment of aneurysmal disease and vascular malformations (Table 45.14). Hence, if you want to avoid the first time you find yourself in this particular tiger country being in the context of carotid artery stenting, it pays to spend a few sessions with the neuroradiologists.

Table 45.14 Carotid arterial imaging depends on the clinical scenario

Scenario	Modality
Elective	
Recent TIA	Ultrasound, CT and MRA to evaluate carotid artery stenosis and also cerebral lesions. Carotid angiography when US/MRA are discordant
Post-dissection aneurysm	MRA/CTA. DSA for carotid stent grafting
Acute	
Suspected CVA	CT/MR perfusion scans and assessment of carotid arteries DSA for thrombolysis (some centres only) or stenting
Suspected carotid dissection	US, MRA, CTA. DSA for stenting in the absence of thrombus

Equipment

- Basic angiography set
- 5F sheath for DSA. A long sheath or guide catheter is essential in carotid artery stenting
- Catheters: non-selective – 90-cm 4F pigtail; selective – personal preference is important, options include Berenstein, Headhunter, Sidewinder and Mani
- Guidewires: 3-mm J and angled Terumo.

Procedure

Consent: In presence of carotid disease, there is an approximately 2% stroke risk associated with selective carotid angiography.

Access: Usually via the right CFA.

Catheterization: To minimize the risk of CVA, scrupulous angiographic technique and attention to catheter flushing are mandatory. Flush catheters in the descending aorta whenever possible; that way, any emboli will not affect the cerebral circulation. Make sure that there are no air bubbles in the flush solution. This is the time to use the double-flush technique – aspirate flowing blood and discard, flush with a fresh syringe with no air bubbles.

 Alarm: Never flush a blocked catheter in the aortic arch!

Arch aortogram: Position a pigtail catheter in the ascending aorta just above the aortic root. An arch aortogram will help to localize the vessel ostia but is not essential if the arch and origins of the great vessels are not diseased. In general, start with an LAO 30 degree projection to 'open up the arch'.

Carotid and vertebral artery catheterization: The difficulty of this procedure depends on the curvature of the aortic arch and the presence of any disease within it. Choose the most suitable catheter for the configuration of the arch; remember the basic rules of catheter selection. The Berenstein catheter is forward facing and can be used for most arch vessels unless they are angled acutely retrogradely. In unfolded arches or when the vessel is awkwardly angulated, use the Headhunter, Sidewinder or Mani catheter.

When selective catheterization is necessary, position the catheter in the common carotid artery (CCA). For a vertebrobasilar problem, start with the catheter in the proximal subclavian artery to show the vertebral artery origin. Then perform selective vertebral catheterization. Cerebral angiography requires selective internal carotid artery (ICA) catheterization.

Runs: The runs performed depend on the clinical indication. Perform the minimum number of runs to achieve a diagnostic examination (Table 45.15). Additional runs may be required to demonstrate specific intracerebral vessels. These are beyond the scope of this book and may be found in textbooks of neuroradiology.

Table 45.15 Typical parameters for carotid angiography

Position	Runs	Contrast volume (mL)	Injection rate (mL/s)	Frame rate (FPS)	Centring	Field size (cm)
Aortic arch	LAO 30 degrees	30–40	15–20	2	Aortic root upwards	40–28
Carotid	AP and lateral	10	Hand	2	Over carotid bifurcation (ant to C4)	28
Internal carotid extracranial	AP and lateral	10	Hand	2	Over ipsilateral carotid	28–40
Internal carotid intracranial	AP and lateral	10	Hand	2–1 for venous phase	Lateral skull and Townes view	28–40
Vertebral	AP and lateral	10	Hand	2–1 for venous phase	Intracranial– lateral skull and Townes view	28–40

Troubleshooting

Catheter 'jumps' around the aortic arch: This is usually a consequence of the catheter being held under tension in the aortic arch (Fig. 45.25). Turn the catheter to face appropriately and pull it back slowly, trying not to 'bridge' the catheter. Occasionally, it may be necessary to use a larger-calibre catheter, particularly if initial attempts were with a 4F. A reverse curve catheter such as the Sidewinder can be useful in this situation.

Unable to catheterize an arch vessel: Perform a run in the LAO 30 degree projection and use this to confirm the anatomy and exclude an origin stenosis. Choose an appropriately shaped catheter.

Unable to advance catheter into arch vessel: Once again, this is usually a consequence of the catheter being held under tension in the aortic arch. Try advancing more wire into the artery to increase stability, perform a run to establish the anatomy and avoid passing the wire up the internal carotid artery. Make use of the subclavian and axillary arteries to get 'a good purchase'. It is rarely necessary to resort to using a larger catheter or a guide-catheter. If you are in trouble, pull the catheter back into the descending aorta and get help!

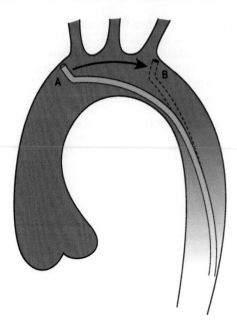

Fig. 45.25 In position A, the catheter is under tension against the inner curve of the aortic arch. As it is withdrawn, it suddenly springs (B) making controlled catheterization impossible.

The external carotid artery superimposes on the internal carotid artery This is fairly common on the AP projection. Try a 15 degree ipsilateral anterior oblique projection. Another common problem is for fillings to project over the ICA. This can also be solved by a suitable oblique projection.

46

Treating arterial occlusive disease

Angioplasty and stenting are cornerstone techniques in interventional radiology and have widespread non-vascular and vascular applications. The key skills and equipment choices remain largely the same, regardless of the site. This chapter assumes that you have already mastered the theory and techniques for getting to and crossing the lesion.

Basic principles

Refer back to the sections on equipment and the basic principles for further guidance on how to plan your case and choose the right gear (Table 46.1).

Table 46.1 Rough guide to balloon and stent diameters

	Diameter (mm)
Aorta	10–15
Common iliac	8
External iliac	7
CFA, proximal SFA	6
Distal SFA	5
Popliteal	4
Crural	2–3

Indications

Indications for treatment vary according to the site of the disease. In most instances, the aim is to increase flow through the artery but in the carotid artery, the aim is almost always to prevent stroke rather than increase cerebral perfusion. A stenosis has to narrow the lumen by 50% before it becomes haemodynamically significant; a 50% diameter reduction results in a 75% reduction in the luminal cross-sectional area.

Remember that atherosclerotic plaque is incompressible and angioplasty works by tearing plaque and stretching the vessel wall.

The key determinants of success of angioplasty are:

- Arterial inflow and outflow
- Lesion morphology: stenosis or occlusion, length, calcification, plaque distribution
- Net lumen gain: a balance between vessel diameter and elastic recoil.

In simple terms, you can expect a good outcome for a focal stenosis in a large vessel with good inflow and run-off and a poor result in a long occlusion of a small, blind-ending vessel.

Consent

The risks of the procedure vary considerably from site to site. Consent always includes:

- **Treatment options:** alternative medical, surgical and interventional radiology options including combined strategies.
- **Outcomes:** probability of technical success, likelihood of the desired clinical result, e.g. relief of symptoms, likelihood of recurrence and subsequent management options. The latter is particularly important if one treatment precludes another option at a later date.
- **Complications:**
  - The 3Bs of arterial access: bruising, bleeding and blockage, at the puncture site. Puncture site haematoma: 2–3%; commoner with larger sheaths, obesity and hypertension
  - Generic angioplasty-related: vessel occlusion ≈1%, rupture or dissection, usually fixed by stent or stent graft, distal embolization 1–4%, often of no clinical importance
  - Site-specific: obviously, emboli to the brain or the kidney are going to be much more important
  - *Remember that you must mention complications that the patient is likely to find significant even if they are uncommon*, e.g. need for reconstructive vascular surgery, amputation and death. About 1% of patients will require emergency surgery as a result of your efforts. The consequences of complications or technical failure are likely to be greater in patients with critical ischaemia and more challenging, distal lesions.

Specific complications will be considered on a site-by-site basis.

Procedure planning

Plan the procedure before starting, try to think through the likely steps and potential problems. Use the preintervention imaging to determine:

Access: This relates to the optimal route to the lesion. The fewer curves the angioplasty balloon has to negotiate the better, so the shortest, straightest route is usually best. However, there may be reasons to choose an alternative approach or to have a back-up plan such as:

- When there is a local problem at the optimal access site
- When there are lesions above and below the common femoral artery (CFA) that require treatment, e.g. combined iliac and superficial femoral artery (SFA) disease.

Fortunately, improvements in equipment make angioplasty and stenting across the iliac bifurcation straightforward and thus facilitate treatment of bilateral lesions via a single puncture. The contralateral approach reduces your ability to 'push' through a very tight lesion. If necessary, simply make an antegrade puncture.

Equipment: This will vary according to the site, indication for and nature of the intended treatment but it helps to consider the following in terms applicable to any case:

- **Access:** needles, wires and sheaths
- **Angiography:** catheters, wires and contrast
- **Catheterization:** catheters and wires needed to navigate to the target, cross the lesion and provide stable platform for treatment
- **Treatment:** angioplasty, balloons and stents- use the non-invasive imaging to estimate sizes
- **Drugs:** heparin, analgesia, etc.
- **Closure:** manual haemostasis or closure device
- **Bail-out intervention:** balloons, stents, stent grafts, thrombolysis and thrombosuction.

Treating arterial occlusive disease at specific sites

This section outlines the clinical and technical steps for successful angioplasty/stenting for the most common indications.

Aorta

Indications for treatment

Symptomatic aortic stenosis and coarctation: Occasionally to allow passage/deployment of a device such as a stent graft or prosthetic aortic valve.

Consent issues

Focal aortic stenoses and coarctation are ideal for angioplasty and have a technical success rate exceeding 95%, with excellent 5-year patency rates. Stents can be reserved for cases of elastic recoil, flow-limiting dissection and recurrent stenoses.

Aortoiliac occlusions can be treated successfully but it should be borne in mind that these are much harder to treat and aortobifemoral grafting and aortic endarterectomy have excellent long-term patency.

 Alarm: Retrograde recanalization of aortoiliac occlusion can lead to passage of the wire deep into the aortic wall, increasing the risk of dissection of important branch vessels and rupture.

Specific equipment

Either a single balloon, if the stenosis is clear of the bifurcation, or kissing balloons when the stenosis involves or is very close to the bifurcation. Remember that it is relatively easy to rupture the aorta (Laplace's law) and a 10–12 mm balloon will often be all that is needed.

There is a predilection for distal stenoses and occlusions to be very close to the origin of the inferior mesenteric artery (IMA).

Procedure

Unless you have ultrasound evidence of haemodynamically significant disease, pressure measurements are essential in the initial assessment of these lesions. Apparently severe stenoses on angiography frequently do not produce a significant pressure drop. As a generalization, if the catheter and wire pass through without a struggle, there is no significant pressure drop.

 Tip: Measure the pressure gradient before placing a very large sheath.

Approach

- **Unilateral femoral access** will usually suffice for uncomplicated aortic stenosis.
- **Bilateral femoral access** is needed for lesions that involve:
  - The aortic bifurcation, which should be treated with bilateral simultaneous common iliac balloons extending into the aortic bifurcation (Fig. 46.1)

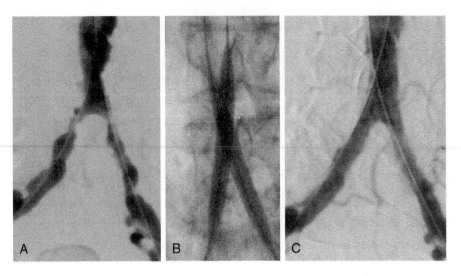

Fig. 46.1 ▪ (A) Stenosis involving the distal aorta and CIAs. (B) Kissing angioplasty balloons. (C) Completion angiography.

- The IMA if a protection wire or balloon is needed; in these circumstances it is sometimes necessary to have brachial access.
- **Brachial access** is sometimes helpful to perform angiography to delineate an aortic stenosis and may be the best approach for traversing the lesion. In this case a rendezvous procedure is performed with angioplasty/stenting via a larger sheath from the femoral artery.

 Tip: If there is a complete aortic occlusion, it sometimes helps to perform a run from the aortic arch to allow collateral perfusion of the distal circulation. Alternatively, inject contrast from both a femoral and a brachial catheter.

Equipment

If a lesion is in the distal infrarenal aorta, either use a balloon with a short taper or use kissing balloons. The taper on some 15–18-mm balloons extends 1–2 cm beyond the balloon marker and will wreak havoc in an iliac artery!

Catheterization These lesions always look easy to cross but, in practice, it can be quite tricky to negotiate a 1–2-mm channel in a 12-mm artery. **Safety first:** once you have traversed the stenosis with a hydrophilic guidewire, this should be exchanged for a stiffer wire, e.g. an Amplatz super-stiff, prior to balloon insertion.

Runs AP may be all that is required to traverse the lesion but consider additional oblique and lateral projections if you need to assess the aorta or identify the visceral vessels. If the IMA is the dominant intestinal vessel, occlusion must be avoided. In this case, use a protection wire or balloon in the IMA from the contralateral femoral artery or the brachial route.

Complications The principal risk is distal embolization secondary to treatment of a large atherosclerotic plaque. Iliac trauma from the balloon is an avoidable risk with good angiographic technique.

Iliac arteries

Indications for treatment

Angioplasty and stenting are effective treatments for iliac atherosclerotic disease and have largely replaced aortofemoral bypass grafting. Indications include:

- symptomatic iliac stenosis and occlusion
- occasionally to improve inflow for a renal transplant or more distal bypass graft
- occasionally to allow passage/deployment of a device such as a stent graft or prosthetic aortic valve.

Consent issues

Initial technical success rates of 90–95% with 80% 5-year patency rates are achievable for stenoses <5 cm in length. Patency rates are lower for occlusions, heavily calcified lesions and stenotic disease that exceeds 10 cm in length, and primary stenting should be considered in these circumstances.

The most feared complications of iliac intervention are:

- Iliac rupture <1% managed using balloon occlusion to control bleeding and then stent grafting to repair the hole
- Symptomatic or potentially important distal embolization 1–2% managed by thrombus aspiration, stenting or surgical embolectomy/bypass.

Equipment

Iliac diameters are usually between 6 mm and 8 mm; however, take particular care in the external iliac artery (EIA) in females, which can be small and is prone to dissection, spasm and rupture. Remember to measure the size of the target vessel before dilation. Following angioplasty, if the EIA is narrowed throughout its length, it may well be secondary to vasospasm (Fig. 46.2). Inject 100 mg of glyceryl trinitrate via the sheath and repeat the angiogram after a few minutes.

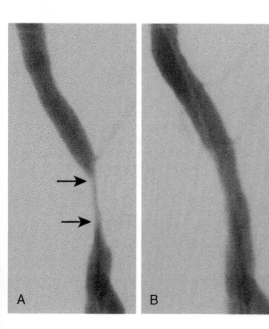

Fig. 46.2 ■ (A) Apparent stenosis of the CFA (arrows). Note the smooth outline characteristic of spasm. (B) Appearance following intra-arterial administration of GTN 200 µg.

A   B

Approach

- **Ipsilateral retrograde femoral access** is the norm for straightforward stenosis/occlusion.

Tip: If the common femoral pulse cannot be felt, use an ultrasound-guided puncture to gain access. If the CFA is severely diseased, consider the contralateral approach with CFA angioplasty or a combined procedure with CFA endarterectomy – this way you do not even need to obtain haemostasis.

- **Contralateral retrograde femoral access:** Used in the presence of:
  - tandem iliac and femoral disease
  - iliac occlusion when the lumen cannot be re-entered retrogradely
  - bilateral lesions if kissing balloons are not required and you do not want to make two punctures.

Tip: You can use your favourite catheter to cross the aortic bifurcation but will need robust support to enter/cross a contralateral iliac occlusion; a braided Sidewinder 2 is a good starting point.

- **Bilateral femoral access** used for:
  - **Bilateral disease.** This is essential for lesions involving the distal aorta and impinging on the origin of the common iliac artery (Fig. 46.3). In this situation, simultaneous inflation of a balloon in each common iliac artery (CIA) origin ('kissing balloons') is needed.
  - **Protection of the internal iliac artery.** The internal iliac artery may be occluded if angioplasty or stenting is performed across its origin. In a male patient with contralateral internal iliac artery (IIA) occlusion, this may cause impotence and you will not have done his buttock claudication any favours! Protect the internal iliac artery by inserting a guidewire into it from the contralateral side. If the internal iliac artery origin is diseased, then angioplasty it as well (Fig. 46.3) – a male patient may be very grateful.

Alarm: If the internal iliac is at risk of occlusion, discuss the risk of erectile dysfunction/buttock claudication in male patients.

- **Brachial access:** seldom required but may be helpful for angiography.

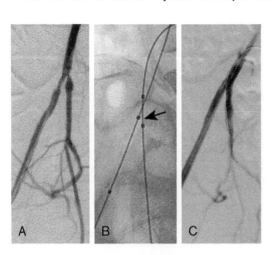

Fig. 46.3 (A) Stenosis involving the external iliac artery (EIA) and the origin of the solitary internal iliac artery (IIA). (B) Angioplasty balloons in situ; the balloon artery (arrow) has been placed from the contralateral approach. (C) Completion angiography.

Procedure

Pressure measurements (Ch. 33) are invaluable for assessing the significance of iliac lesions before and after treatment. Pullback pressure measurements are particularly useful in multifocal disease, remember to keep an 0.018-inch wire across the lesion.

Catheterization If you cannot negotiate a lesion from the retrograde approach use a Sidewinder or SOS catheter to manipulate over the bifurcation and try to cross the lesion from above (see Fig. 31.5). If successful, the wire can either be snared or manipulated through the sheath (see Fig. 36.4) or permit ipsilateral passage of balloons.

Runs: When treating iliac occlusions perform a run with simultaneous injections from both the aorta and the ipsilateral sheath. Always perform obliques and use the run that shows the lesion in profile during attempted catheterization. When it comes to stent deployment use the projection which best delineates the anatomy, e.g. common iliac and IIA origins.

Complications

Complications are more frequent in occlusions than stenoses and probably more frequent in the external iliac artery.

Distal embolization may be impossible to treat by clot aspiration because of the pre-existing 6–7Fr retrograde puncture used to perform the angioplasty. Primary stent insertion minimizes the risk by trapping atheroma and thrombus against the vessel wall.

Iliac rupture (see Fig. 32.6) can occur after angioplasty, particularly of the external iliac artery. Blood loss can be very rapid and prompt balloon tamponade is essential. It is now that you realize the importance of having a stent-graft available for 'endovascular rescue'. If this fails, seek immediate surgical assistance.

Common femoral artery

Indications for treatment

CFA stenoses are often the result of large calcified eccentric plaques. As the CFA is superficial, lesions are often treated by endarterectomy rather than angioplasty. If the stenosis is post-surgical, try angioplasty instead. CFA angioplasty is sometimes performed in association with iliac/SFA intervention on the grounds that it will not preclude subsequent endarterectomy.

Approach

Access is usually from the contralateral groin or the arm but occasionally retrograde access will be obtained from the popliteal artery usually in the context of treating a chronic SFA occlusion.

Procedure

Consider using a protection balloon for complex lesions involving the profunda origin. Kissing balloons may occasionally be required in this context.

Alarm: Try to avoid stents in the CFA as they will be prone to repeated flexion (Fig. 46.4) and will preclude arterial access and complicate any future surgery.

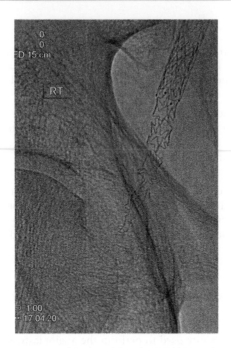

Fig. 46.4 ■ Stent fracture due to repeated flexion of the distal EIA/CFA. (Courtesy Dr Sapna Puppala.)

Outcomes

These are not well documented but would be expected to be similar to the external iliac artery.

Femoropopliteal segment

Indications for treatment

- Symptomatic femoropopliteal stenosis and occlusion
- Occasionally to improve inflow in more distal bypass graft.

Angioplasty of the SFA/popliteal for claudication is bread and butter for most radiologists. Treatment is increasingly undertaken for patients with critical limb ischaemia. Stenting is gaining widespread acceptance for long segment disease but restenosis remains problematic. Stent-grafts in the SFA remain largely unproven compared with endovascular and surgical alternatives.

Equipment

- Angioplasty balloons: Most patients are treated with primary angioplasty, 20–30 cm-long balloons are helpful when treating patients with long segment disease.
- Drug-eluting balloons are sometimes used when there is a high risk of re-stenosis.
- Stents use is usually reserved for when primary angioplasty fails or in re-stenosis. Use stents specifically designed for use in the distal SFA/popliteal segments to reduce the risk of fracture due to flexion.

Approach

- Ipsilateral antegrade femoral approach: used for the majority of cases
- Contralateral retrograde femoral approach: used for tandem iliac and femoral lesions and occasionally when ipsilateral access is challenging

- Other approaches: SFA, popliteal artery or even pedal access, these are much less commonly used and are generally reserved to traverse long occlusions when other approaches have failed.

Outcomes

Angioplasty confers immediate benefit and appears to improve outcome in the mid-term compared with best medical therapy and exercise. Overall patency rates for SFA disease are around 50% at 3 years. As always, short non-calcified stenoses offer the best long-term results; 5-year patency is up to 70%. The results of angioplasty in stenoses or occlusions >10 cm are much poorer but angioplasty/stenting may be appropriate if the patient is not a surgical candidate and has rest pain or tissue ischaemia.

Procedure

Catheterization Stenoses are usually negotiated with a hydrophilic guidewire. Occlusions may be more readily traversed with a straight wire and shaped catheter. Always perform a run after successfully crossing the lesion to confirm re-entry into the target vessel. Dilating a collateral will cause havoc and few things are more embarrassing than creating a 5-mm hole through the side of the SFA.

Runs In difficult lesions, manipulate a catheter and guidewire to the target lesion, then perform a magnified view to optimize the chances of steering through the lesion. Choose the largest magnification that allows visualization of the lesion and the target run-off vessel, as this keeps the wire in view at all times.

Calf vessels (*aka* below knee, BTK, tibial or crural)

Indications for treatment

Below knee angioplasty is usually reserved for patients with critical limb ischaemia and is particularly useful in the presence of ulceration where relatively short-lived improvement in flow may be sufficient for healing. Conversely, it is less useful in patients with rest pain, as this recurs with re-stenosis.

Consent issues

It is essential to be realistic regarding the possibility that ulceration may not heal despite successful angioplasty and also the likelihood of restenosis. In advanced disease, particularly single-vessel disease, there is no margin for error and a complication such as thrombosis may result in amputation – it is essential that this is explained beforehand.

As always, the elusive single focal non-calcified stenosis does best, but you are very unlikely to be treating that disease pattern. More diffuse disease is common and can be successfully treated and may stay open long enough to permit ulcer healing. Extraluminal angioplasty can be particularly effective in crural vessel occlusion (Fig. 46.5).

Equipment

In the last few years, the quality of equipment available for crural angioplasty has improved markedly. Low-profile crossing catheters, specialized occlusion wires and supportive sheaths are all available and can make a huge difference. Small-calibre, low-profile balloons (2–4 mm) usually in longer lengths and 0.014–0.018-inch guidewires are required. These vessels are extremely prone to vasospasm and the use of antispasmodic agents is essential.

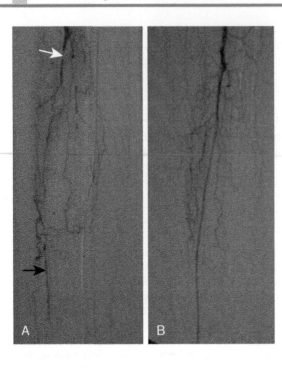

Fig. 46.5 Extraluminal angioplasty of the posterior tibial artery. (A) Diseased tibioperoneal trunk (white arrow) and posterior tibial artery (black arrow). (B) Following extraluminal recanalization of the posterior tibial artery, in line run-off is restored.

Approach

Ipsilateral antegrade femoral artery: This remains the access of choice.

Alternative approaches

Popliteal and pedal access: This is reserved for cases where all other approaches have failed.

Procedure

The techniques for treating stenoses are much the same as for those anywhere else, except for the use of low-profile platforms. There is increasing interest in the angiosome concept of treating the 'ulcer-related' vessel, e.g. posterior tibial for the medial heel and sole of the foot, anterior tibial for the dorsum of the foot and anterior shin, peroneal for lateral heel and ankle. Crossing occlusions requires more specialist equipment; special 'weighted' shapeable guidewires are available and these should be used with low-profile crossing catheters to navigate the occlusion. Retrograde access via the pedal arteries can be invaluable when antegrade access has failed.

Outcomes

Long-term patency is not well established for below-the-knee angioplasty but there is no doubt that calf vessel angioplasty is a useful tool in the armamentarium for treating critical limb ischaemia.

Renal artery

Indications for treatment

Renal artery angioplasty and stenting are performed relatively infrequently due to a lack of proven benefit in the management of ischaemic chronic kidney disease or hypertension. It is worth noting that without revascularization, only about one in six patients with severe renal artery stenosis will ever need dialysis; many more will succumb to other complications of cardiovascular and cerebrovascular disease.

There are five groups of patients most likely to benefit from renal angioplasty/stenting:

- **Patients with symptomatic transplant renal artery stenosis**
- **Flash pulmonary oedema** – the aetiology of this condition is incompletely understood but treating the underlying renal artery stenosis is usually effective
- **Hypertension refractory to treatment.** A few patients have hypertension which is poorly controlled, despite maximal drug therapy, or malignant hypertension, or do not tolerate the antihypertensive medication. In these patients, it is worth trying renal artery angioplasty and stenting, with the caveat that there will be no improvement in about one-third of patients
- **Hypertension in children** with fibromuscular dysplasia or neurofibromatosis
- **Rapidly decreasing renal function with preserved renal size.** These patients are going to require renal replacement therapy in the near future and have nothing to lose. This group of patients is least likely to benefit from revascularization therapy. Remember that renal artery stenosis must affect the entire functional renal mass to be a significant contributory factor in chronic kidney disease.

Pathology of renal artery stenosis The majority of renal stenoses are secondary to atherosclerotic lesions that tend to involve the proximal renal artery or its ostium (Fig. 46.6A). Fibromuscular dysplasia can affect any part of the renal artery and has a characteristic beaded appearance at angiography (Fig. 46.6B). Angioplasty success rates are highest with fibromuscular dysplasia, moderate with non-ostial atherosclerotic stenoses (Fig. 46.7) and poorest with ostial lesions. Ostial lesions are due to aortic wall atheroma and are prone to elastic recoil. Most angiographers will opt for a primary stent placement when dealing with an ostial lesion (Fig. 46.8).

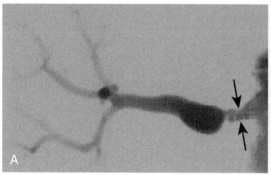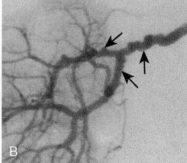

Fig. 46.6 ■ (A) Atheromatous ostial renal artery stenosis (arrows) with post-stenotic dilation. (B) Typical beaded appearance of fibromuscular dysplasia (arrows) involving the distal renal artery and its branches.

Consent issues

Renal artery angioplasty and stenting is a complex procedure; access can be difficult and when there is a problem, the consequences are rapid and serious and the kidney may be lost, resulting in the need for dialysis in approximately 2–5% patients. Patients with transplant kidneys are likely to be particularly concerned about this.

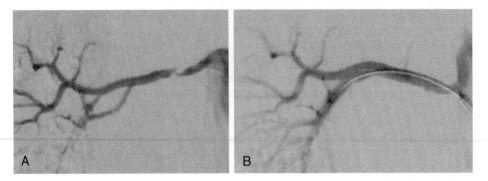

Fig. 46.7 ▨ Atheromatous stenosis in the mid-renal artery. (A) Before and (B) after angioplasty. Hypertension was cured but returned 2 years later and was again successfully treated.

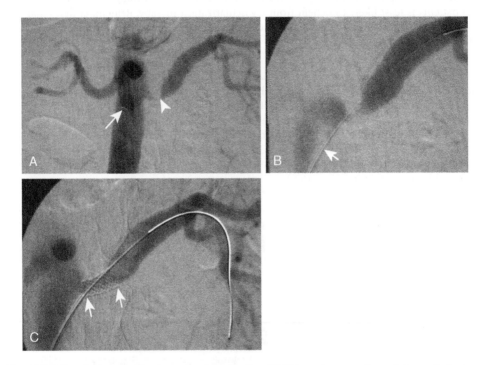

Fig. 46.8 ▨ Renal artery stenting for severe hypertension. (A) CO_2 angiogram using a Cobra catheter in the aorta (arrow), high-grade ostial stenosis (arrowhead) with poststenotic dilatation affecting the entire renal artery. (B) The stenosis has been crossed, angiography performed by injection through the Cobra catheter (arrow) around an 0.018-inch guidewire. (C) Completion angiogram obtained as in (B). Note that the stent (arrows) has been dilated to 6 mm to match the diameter of the contralateral renal artery.

Equipment

- **Selective catheters and guide catheters**: most native renal artery stenosis can be traversed using Cobra or renal double-curve catheters, occasionally a reverse-curve catheter, e.g. a SOS OMNI, will be required. A multipurpose shape guide catheter will normally provide sufficient support

- **Wires**: crossing the stenosis angled hydrophilic wires or steerable 0.018-inch wire, e.g. V18. Support wires – depends on the balloon platform, typically supportive 0.018-inch wire, e.g. platinum plus or V18
- **Balloons and stents**: low-profile balloon expandable stent system 3–6 mm diameter, 12–15 mm length
- **Antispasmodic agents**: nifedipine, GTN
- **Closure device**: recommended.

Approach

Native kidneys: The majority of native renal artery lesions can be crossed from the femoral approach. The contralateral femoral may offer a slight advantage. If the renal artery passes steeply caudal, then consider the brachial or radial approach and use a forward-facing catheter, e.g. Berenstein.

　　Transplant renal artery stenosis: the approach should be decided based on the location of the proximal anastomosis and course of the proximal renal artery. The contralateral femoral approach is sometimes best, especially if the transplant has been anastomosed to the internal iliac artery.

Dilation Always measure the required balloon size, this can usually be assessed on the diagnostic imaging, take care not to measure an area of post-stenotic dilation. If the entire renal artery is dilated, measure the contralateral renal artery. In practice, most males require a 5–6 mm balloon, with small female patients needing 4–5 mm dilation. Warn the patient that it is normal to experience mild loin pain during angioplasty. Ask the patient to let you know when discomfort is felt and be careful if dilating more than this.

Outcomes

Primary technical success rates for renal artery angioplasty exceed 90% in most series; clinical success is considerably poorer and notoriously difficult to predict. Hypertensive patients are only 'cured' in 15–20% of cases, although blood pressure control is often improved. Typically, young patients with hypertension due to fibromuscular hyperplasia respond well and patients with unilateral disease do better than those with bilateral disease.

Complications

- **Transient renal insufficiency**: prevention is better than cure. Pre-hydrate the patient, give *N*-acetylcysteine; use carbon dioxide or iso-osmolar non-ionic contrast (Iodixanol) and minimize contrast volume; perform diagnostic and therapeutic examinations separately.
- **Flow-limiting dissection**: readily treated with stent insertion.
- **Vasospasm**: use oral nifedipine 10 mg as a pretreatment and intra-arterial GTN 100-mg aliquots.
- **Intrarenal embolization**: thrombus may be treated with in situ thrombolysis.
- **Renal artery rupture**: either secondary to overdilation or subintimal balloon passage. Re-inflate the balloon within the renal artery to tamponade the hole. Sometimes this is sufficient to allow a small defect to close. When this fails, reach for your friend the stent-graft and deploy it over the defect. If this does not work, leave the balloon inflated. It is good to have a strategy for this rare eventuality worked out before starting the procedure. Either embolize the kidney or call your ex-friend, the vascular surgeon. The warm ischaemia time for a kidney is fairly short (approximately 40 min) and therefore renal loss is likely.

- **Aortic dissection:** has been described. By this time, your nerves will be jangling. Call for back-up and if the dissection is symptomatic or flow-limiting, it should be treated with a stent.

Supra-aortic angioplasty and stenting

Roughly speaking, supra-aortic angioplasty and stenting can be divided into treatment of upper limb ischaemia and treatment of cerebral embolic disease and occasionally flow-limiting ischaemia (carotid and vertebral arteries). Each carries a risk of stroke. This is not the vascular territory to learn angioplasty and stenting.

Supra-aortic angioplasty consent issues

- Risk of causing cerebrovascular accident; approximately 5% for carotid angioplasty and stenting. Probably less for arm ischaemia. As with carotid endarterectomy, the patient may prefer medical treatment alone.

Upper limb angioplasty

Indications for treatment

Improved flow is required for patients with symptomatic arm ischaemia and in those requiring flow improvement for haemodialysis access.

Equipment

If working from the femoral approach check that balloons, stents, catheters and wires are long enough to reach. Typically this means ≥80 cm.

Approach

Stenoses are usually managed from the femoral approach, unless the morphology of the aortic arch looks challenging.

Occlusions are best approached from the brachial route and are frequently stented to minimize the risk of cerebral embolization. If you are concerned about placing a large sheath in the brachial artery, then consider a combined procedure, cross the occlusion using the brachial puncture but stent from the femoral artery.

Procedure

As with all procedures involving catheter and wire manipulation in the aortic arch, there is a risk of stroke, to keep this to a minimum:

- Make sure the patient is adequately heparinized.
- Use double-flush techniques and make sure never to inject unless there is free back flow of blood.

Patients with subclavian steal usually have retrograde flow in the vertebral artery; this might confer some degree of protection against cerebral embolization, at least until the lesion is treated. Some angiographers opt to protect the vertebral circulation with an additional balloon but there is no evidence for or against this practice.

Outcomes

Subclavian stenoses and occlusions can be successfully treated in 90% of patients and over 80% of patients have sustained clinical improvement at 3 years.

Carotid angioplasty

Indications for treatment

Evidence suggests that, in experienced hands, carotid stenting (CS) and carotid endarterectomy (CE) have similar outcomes in terms of prevention of stroke and similar complication rates of major stroke and death. It is essential to regard the two approaches as complementary to each other. Carotid stenting probably has the advantage when there is a 'hostile neck' due to surgery, local pathology or radiotherapy. Major complications of CS are more frequent in elderly patients.

Patients should be assessed in conjunction with a neurologist and carefully worked-up. Remember that carotid intervention is of the greatest benefit in those patients with recently symptomatic stenosis (within 2 weeks); clearly these patients also have the greatest risk of embolic events. Patients with crescendo transient ischaemic attack (TIA) or with visible thrombus are not suitable for carotid artery intervention.

Consent issues

The risk of major stroke or death is around 5% and this must be discussed in advance. Minor stroke is more common with CS but neck complications are more common with CE.

Equipment

All CS procedures should be performed using dedicated equipment intended for CS. Most systems use low-profile monorail balloons and stents and may incorporate a protection device such as a filter. Essentials include:

- Long sheath or introducer guide
- Angioplasty balloons for pre-dilatation of tight lesions and post stent dilation
- Carotid stent system
- ± Cerebral protection device.

Cerebral protection devices

There are a variety of devices on the market, they prevent cerebral emboli during CS procedures by:

- filtering the blood downstream of the stenosis catching major embolic material
- reversing flow in the internal carotid artery and returning any emboli to the venous circulation.

Each device has unique features and they are really far beyond the remit of a survival guide (Table 46.2).

Procedure

The key to success is obtaining a stable position in the common carotid artery. Before starting, obtain an MRA or CTA to assess the aortic arch and carotid arteries. If the aorta is unfolded and the carotid arteries are tortuous, seek expert guidance, as not all carotids can be treated by endovascular means.

Alarm: Patients should be started on clopidogrel (75 mg/day), a week before the procedure.

Table 46.2 Cerebral protection devices: pros and cons

Technique	Pros	Cons
Filter wire	Flow preserved throughout unless the filter becomes clogged, in which case it has done its job! Simple to deploy	No protection until the lesion is crossed with the device and it is fully deployed Needs to be appropriate size for the vessel Will still allow small emboli Can snag on the stent during retrieval, causing anxiety all round
Flow reversal	Actively prevents emboli travelling forward up the ICA to the brain	Requires intact circle of Willis (at least anterior communicating artery). This should be assessed on pre-procedure imaging Not tolerated by all patients; test occlusion of the ICA gives an indication of which patients may be suitable Cumbersome to deploy Requires increased sheath size

The basic principles of carotid angioplasty and stenting are set out below.

Ten key steps to carotid intervention

1. Obtain CFA access, fully heparinize the patient.
2. Catheterize the symptomatic common carotid artery and perform a lateral carotid angiogram.
3. Catheterize the distal external carotid artery and introduce a 260-cm length Amplatz wire (1-cm tip).
4. Introduce an 80-cm guide-catheter or reinforced sheath into the common carotid artery (CCA) and perfuse this from a bag of pressurized, heparinized saline, which is run slowly.
5. Place a coin of known diameter over the ipsilateral mandible close to but not obscuring the ICA. This is used to measure the diameter of the carotid artery. Perform another lateral carotid angiogram and measure the diameters of the ICA and CCA and the length of the diseased segment (Fig. 46.9).
6. Give atropine 1.2 mg into the sheath. This will cause the ipsilateral pupil to dilate. Warn the patient and ward staff that this is not a cause for concern.
7. Cross the stenosis with a steerable 0.014- or 0.018-inch guidewire. This may be part of the cerebral protection device if one is being used. Use a 3-mm balloon to pre-dilate lesions with a very tight stenosis.
8. Pass the stent across the lesion and deploy it and dilate to an appropriate diameter, usually 4–6 mm.

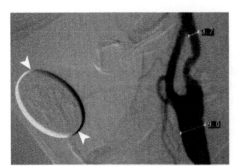

Fig. 46.9 ▦ Lateral view from a selective carotid angiogram. A 26-mm diameter metal disk (21p coin) is taped on the ipsilateral mandible (white arrowheads). This is used to calibrate the angiography machine for accurate measurement of the carotid artery for sizing the appropriate protection device and stent.

9. Perform a check angiogram to demonstrate the treatment site; carefully remove the cerebral protection device if one was used.
10. Use a closure device at the common femoral artery puncture site. This is a prime indication to use a closure device; large sheath, heparinized patient, clopidogrel.

Vertebral artery intervention

Indications for treatment

Vertebrobasilar insufficiency, this is usually a flow-related phenomenon. The lesions are typically short and focal; the proximal vertebral artery is by far the commonest site for disease, but occasionally stenoses are seen in the mid-vertebral or basilar arteries.

 Alarm: MIP images from carotid MRA tend to overcall vertebral artery stenosis, due to the orientation of the vessel orthogonal to the scan plane (check the next few you look at if you don't believe us). Always review the source images, which are much more reliable.

Consent issues

The risk of stroke is not well quantified and is probably in the range of 2–5%. Technical success rates are high for suitably chosen lesions. Clinical success is almost wholly dependent on the skill of the referring neurologist making the correct diagnosis of vertebrobasilar insufficiency.

Equipment

- Guide catheter or long sheath
- Low-profile angioplasty 3–5 mm balloons and stents – coronary artery stents are ideal for this as the vertebral artery origin is often tortuous.

Approach

The vertebral artery can be approached from the femoral or brachial approach.

Outcomes

Re-stenosis is not uncommon but can usually be treated again.

47

Treating acute limb ischaemia

Acute limb ischaemia describes a sudden reduction in perfusion of <3 days' duration. The ischaemia is usually due to thrombosis in native arteries or bypass grafts secondary to an underlying stenotic lesion. The severity of ischaemia is categorized using the Rutherford classification (Table 47.1). Patients with rest pain without neuromuscular complications (Rutherford grade IIa) are the optimal candidates for thrombolysis in terms of time available to restore flow and risk–benefit ratio.

The aim of thrombectomy and thrombolysis is to restore perfusion, and reveal the vascular anatomy by breaking down or extracting the blood clot. When the vessel has been cleared, an underlying lesion should be carefully looked for and treated or re-thrombosis is inevitable. The use of thrombolysis and thrombectomy in the management of dialysis access salvage and venous thrombosis (especially axillary vein and massive iliofemoral vein thrombosis) will be discussed elsewhere. The use of thrombolysis and thrombectomy in the specialist management of myocardial infarction and stroke is beyond the scope of this book.

Table 47.1 Clinical categories of acute limb ischaemia

| Category | Description | Capillary return | Muscle paralysis | Sensory loss | Doppler signal | |
					Arterial	Venous
I Viable	Not immediately threatened	Intact	None	None	+	+
IIa Threatened	Salvageable, if promptly treated	Intact/ slow	None	Partial	–	+
IIb Threatened	Salvageable, if immediately treated	Slow/ absent	Partial	Partial	–	+
III Irreversible	Amputation regardless of treatment	Absent	Complete	Complete	–	–

Modified from the Consensus Report on Thrombolysis. J Intern Med 1996; 240:343–355.

Thrombolysis

This is the use of drugs to break up a blood clot by breaking down the fibrin holding the clot together. Acute thrombosis is particularly likely to clear, thrombolysis is not usually clinically indicated >6 weeks after the thrombotic event. Several agents are licenced for use in thrombolysis and there is no randomized evidence of clinical superiority for any of these. In practice, the majority of thrombolysis is undertaken with tissue-plasminogen activator (rt-PA).

Indications for treatment

Acute or acute-on-chronic critical limb ischaemia due to:

- Acute native vessel thrombosis
- Bypass graft thrombosis.

Thrombosed popliteal aneurysm: the aim here is to clear the run-off vessels to allow bypass grafting.

Peri-procedural thrombolysis: thrombosis may occur during interventional procedures and surgery. Acute thrombus is particularly likely to clear, and thrombolysis may salvage the procedure.

Contraindications

Thrombolysis is not without risk, particularly bleeding and CVA; the risk–benefit ratio is so unfavourable in some patients that thrombolysis is contraindicated.
   Absolute contraindications:

- Irreversible ischaemia (Rutherford class III)
- Major trauma, surgery or cardiopulmonary resuscitation within the past 2 weeks
- Stroke within the last 2 months, primary or secondary cerebral tumour. Risk of cerebral haemorrhage. Note: this does not apply to hyperacute cerebrovascular accident (CVA) where the intention is to restore cerebral perfusion
- Active bleeding diathesis with the potential for major haemorrhage
- Pregnancy.

   Relative contraindications:

- Age >80 years; these patients have the highest risk of stroke and haemorrhagic complications
- The white limb (Rutherford class IIb) where urgent revascularization is required
- Graft thrombosis within 4 weeks of surgery. Early graft failure is almost always due to a technical problem with the surgery, e.g. poor-quality vein, graft kinking.
- Anticoagulation
- **Knitted Dacron grafts:** these rely on deposition of thrombus to be impermeable; hence they become porous during thrombolysis and marked extravasation may occur.
- **Vein graft:** the vein relies on perfusion for its viability, and after about 3 days, the vein is irreversibly damaged. However, the run-off may be cleared, allowing subsequent re-grafting. Recent thrombolysis with no underlying cause demonstrable. Re-thrombosis is very likely. Thrombolysis with streptokinase within the previous 5 years. This is only relevant if using streptokinase, as antibodies persist for many years and limit the effectiveness of the treatment, while increasing the risk of adverse reaction.
- **Cardiac emboli:** thrombolysis may lead to further embolization.

Consent issues

It is essential to discuss the risks of haemorrhage requiring transfusion or surgery in up to 7% of patients and CVA due to haemorrhage or thrombosis in 1–3%. There is some evidence that the risks are lower in younger patients but this reduction has not been quantified.

Equipment

There are different techniques for performing thrombolysis, and the equipment varies according to the strategy being used:

- Ultrasound to guide puncture
- Mini access kit
- Basic angiography set
- Infusion catheters: a 4F straight catheter with sideholes is suitable in most cases
- A pump suitable for arterial infusion
- Co-axial systems or microcatheters may be helpful
- Pulse spray techniques require special catheters and pumps.

Procedure

The key to thrombolysis is to establish the vascular anatomy; before starting, perform magnetic resonance angiography (MRA) or computed tomography angiography (CTA) to demonstrate the extent of the thrombosis, inflow anatomy and, with luck, the run-off vessels. Remember that you may need to obtain delayed images to see the distal circulation.

 Tip: Avoid unpleasant surprises by clarifying what bypass grafts are in situ. Look for operation notes and talk to the patient and a senior surgeon.

Approach

As always, the shortest most direct approach is usually the best, as it affords the greatest scope for adjunctive intervention. In some cases, the best approach will involve direct puncture of a bypass graft. Table 47.2 provides suggestions but these are not set in stone and you should consider the pros and cons of each approach in the context of the individual patient. If possible, avoid the brachial approach, as there is a risk of peri-catheter thrombus embolizing to cause CVA.

Table 47.2 Guidelines for best arterial access

Site of occlusion	Optimal arterial access
Iliac artery	Ipsilateral CFA if patent, otherwise contralateral CFA
CFA	Contralateral CFA or exceptionally brachial
SFA, PFA or femoropopliteal graft	Ipsilateral CFA
Femoro-femoral cross-over	Direct graft puncture or inflow CFA
Axillo-femoral graft	Consider surgery

Arterial puncture: At the risk of stating the obvious, try to make a single arterial puncture. Thrombolysis is sure to lead to bleeding from any extra puncture sites. This is a good time to use ultrasound to ensure safe arterial puncture. Use a mini access kit to keep the size of any unwanted holes to a minimum. Infra-inguinal grafts almost invariably arise from the anterior aspect of the common femoral artery (CFA). Arterial puncture must be sufficiently proximal to allow manipulation of a shaped catheter (Cobra or RDC) to direct a straight guidewire toward the graft origin.

 Tip: To catheterize the graft origin, it is often helpful to obtain an angiogram in a steep oblique projection. Use roadmapping or fluoroscopy fade if these options are available.

Direct prosthetic graft puncture: Ultrasound guidance is still the preferred option. When the graft is palpable, fix it between forefinger and thumb and then perform a single wall puncture in the conventional manner. There is a very distinctive give and fall in resistance as the needle enters the graft lumen. Depending on the direction of catheterization, direct graft puncture will preclude accessing either the origin or the outflow. Retrograde lysis often occurs but sometimes it is necessary to make a second puncture from the other end of the graft – the 'crossed catheter technique'.

Techniques and regimens

There are several different techniques used for performing thrombolysis, none has been shown to be superior to any of the others. Accelerated regimens may restore flow more rapidly but at the price of increased complication rates.

All the techniques share a common principle; the thrombolytic agent is delivered directly into the thrombus and this requires the delivery catheter to be embedded in the thrombus. This is only possible if a guidewire can be passed through the thrombus. Failing this 'guidewire traversal test' indicates that the thrombus is organized and hence is much less likely to clear with thrombolysis.

Infusion techniques

The simplest technique is to infuse the lytic agent through a straight catheter. The dosages given below are for rt-PA. Heparin (250 IU/h) is usually administered via the sheath to minimize the risk of peri-catheter thrombosis.

Low-dose infusion. rt-PA is infused directly into the thrombus at a rate of 0.5 mg/h (10 mg rt-PA in 500 mL of normal saline [0.02 mg/mL] run at 25 mL/h). The catheter tip is embedded into the proximal thrombus and the infusion started. Check angiography is performed every 6–8 h and the catheter is repositioned distally as necessary. This form of thrombolysis often takes 24–72 h.

 Tip: There is no need to perform check angiography overnight unless there is a clear clinical deterioration.

Bolus lacing followed by low-dose infusion. The catheter is advanced to the distal portion of the clot and then 5 mg of rt-PA is injected at high concentration (rt-PA 1 mg/mL) as the catheter is pulled back through the proximal clot. The bolus lacing is performed up to a total of three times (15 mg of rt-PA). A check angiogram is performed every 15–30 min. If thrombus persists after this, a low-dose infusion is initiated as above.

Bolus lacing followed by high-dose infusion. The technique is performed as above, but a high-dose infusion (rt-PA 10 mg in 100 mL, i.e. 0.1 mg/mL) is set up and run at 40 mL/h (4 mg/h) for up to 4 h. Check angiography is performed every 60–90 min. After this, a low-dose infusion is used if indicated.

Pulse spray techniques. These use special catheters with multiple sideholes or slits. The catheter endhole is occluded with a guidewire and the drug is injected through the side-arm of a Tuohy–Borst adaptor. Manual injections can be made using a 1-mL syringe but most operators favour using a dedicated pump to generate low-volume (e.g. 0.5 mL = 0.05 mg rt-PA) high-pressure pulses every 30 s. The theory is that the 'jets' macerate the thrombus and introduce the drug deeper into the clot and therefore speed up lysis.

Coaxial lysis. When there is extensive thrombus, a coaxial system allows the lytic agent to be delivered at more than one site. The simplest method is to infuse the drug through the arterial sheath into the proximal clot and through the catheter into the distal thrombus (Fig. 47.1). Microcatheters can be used to deliver the drug to the crural circulation.

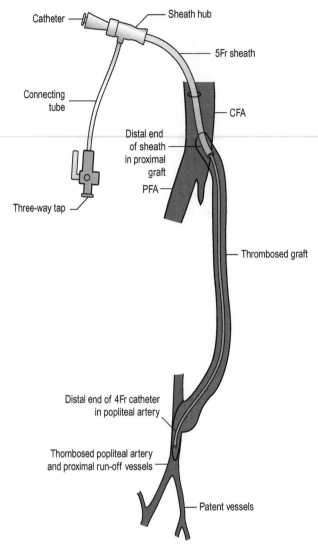

Catheter
Sheath hub
5Fr sheath
Connecting tube
CFA
Distal end of sheath in proximal graft
PFA
Three-way tap
Thrombosed graft
Distal end of 4Fr catheter in popliteal artery
Thombosed popliteal artery and proximal run-off vessels
Patent vessels

Fig. 47.1 ■ In the presence of extensive thrombus, the distal catheter is used to clear the run-off vessels, while the sheath delivers the lytic agent to the graft. It is essential to secure the catheter and sheath. Failure to do so invariably leads to inadvertent removal, and the subsequent haemorrhage is extremely difficult to control.

Procedural care

It is essential to liaise closely with the surgical team. Keep the treatment plan under review and be alert to the need for surgical or radiological intervention.

The patient is nursed in bed as flat as possible and may have a light diet unless surgery is imminent.

Close observation is essential to detect complications, most patients are cared for in a high-dependency area where their condition can be closely monitored. Confusion, agitation, tachycardia and hypotension indicate bleeding; if there is a change in the patient's mental state, the infusion should be stopped pending a thorough assessment.

The following must be checked:

- Arterial puncture sites every 15 min, looking for bleeding/haematoma
- Limb viability – perfusion, pulses, Doppler signal, movement and sensation

- Urine output – the patient must be kept adequately hydrated. If necessary, IV fluids should be given and the patient catheterized
- Pulse, BP and temperature – 4-hourly
- Daily full blood count (FBC), coagulation screen and fibrinogen, urea and electrolytes, glucose
- Analgesia should be reviewed regularly. Intramuscular injections must not be given.

Endpoints:

- If the patient's condition allows, thrombolysis is continued until the clot has cleared and flow has been restored. Try not to continue for more than 48 h.
- Lytic stagnation is when there is no clearing of thrombus in between check angiograms and is an indication to stop the procedure.
- Deterioration in the clinical status of the limb mandates urgent review and discussion and, depending on the cause, may necessitate urgent surgical revascularization.
- Significant bleeding is most common at the puncture site but most devastating when intracerebral (Fig. 47.2). If bleeding occurs, stop the infusion and review the patient immediately.

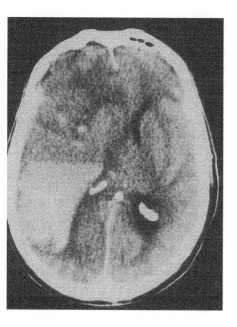

Fig. 47.2 ▪ Fatal acute haemorrhagic cerebral infarct during thrombolysis.

Adjunctive techniques

Successful thrombolysis usually reveals an underlying stenosis or occlusion. Failure to correct these lesions by endovascular or surgical means condemns the patient to re-thrombosis. Thrombolysis alone may not be sufficient to restore flow. The following techniques may be helpful:

- **Angioplasty and stenting**: used to treat stenoses and occlusions following thrombolysis. In high-risk patients it is worth considering directly stenting over thrombus (Fig. 47.3).
- **Thrombo-aspiration**: see later.
- **Surgical intervention**: embolectomy may be needed if there is distal embolization during thrombolysis. Fasciotomy is indicated if a compartment syndrome develops; this is most likely when there has been prolonged ischaemia and is recognized by painful swollen muscle, often with paralysis. If there is any suggestion of a compartment syndrome, make sure that the surgical team is aware and that they measure the compartment pressures.

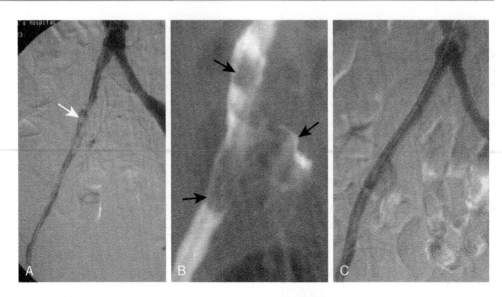

Fig. 47.3 ▪ (A) Acute critical limb ischaemia with near occlusion of the right iliac artery (white arrow). (B) Non-subtracted view clearly demonstrates saddle embolus (arrows) at the right iliac bifurcation. (C) The patient was warfarinized and had recently had a CVA, hence primary stenting was performed and a closure device used.

Bypass grafting or graft revisions are performed when thrombolysis reveals underlying disease that is not amenable to endovascular treatment.

 Tip: Be very, very careful if considering angioplasty when residual thrombus can still be seen. It is very easy to embolize loosely adherent residual thrombus with disastrous consequences. It may be better to anticoagulate the patient and wait for the residual thrombus to clear before angioplasty.

Complications

Unfortunately, complications of thrombolysis are not rare and may be life-threatening. Complications increase with the age of the patient, the duration of treatment and the dose of the lytic agent. Stop the infusion and the heparin if a complication develops.

- **CVA:** perform an urgent CT scan if there are signs suggestive of CVA (Fig. 47.2). If there is thrombotic CVA, seek expert neurological opinion and discuss whether to continue with thrombolysis; haemorrhage means game over.
- **Puncture site haematoma:** perform manual compression, check that the sheath has not been displaced and consider exchanging for a larger sheath.
- **Significant bleeding:** consult a haematologist for advice if bleeding persists after the infusion is stopped. Check the clotting and try to intervene early before the patient becomes unstable. Resuscitate the patient with blood and fresh frozen plasma (FFP) as necessary. Surgical intervention may be required.
- **Acute clinical deterioration with increased pain:** reassess, this is often due to distal embolization of thrombus which occurs in up to 5% of patients. Macroemboli may lyse spontaneously or can be aspirated. Microemboli are much more serious and may cause trash foot.
- **Reperfusion syndrome:** this is caused when there has been prolonged and severe ischaemia. Adult respiratory distress syndrome and renal failure are common sequelae and there is a high mortality.

Thrombosuction

Thrombus aspiration is the endovascular equivalent of balloon embolectomy, thrombus/embolus is sucked into a catheter and removed. The technique is limited by the size of catheter and sheath.

Indications

Typically, the technique is used to clear small distal emboli but may be used as an adjunct to thrombolysis to accelerate reperfusion when there is a large volume of thrombus to clear.

Thrombosuction is relatively safe in prosthetic grafts that have a large smooth lumen and do not collapse when they thrombose (Fig. 47.4). The catheter can be safely manipulated without a guidewire. The situation is different in diseased native vessels where repeated catheter passage is undesirable.

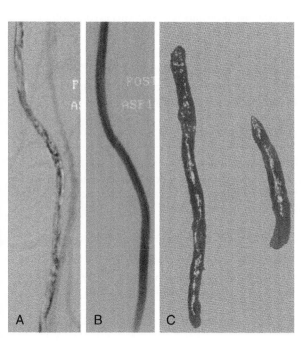

Fig. 47.4 ▣ (A) Thrombosed PTFE graft following thrombosuction with an 8F catheter (B). (C) Some of the thrombus removed.

Equipment

- Sheath with removable haemostatic valve, otherwise the thrombus simply gets stripped off by the valve of the sheath during catheter removal.
- Large lumen catheters, e.g. 7F straight guide-catheter (6F lumen) for prosthetic graft and native SFA; 5F catheter (4F lumen) for native popliteal and crural vessels.
- 50-mL syringe.

Procedure

Access: Ipsilateral arterial access is essential.

Catheterization: The vessel is catheterized in the conventional manner but a removable hub sheath is used.

Technique: The aspiration catheter is embedded into the proximal occlusion and then the 50 mL syringe is attached. Pull back the syringe plunger to create a vacuum and advance the catheter until it occludes with thrombus. Maintain suction and withdraw the catheter. When the catheter reaches the sheath, the hub is removed; this prevents thrombus trapping on the haemostatic valve as the catheter is taken out. Brisk arterial backflow immediately follows, so quickly put a finger over the sheath until the valve is replaced. Flush the contents of the catheter/syringe through a gauze cloth to allow examination. The procedure is repeated as often as necessary until the vessel is clear.

Troubleshooting

Thrombus cannot be aspirated: There are two main causes:

- The thrombus is old; try again after a bolus of thrombolysis to soften the thrombus
- The catheter/sheath is kinked at the arterial puncture site: replace the sheath and try again, keeping it under slight tension as the catheter is pulled back.

A central core of thrombus is removed but extensive thrombus remains: This is common in artificial grafts and is a limitation of the technique; use adjunctive thrombolysis to clear residual thrombus.

Thrombus embolizes distally: This is a pitfall of the technique; advancing a large catheter can 'bulldoze' thrombus distally and may even impact it in a distal vessel. Try thrombolysis to clear the blockage and consider surgical embolectomy if necessary.

Mechanical thrombectomy

Mechanical thrombectomy uses special catheters to macerate the thrombus (Fig. 47.5). The residue is either small enough to pass through the distal circulation or is aspirated. The catheter has to be appropriately sized for the vessel and large sheaths may be necessary. These devices work best with fresh thrombus and small acute emboli.

Equipment

There are several commercially available devices:

- **Rheolytic catheters** (Fig. 47.5): these devices utilize an injection pump to create a high-velocity saline jet, which produces a zone of low pressure at the catheter tip. Thrombus is

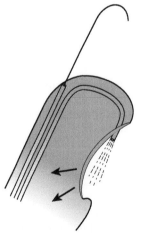

Fig. 47.5 ■ Rheolytic mechanical thrombectomy catheter. A high-pressure jet creates a vortex, sucking in thrombus and removing the slurry via the exhaust port.

sucked into the jet and is broken up. The resultant slurry is cleared through the catheter into a drainage bag. Some of these devices do not operate over a guidewire and hence they cannot be steered except with a guide-catheter.

- **Fragmentation baskets**: these devices are essentially like a miniature egg whisk powered by battery, that breaks up thrombus. The basket is made of nitinol and inserted collapsed within a covering catheter through a short 7F sheath over a 0.014-inch wire. The most common application is in dialysis grafts. Use only in larger veins and be careful as vein size reduces, or near stents, etc., as these can easily get tangled up in the device with disappointing results.
- **Catheters combining ultrasound and thrombolysis**: these specialized catheters deliver lower-dose lysis with ultrasound to aid drug penetration through clot fibrin. The evidence base for this technology and its role compared with conventional systemic lysis and catheter lysis is still developing.

Procedure

Access: Ipsilateral puncture is necessary.

Catheterization: A standard vascular sheath is used.

Technique: Rheolytic devices are switched on just proximal to the thrombus and then advanced slowly into the occlusion. It helps to advance the catheter only a few centimetres and then pull it back and repeat the procedure. This is continued until the vessel is clear. Some manufacturers advocate inflating a blood pressure cuff around the limb distal to an occlusion to prevent distal embolization.

Fragmentation baskets are confusingly the reverse in use. The catheter containing the constrained basket is advanced beyond the thrombus then the catheter pulled back to allow the basket to open. The battery-powered impeller is started and the device slowly withdrawn. It is vital that you slowly withdraw the rotating basket – advancing while the basket is rotating is not recommended. If you want a second run at it, collapse the basket by carefully advancing the outer catheter before advancing the device.

Troubleshooting

The catheter will not pass down the vessel: If there is stenosis or occlusion blocking the way, treat with angioplasty. If the vessel is tortuous, try directing the catheter with a guide-catheter.

The catheter has been kinked and the drive shaft has fractured: Keep the catheter as straight as possible because once kinked, it is useless.

The catheter clears a central core but leaves residual thrombus: This is a limitation of the technique. Ensure that the catheter is correctly sized for the vessel – an 8F Amplatz thrombectomy device is necessary for the SFA and most grafts; the 6F device is suitable for the popliteal artery. Consider adjunctive thrombolysis to clear any remaining thrombus and distal emboli.

The device does not clear the thrombus: Unfortunately, this is not rare – check that the device is activated properly. If it is, then the thrombus is probably too organized to break down; consider other techniques.

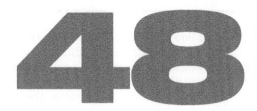

Treating aneurysmal disease

Aneurysms can affect vessels of any size. Clearly, not every aneurysm requires immediate treatment but, when indicated, successful endovascular management requires exclusion of the aneurysm from the circulation. The main options can broadly be thought of as:

Embolization techniques which sacrifice the target vessels: This is only used when it is safe to occlude part of the circulation, i.e. there is a collateral pathway or the end target can be sacrificed; this will be covered in detail in the management of haemorrhage section.

Techniques that preserve flow through the target vessel:
- Stent-grafting to restore a normal-calibre lumen. Most often used in larger-calibre vessels (>6 mm)
- Packing the sac with coils sometimes combined with stenting across the aneurysm. This technique is most commonly used to manage aneurysms in the cerebral circulation and is a useful adjunct in the visceral arteries where flow must be preserved and a stent graft cannot be used.

Each of these strategies has its place and, as always, the real skill lies in choosing who, when and how to treat. There is not enough space to cover the nuances of every clinical scenario and each device, so the emphasis here is on the generic aspects of terminology, assessment for stent-grafting and the basic principles of deployment of devices.

Aneurysm terminology

As a general rule, a region is deemed aneurysmal when it is at least 1.5× greater than the adjacent, normal arterial segment. When commenting on less dilated vessels, consider using 'ectatic' rather than 'aneurysmal'; this generates less alarm and work. Aneurysms are classified and discussed in several ways.

Morphology: Useful really only as a descriptive term.
- Fusiform – a roughly symmetrical swelling of an artery
- Saccular – an asymmetric outpouching from the artery wall.

Aetiology: An important consideration when deciding treatment.
- Degenerative/atheromatous: commonest type, usually age-related
- Infective/mycotic: often irregularly shaped with adjacent inflammatory change
- Inflammatory: classically abdominal aorta with evidence of thickening of vessel wall and lack of separation between aneurysm and adjacent structures

- Traumatic: more often saccular and associated with other injuries, presentation may be delayed
- Abnormal connective tissue: often multiple sites, e.g. Ehlers–Danlos.

Structure: 'True' or 'False' aneurysm?

True aneurysms involve all the layers of the artery wall, these have a more predictable prognosis, e.g. risk of rupture of an abdominal aortic aneurysm (AAA) increases with increasing diameter.

False aneurysms (*aka* pseudoaneurysms) form due to a defect in the artery wall and the blood is constrained only by adjacent soft tissue, e.g. following trauma such as arterial puncture. The absence of a wall makes a false aneurysm prone to catastrophic rupture.

 Alarm: Improved technology makes more aneurysms amenable to treatment by endovascular means; it does not follow that all aneurysms need to be treated or that the endovascular approach is the best option for the patient.

When to treat aneurysms?

Aneurysms are more frequently detected now due to the prevalence of multislice computed tomography (CT). Many will be incidental findings. The threshold for intervention varies depending on the size, site, the anticipated impact of rupture and our level of knowledge about the benefits and risks of intervention. Diameter thresholds for treating aortic and thoracic aneurysms are well established, fairly well agreed for visceral aneurysms and some larger vessel peripheral aneurysms but for smaller aneurysms, the natural history is often uncertain. Guidelines and treatment thresholds (Table 48.1) are a useful starting point but management decisions will also reflect other factors including aetiology, symptomatology and speed of aneurysm growth. Patients with a symptomatic, very large or rapidly growing aneurysms are at increased risk of rupture and may have a greater benefit from treatment. Case-by-case discussion is essential, especially for less common scenarios.

Table 48.1 Accepted thresholds for intervention[a]

Thoracic aorta	55 mm if atherosclerotic; 45 mm if Marfans[b]
Abdominal aorta	55 mm or growth rate >10 mm year
Iliac	40 mm
Popliteal	12 mm
Visceral aneurysms	20 mm in diameter or larger in women beyond childbearing age and in men

[a]*Excludes cerebral/cardiac aneurysms*
[b]*From European Guidelines.*

Guidance for imaging prior to endovascular repair

Endovascular aneurysm repair requires far more detailed assessment than is necessary for open surgery. Computed tomography with multiplanar reconstructions is the method of choice and is able to accurately measure the diameters, lengths and angulation of the aneurysm, anchorage sites and the access vessels (Figs 48.1, 48.2).

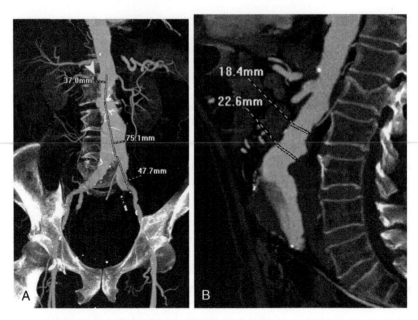

Fig. 48.1 ▦ Use of CT to assess AAA suitability for EVAR. (A) Coronal MIP allowing lengths to be assessed. The yellow arrowhead indicates level of the renal arteries. (B) Sagittal MIP showing angulation of the neck.

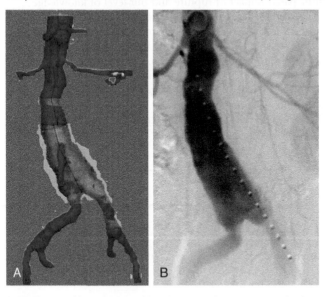

Fig. 48.2 ▦ (A) CT reformat and (B) calibrated angiogram of a patient with AAA.

Tip: Use suitably wide windows when reviewing the images to allow you to distinguish between calcification in the vessel wall and contrast enhancement in the lumen.

Imaging assessment

What to look for?

The variety of scenarios and devices makes it impossible to be dogmatic and each manufacturer has their own restrictions in the 'indications for use' for the device; if in doubt check with the 'sizing chart'. There are however some general points to consider:

Access: Usually the common femoral and iliac arteries.

Stent grafts are relatively large and inflexible devices. Check the size (≈French size/3), currently available devices for endovascular abdominal aortic aneurysm repair (EVAR) are introduced via ≈18–28F (6–9 mm) sheaths. Ask yourself whether it will be possible to introduce the device (percutaneously or by surgical cut down) into the chosen access vessel and advance it from there to the target. Normal vessels will usually straighten with a stiff wire but heavily calcified, narrow and tortuous vessels are unlikely to be winners. In the presence of significant disease, review alternative points of access.

 Tip: If there is uncertainty whether a calcified artery will straighten, perform a test catheterization using the stiff wire needed for EVAR.

 Alarm: Severe disease in the common femoral artery (CFA), iliac arteries or anywhere else en route is likely to be problematic for either introducing or removing the delivery system.

Anchorage: *At either end of the aneurysmal segment (aka neck).* Secure fixation is essential to forming a seal. Failure to achieve this will lead to type I endoleak or graft migration! The ideal neck is straight, parallel-sided, disease-free and of suitable diameter and length to allow a seal. Atheroma, calibre discrepancy and tapered necks will make deployment more challenging. Too short and you will risk occluding branch vessels or landing in the sac.

 Alarm: Significantly oversized grafts may not seal due to folds in the graft material.

Target site: *Is the target artery straight or tortuous?* Ask yourself whether the graft can be delivered to the target and whether it is sufficiently flexible to conform to the arterial anatomy. If not, ask yourself what will happen if the stent graft straightens out the vessel?

 Alarm: There is a real risk of kinking at the end of the stent graft leading to occlusion.

Aneurysm sac

Wall: Look for evidence of inflammatory change including thickening and loss of fat planes.

Diameter: This will serve as a baseline for comparison with evolution during follow-up.

Thrombus: It is also customary to note the degree of thrombus within the sac. In general, the greater the amount of thrombus, the fewer branch vessels arising from the sac.

Branch vessels: *Are there any branch arteries arising from the target area?* As the stent graft will cover them they will either occlude, leading to ischaemia, or alternatively they may compromise repair by retrograde perfusion of the aneurysm (type II endoleak). In either case, ask yourself: can these be safely sacrificed if they are occluded or by pre-emptive embolization?

Aortic disease

Endovascular abdominal aortic aneurysm repair (EVAR) and thoracic EVAR are the commonest stent-graft procedures. Ruptured abdominal aortic aneurysm (AAA) carries a 75%

mortality, roughly half the patients die within 30 min and a further 50% will die despite undergoing repair. Hence, the management strategy aims to prevent rupture by screening to identify patients with asymptomatic AAA and then following up until they reach a diameter of 5.5 cm, show accelerated growth or become symptomatic.

The majority of infrarenal abdominal aortic aneurysms are secondary to atherosclerotic disease. Rarer, but still seen with reasonable frequency, are inflammatory aneurysms; surgical dissection can be difficult in these patients and endovascular repair is often preferred if possible. Even rarer are mycotic aneurysms; they are often diagnosed by a combination of unusual site/morphology and a good history. Decision-making is complex and will depend on the underlying cause and prognosis. Treatment is usually considered when aneurysm diameter is >55 mm or becomes symptomatic or fast-growing (10 mm/year). As well as CT, the patient should undergo physiological assessment of cardiorespiratory function to assess suitability for EVAR. Patients with an asymptomatic infrarenal AAA >5.5 cm in diameter who are deemed 'fit enough for surgery' should be offered treatment by EVAR or open surgery. Patients who are judged unfit for surgery are unlikely to live long enough to benefit from aneurysm repair and should be managed conservatively.

Assessment for EVAR

When assessing the aorta, before making measurements, use the guidance for imaging and make a rapid review of factors that will preclude or may complicate EVAR and consider possible solutions. These include:

Access issues

Small CFA/iliac artery <7 mm
Solutions: Consider the use of a temporary graft conduit to allow device delivery.

Tortuous, calcified vessels especially with more than one ≥90 degree angulation
Solutions: Angioplasty for focal stenosis, consider alternative access for more extensive disease, e.g. cutdown onto the iliac arteries ± placement of a temporary conduit.

Narrow distal aorta This can prevent access for a contralateral iliac limb or cause narrowing of both limbs of a bifurcated graft. Prevention is better than cure!

Solutions: Consider an aorto-uni-iliac (AUI) graft and femoro-femoral cross-over graft, but do not forget to occlude the contralateral common iliac with an Amplatzer plug to prevent type II endoleak.

Short, angulated, tapered and diseased anchorage sites
Length: Should be ≥10 mm for the proximal neck but limits vary from device to device.

Configuration
- Angulation: Ideally should be ≤60 degrees, though some devices will cope with greater angles

 Tip: If the neck is short and angulated, then use reformats to assess the optimal obliquity to use for angiography/fluoroscopy during graft deployment.

- **Shape:** Ideally the neck should be parallel-sided. If conical, does the diameter increase or decrease towards the aneurysm?

Alarm: Short cone-shaped necks which enlarge towards the aneurysm increase the risk of migration.

- **Neck quality:** Thrombus, eccentric calcification or atheroma can impact on sealing. Usually recorded as 25%, 50%, 75% of the circumference.

Solutions: In theory, most issues with the proximal neck can be remedied by the use of grafts with suprarenal fixation (Fig. 48.3), fenestrated grafts which have a greater contact with the wall or branched grafts, which anchor proximally in the 'normal' aorta. In practice, consider whether this will be better for the patient than an open repair.

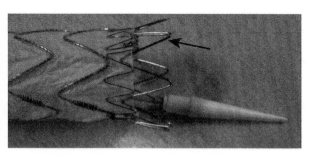

Fig. 48.3 ■ Graft with anchor stent (arrow) proximal to graft material.

Branch vessels

Review the imaging, looking for expected and variant anatomy:

- **Important branches:** decide whether the vessel is essential, e.g. hypertrophied inferior mesenteric artery (IMA) in the presence of superior mesenteric artery (SMA) disease or if it can be sacrificed, e.g. a small accessory renal artery.
- **Unwanted vessels:** decide whether pre-procedure embolization will improve outcome and treat as required.

Measurements for EVAR

With conventional bifurcated and aorto-uni-iliac (or AUI as the 'cool' operators term them) devices, roughly one-third of patients with AAAs will be straightforward to treat. A further 30–50% will be treatable but would be expected to be more challenging with limited implantation sites, awkward angulations or difficulty with access. Such cases will be higher risk with less certain long-term outcomes. These should only be undertaken after careful consideration by the clinical teams and discussion with the patient. Juxtarenal, suprarenal and thoracoabdominal aneurysms are treatable but their management should be undertaken in tertiary centres and is beyond the scope of this book.

For AAA repair, it is conventional to know the following measurements:

Aorta proximal neck

Remember to note any thrombus/atheroma.

Diameters (mm): Check whether your device recommends inner wall to inner wall or outer wall to outer wall. Remember to obtain these perpendicular to the centreline or you will overestimate. Form an opinion whether the neck is parallel-sided or if it tapers.

Centreline length (mm): This is measured in the centre of the lumen from the level of the bottom edge of the lowest renal artery you intend to preserve to the point at which the neck starts to expand into the aneurysm. This can be difficult to determine on a conical neck which expands distally. If <10 mm long, this is probably not suitable for conventional EVAR. Longer than 15 mm is straightforward.

Angulation (degrees): This is deviation measured from the centreline of the upper abdominal aorta.

Aorta

Remember to note the presence of patent vessels and thrombus.

Length from lowest renal artery to aortic bifurcation (mm): This is the sum of the neck length plus the centreline from the neck to division of the aorta.

Distal aortic diameter (mm): Remember there needs to be enough space to accommodate either an AUI or both limbs of a bifurcated stent graft.

Sac diameter (cm): As long as there is an indication for treatment, this has little relevance other than as a baseline to measure subsequent evolution.

Distal anchorage sites

Diameters (mm): Both common iliac arteries for a bifurcated device. Measured proximal, mid and distal. If the CIA is aneurysmal, then the target site becomes the EIA.

Length (mm): Both common iliac arteries from their origin to the internal iliac artery or to the EIA if the CIA is aneurysmal.

Access

Diameters (mm) of CFA and EIA: Remember to note if the vessels are calcified as well as diseased.

Specific consent issues

Remember that the principal advantage in using stent-grafting to treat AAA is reduced physiological stress during the procedure (no aortic cross-clamping, less peripheral ischaemia, reduced blood loss) and also a shorter convalescence (no abdominal wound).

Death: The operative mortality for conventional EVAR in a 'fit' patient is 1–2%, approximately one-third that of open surgery. This initial survival benefit decreases with time, largely due to cardiovascular mortality.

Occlusion of important vessels: This may result in the need for dialysis, bowel or pelvic ischaemia and may require emergency surgery to restore flow or explant the device.

Durability: Improved stent-graft technology has resulted in increased durability, however, EVAR patients still require imaging follow-up to detect complications, such as endoleak, device migration or stent fracture. The benefits conferred by improved durability may be offset by the fact that patients with more challenging anatomy are now selected for EVAR.

Aneurysm exclusion with a straight stent graft

Less than 10% of AAA will be suited to a straight graft. The main use for tube grafts will be the treatment of thoracic aortic pathologies, arterial rupture, iliac aneurysm and false aneurysm repair (Fig. 48.4). If you are considering using a tube graft, as opposed to an AUI device, it is worth reviewing the case again as repair with a bifurcated device may prove more durable.

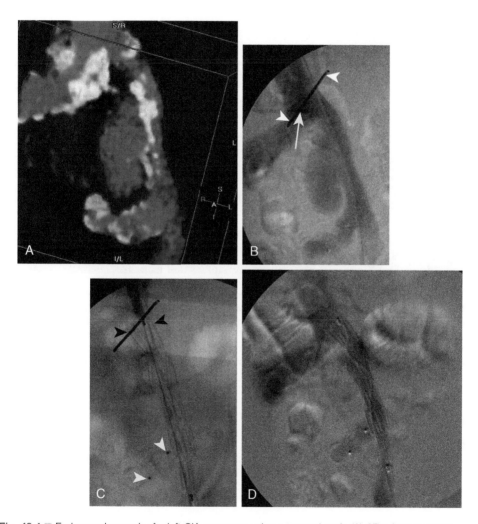

Fig. 48.4 ▪ Endovascular repair of a left CIA aneurysm using a tapered graft. (A) CT reformat shows morphology, allows accurate sizing and appropriate view. (B, C) Photographs of the angiographic display showing chinagraph pencil (white arrowheads) marking the target drop zone; the proximal CIA is shown by the yellow arrow. (C) A stent graft has been deployed according to the marker. Note the Amplatzer device (yellow arrowheads) occluding the IIA. (D) Completion angiogram showing exclusion of the aneurysm. Note that the graft is flush with the origin of the CIA and only appears to overlap the contralateral CIA.

The principles for deploying a stent graft in the aorta are no different from accurately deploying a stent. The safest place to learn positioning and deployment technique for a specific device is to insert the contralateral iliac limb during a bifurcated stent graft.

Deployment of a modular bifurcated stent graft

This is a complex practical procedure (Fig. 48.5) that requires a well-integrated team of vascular surgeons and radiologists and cannot be learnt from a book. Training usually commences on a simulated aneurysm before performing in vivo deployment. The general concept of graft deployment will be considered but details of individual devices will not be included.

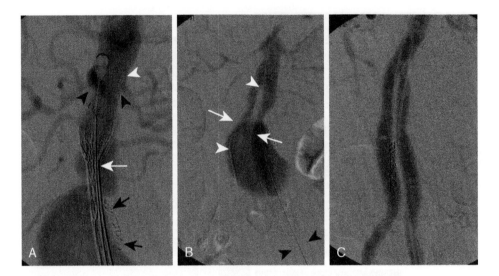

Fig. 48.5 ■ Stages in deployment of an aortic stent graft. (A) CO_2 angiogram through a Cobra catheter positioned just above the renal arteries (white arrowhead). The graft is partly open, the upper stent crowns (black arrowheads) are immediately below the renal arteries and the graft has been deployed as far as the white arrow. Note coils in the IMA (black arrows). (B) Angiogram following deployment of the body and ipsilateral limb (black arrowheads). The catheter (white arrowheads) has been pulled back and used to cannulate the contralateral limb (white arrows) of the stent graft. (C) Completion angiogram showing aneurysm exclusion.

 Stent-graft deployment: a step-by-step guide

Phase 1: Surgical pause

Confirm the plan for deployment, approach, choice of graft/s, and any anticipated difficulties. Confirm that you have all the kit you anticipate needing and any back-up equipment – balloons, wires, snares, stents, catheters and additional stent grafts/extensions.

Phase 2: Access

Percutaneous treatment requires initial placement of a suture closures (see Ch. 37). Surgical cutdown is the commonest approach to access the CFA to allow introducer placement. Vascular slings are placed around the upper CFA, the superficial femoral artery (SFA) and profunda femoris artery (PFA), as well as any large branches. Tightening these maintains haemostasis.

A 6F sheath is inserted into each CFA. Ensure that there is room for you to hold the artery between two fingers above the puncture. This will allow you to support the vessel during graft insertion and compress it for haemostasis during exchanges. A catheter is passed from the ipsilateral CFA into the thoracic aorta; negotiating out of the aneurysm can be harder than you might expect. A highly supportive 260-cm guidewire is passed into the thoracic aorta just distal to the arch (note the position of the back end of the wire on the drapes), as this will give you an indication that the tip remains in the correct place as opposed to the left ventricle or carotid artery! This wire will be used to insert the stent graft.

Phase 3: Positioning

Place a pigtail catheter at the level of the renal arteries from the contralateral sheath and perform initial angiography to demonstrate the neck and renal arteries. Use the predetermined oblique projection from the preoperative CT.

Before you insert the stent graft into the patient use fluoroscopy to demonstrate the graft markers and ensure that it is correctly oriented – it can be almost impossible to rotate the delivery system once it is in the patient! Insert the delivery system until the top of the graft (covered stent) is just above the renal arteries. Perform a magnified angiogram to demonstrate the position of the renal arteries. The table is locked in position and the exact level of the lowest renal artery is marked on the monitor.

Tip: Make sure that you support the femoral artery with your fingers while introducing the stent graft or large sheaths.

Phase 4: Deployment of the body

Using continuous fluoroscopy, start deployment of the stent graft just above the renal arteries. As the graft starts to open, perform fine positioning so that deployment of the upper graft fabric will be immediately below the lowest artery you are intending to preserve. Perform additional runs as needed, to confirm position. Remember you can still do this if you are using the catheter and wire in the renal artery. Fully deploy the aortic component of the graft; this will normally include the ipsilateral iliac arterial limb.

Phase 5: Removal of the delivery catheter

Re-sheath the nose cone of the delivery device in accordance with the manufacturer's instructions – this often requires advancing the delivery system a few centimetres above the graft to avoid entanglement. Remove the initial introducer system and use your fingers to control haemostasis. Either leave a sheath in position or immediately insert a secondary device if required. Remember, haemostasis can be achieved around smaller devices by tightening the arterial sling.

Phase 6: Deployment of the contralateral limb

The contralateral iliac limb stump must now be catheterized. If you are intending to preserve the IIA, now is the time to check where it is by performing a suitably angulated angiogram. Insert the contralateral limb deployment system and line up markers to ensure sufficient overlap with the body of the graft and avoid covering the IIA. Deploy the contralateral iliac limb.

Phase 7: Completion angiography

This is sometimes a misnomer, as this can be the *start* of all the trouble! Perform check angiography with a regular guidewire in situ to allow the arteries to revert to their normal configuration.

Troubleshooting

There are four categories of problem: malposition, poor flow, stenoses and endoleak.

Malposition of the graft

Graft too high: This usually means that the graft covers one or both of the renal arteries. If both renal arteries are occluded, there is little time to re-establish flow before irreversible damage ensues. Here are the options – none are attractive:

- Accept the situation and the need for lifelong renal replacement therapy.
  Generally do not give up without a fight unless it is clear that there is no realistic chance of recovering renal function.
- Endovascular treatment: Place a catheter from the arm and try to probe around the graft to access the renal artery. If you are successful, place a stent to hold the graft away from the ostium. Set a time limit of 10 min for this, with the option of trying surgery if unsuccessful. If surgery is not an option, then continue for up to 30 min.

 Tip: If there is a protection wire in the renal artery, you may be able to use this to inflate a balloon between the graft and the aortic wall to allow some flow and buy time.

- Surgical bypass: this may be the best option in expert hands but there is a high morbidity. This will probably only be attempted if both renal arteries are covered. Do not return to try endovascular techniques if the kidney is dead.

Graft too low: This causes two problems:

- *Insufficient anchorage*: this is associated with early failure due to migration or type I endoleak and late failure due to further expansion of the neck and endoleak. Unless the neck is several centimetres long, it is normal to deploy a cuff to extend to the desired position just below the renal arteries.
- *Distal coverage of the internal iliac artery origin*: if this is unilateral, it can probably be left as it is. If there is no flow in either internal iliac artery, then intervention may benefit to prevent buttock claudication. It may be possible to pass a wire alongside the graft and into the artery to allow a stent to be placed.

Abnormal flow through the graft

In practice, this means flow is very slow, which is almost always due to lack of outflow around the large sheaths. This is inevitable if the internal iliac arteries have been occluded. The easiest trick here is to simulate run-off, simply attach a 20-mL syringe to the side-arm of the sheaths and aspirate during the contrast injection. Occasionally close the arteriotomy leaving a smaller sheath in situ to perform angiography and stenting.

Stenoses

Problems occur at three sites: in the renal arteries, in the graft limbs in the distal aorta and in the run-off vessels.

Renal artery stenosis: This is almost always due to the graft being too high. Unless the coverage is minimal stent the origin open.

There is significant narrowing of the iliac limbs in the distal aorta: This is a consequence of the aorta being too narrow to accommodate both graft limbs. Measure pressures and if there is a gradient, then perform kissing balloon angioplasty and consider stenting with strong balloon-mounted stents.

Tight bend/kinks just beyond the stent graft: These occur in tortuous vessels which have been straightened by the stiff guidewires. Kinking can restrict flow and lead to thrombosis, in which case stenting is mandatory.

 Tip: Investigate stenoses or kinks with pressure measurements and treat significant pressure gradients to prevent subsequent thrombosis.

Distal run-off: Sometimes stenoses have not been appreciated on the pre-procedure imaging but mostly this is a result of damage due to passage of sheaths and the stent-graft delivery system. Treat by stenting as you would any iliac artery disease.

Endoleaks

This is contrast seen outside the graft within the sac. Decide whether it is:

- **Type I:** Leak around the graft anchorage points. If the graft is too low, then an extension cuff will probably be needed to create a seal. If the graft is in the correct position, initial management is to try moulding a balloon. If this does not work, large leaks are usually treated by placing a large balloon-expandable stent in the neck. If a large leak persists, the aneurysm has not been treated and conversion to an open repair will be needed. Smaller type I leaks may be left, as they will sometimes seal once the anticoagulation wears off. Early follow-up imaging is required to confirm this; intervention will be required for persistent leaks.
- **Type II:** Via collateral vessels, lumbar arteries and IMA. You knew about these from the pre-procedure imaging and chose not to embolize, so can safely ignore them now. If they persist at follow-up they can be dealt with if required.
- **Type III:** Limb dislocation. This is uncommon but easily rectified as long as you still have a wire access, simply insert another limb to bridge the gap. If the wire has been removed it may be challenging to re-catheterize, particularly if the two ends overlap.
- **Type IV:** Leakage through the graft material due to porosity. This will settle when the heparin wears off.

Aorto-uni-iliac systems

AUI systems are used less frequently than bifurcated grafts. They are still used occasionally:

- In the presence of unilateral iliac artery occlusion
- When the CIAs are so aneurysmal that a seal is not possible (see below)
- In a small-calibre distal aortic neck
- In emergency EVAR, as they allow more rapid control of the leaking AAA (Fig. 48.6).

Procedure

The graft deployment steps are similar to deploying the body of a bifurcated system. Unless there is unilateral iliac occlusion, the patient normally also requires femoro-femoral cross-over grafting and occlusion of the contralateral common iliac artery.

EVAR in patients with common iliac artery aneurysms

When it is impossible to achieve a seal in the CIA but EVAR is still judged to be the best option for the patient, this can be managed in several ways.

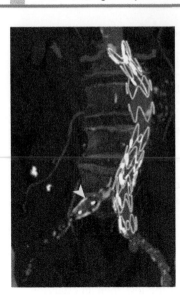

Fig. 48.6 ▓ AUI stent graft in a patient with a narrow distal aorta. Note the Amplatzer plug in the contralateral CIA (yellow arrowhead). A left-to-right cross-over graft supplies the right leg.

- Using branched grafts to preserve internal iliac artery flow. Elegant and attractive but more expensive and less commonly used.
- Ipsilateral internal iliac artery sacrifice; femoro-femoral cross-over and contralateral external-to-internal iliac artery stent graft.

Emergency endovascular abdominal aortic aneurysm repair (E-EVAR)

This is the repair of ruptured aneurysms, and traumatic aortic injury is a specialist service and is only practicable in centres with rapidly available experienced teams, appropriate facilities and extensive stock. The only difference between E-EVAR and conventional EVAR is having an occlusion balloon to control bleeding. The trick is to be able to maintain/obtain balloon occlusion at any time during the procedure. This requires initial placement of an occlusion balloon through a long sheath into the aorta above the aneurysm.

There are two distinct scenarios in the context of rupture:

The patient is haemodynamically unstable: in which case the balloon must be inflated urgently to 'cross-clamp' the aorta.

The patient is haemodynamically stable: If the patient is stable, bleeding has stopped and the blood pressure is 'acceptable', this usually means the patient is hypotensive but not shocked. In this case, the procedure steps are similar but the balloon is not inflated unless there is a deterioration.

Balloon deployment: a step-by-step guide: There is no definitive procedure, just a set of steps to maintain balloon access above the rupture.

Phase 1: Position the occlusion balloon

Access is obtained and a supportive wire inserted into the aorta to the level of the distal thoracic aorta. A long sheath large enough to accommodate the occlusion balloon is inserted. A 40-cm-long 12F sheath is often used. The occlusion balloon is positioned just above the sheath.

Phase 2: Inflate the occlusion balloon

If the patient is unstable: Inflate using one-third-strength contrast until the sides of the balloon conform to the aortic wall – they will look to be straight and parallel. The combination of the stiff wire and the sheath should stop the balloon from migrating. Ask the anaesthetist to record the time of 'cross-clamping' and to notify you every 5 min.
  Either:
- the blood pressure stabilizes, in which case give 5000 U heparin to prevent thrombosis
  or
- The blood pressure does not stabilize. If the balloon is sealing and the blood pressure does not recover, this means either that aggressive fluid resuscitation is required or that there is severe cardiac compromise. Correct the former and review the latter with the anaesthetist and surgeon; it may be time to stop.

Phase 3: Deployment of the stent graft

From the contralateral access, perform angiography to establish the position of the key branches. Position and deploy the body of the graft as normal. Remove the delivery system and exchange for a similar-sized sheath. Introduce a second balloon to just above the graft and inflate.

Phase 4: Removal of the original occlusion balloon

Deflate the balloon and pull back into the long sheath. Slightly deflate the second balloon while you pull the sheath back into the aneurysm sac. Remove the original balloon.

Phase 5: Deployment of the contralateral limb

Catheterize the contralateral stump, you may need to deflate the occlusion balloon to allow the wire to pass. Deploy as normal.

Phase 6: Completion angiography

Deflate the occlusion balloon and perform as normal.

Thoracic aortic aneurysms, aortic trauma and acute aortic syndromes

Indications for treatment of thoracic aortic disease

This is a very complex and evolving subject due to the range of pathologies, symptomatology and location/extent of the disease. The first step in all but the direst emergency, is instituting correct medical management to reduce blood pressure and pulse rate. In acute cases, focus should be on resuscitation, control of hypertension and pain. Management of disease of the ascending aorta, aortic arch and thoracoabdominal aneurysm is complex and beyond the scope of this book.

Thoracic aorta stent-grafting

Stent-grafting can be used to treat a wide range of conditions, including thoracic endovascular aortic repair (TEVAR) for a thoracic aortic aneurysm. The benefit from thoracic stent-grafting is potentially greater than with abdominal aortic disease, due to the high morbidity and mortality associated with thoracotomy and open repair. As the natural history of some of the pathologies is uncertain, the indications for treatment are evolving. Therefore, we must be careful to avoid mission creep by subjecting patients to 'unnecessary' stent-graft procedures. Patient selection aside, the basic principles of assessment and deployment of stent grafts in the thoracic aorta are similar to those in the abdominal aorta.

Indications for treatment of thoracic aortic aneurysm

For asymptomatic aneurysms of the descending thoracic aorta, the indications for treatment are broadly the same as for infrarenal AAA, i.e. >5.5 cm diameter should be considered for treatment. The extent, location and underlying pathology also have a bearing on the decision, e.g. in Marfan's disease, a lower-diameter threshold is usually considered. When the thoracic aorta is extensively diseased and a longer graft is indicated, there is an increased risk of spinal cord ischaemia following EVAR or surgery.

Acute aortic syndromes

Acute aortic syndromes include intramural haematoma, penetrating ulcer and dissection, and are a spectrum of conditions which may lead to aneurysm or rupture. Indications for treatment are:

Type B aortic dissection: There is evidence to support early intervention in acute dissection for patients in whom the dissection is causing ischaemic symptoms, there is evidence of propagation, development of aneurysm or intractable pain or hypertension, despite medical treatment.

Penetrating ulcer and intramural haematoma: These conditions may be the precursor of aortic dissection. Intramural haematoma may result from bleeding into the wall from the vasa vasorum. The evidence base is weak and treatment is usually reserved for symptomatic patients in whom there is progression of the disease, despite best medical therapy.

Traumatic aortic injury (TAI): This is probably the situation where stent-grafting has the most to offer but there is a spectrum of disease from minor intimal tear through to complete disruption of the aortic wall. In addition, TAI frequently affects young patients in whom there are implications for lifelong follow-up. Many of the lesser injuries are only detected through high-quality CT. Intimal injury may not require treatment but if there is significant intramural haematoma or dissection, then stent-grafting should be considered. Full-thickness tears mandate treatment.

Imaging assessment

The principles of assessment for AAA apply in the thoracic aorta. CT with multiplanar reformats is central to diagnosis and assessment. There are a few additional considerations relating to the proximal neck. Thoracic aortic aneurysms (TAA) often start adjacent to the left subclavian artery, a proximal seal zone of 10–15 mm is usually advised and sometimes the landing zone is increased by debranching one or more of the arch vessels. This simply means occluding the artery either by surgical ligation or embolization. Clearly, some of these vessels are essential, so thoroughly assess the right subclavian, carotid and vertebral arteries prior to embarking on this treatment. It also pays to review the circle of Willis with a neuroradiology colleague, as absent communications could be a disaster. Once you have worked out the vascular anatomy, discussion with your vascular surgery colleagues is essential.

The simplest debranching involves just the left subclavian artery; this may be combined with carotid subclavian bypass grafting to preserve flow in the vertebral artery and arm.

Grafting will be required if the ipsilateral vertebral artery is dominant or the contralateral artery is diseased or if there are issues with the cerebral circulation making the left vertebral territory vulnerable. More extensive debranching simply escalates the procedure and involves bypasses to the left common carotid and left subclavian arteries.

Consent

Manipulating catheters, wires and stent grafts in the aortic arch carries a risk of stroke of the order of 1–2%. The feared complication of TEVAR is paraplegia due to spinal ischaemia. The risk of permanent paralysis due to cord damage is difficult to quantify given the heterogeneity of the underlying conditions. For TEVAR, some degree of ischaemia will occur in 5–10% of patients. This is most likely if there is extensive coverage of the dorsal aorta and previous AAA repair. Prophylactic cerebrospinal fluid (CSF) drainage is often performed, particularly for longer stent grafts and the patient must be informed that they will be monitored for neurological signs and that CSF drainage will be instituted immediately if there is any sign of paraplegia developing.

Tube graft deployment: a step-by-step guide: The procedure is essentially deployment of one or more tube grafts. TEVAR should only be performed on angiographic units, which allow steep LAO projections (at least 60 degrees) to demonstrate the proximal neck relative to the arch vessels.

Phase 1: Placement of CSF drain

This is not routine but prophylactic drainage should certainly be considered in high-risk patients and the discussion and decision must be documented in the patient record.

Alarm: Consider prophylactic drainage in those requiring extensive coverage extending to the low thoracic aorta, especially if there has been previous abdominal aortic aneurysm surgery.

Phase 2: Placement of a support wire around the aortic arch

Successful TEVAR is reliant on having an extremely stiff wire in place across the aortic arch. Failure to have sufficient support will result in the nose cone of the delivery catheter prolapsing into one of the arch vessels as it is advanced around the arch.
- Obtain angiography via a pigtail catheter in the proximal ascending aorta.
- Advance a Terumo wire through the pigtail so that it loops back off the aortic valve.
- Advance the catheter so that it forms a loop in the ascending aorta.
- Exchange the Terumo for a very supportive wire with a flexible J-tip, e.g. the 10-cm J-tip Meier wire.
- Carefully advance the wire until the supportive portion is in the ascending aorta and the J-tip starts to from a loop at the aortic valve, then remove the catheter.
- Note the position of the rear end of the wire and mark this on the drape and maintain this position when advancing the stent graft.

Phase 3: Deployment of the stent graft

The techniques are the same as for EVAR but, as there is higher flow in the thoracic aorta, even more attention must be paid to maintaining graft position during deployment to avoid distal migration.

Phase 4: Completion angiography

This is the same as for EVAR, incorrect position and endoleak are the main challenges and the treatment options are the same.

Phase 5: Monitoring

Aftercare must be in a ward competent to carry out neurological assessment to check for motor or sensory signs suggesting spinal cord ischaemia.

Aneurysms, which involve the ascending aorta, aortic arch or extend to involve the visceral arteries, are likely to require branch grafts or surgical bypass to maintain perfusion of the coronary, cerebral and visceral circulation and are beyond the scope of this book.

Renal and visceral aneurysms

Visceral aneurysms are more commonly detected with modern imaging and are often referred to interventional radiology for treatment. Most of us should see and assess many more aneurysms than we treat. Rupture of visceral artery aneurysms can be fatal and urgent treatment is needed. Treatment is also warranted if there is a high risk of rupture, e.g. false aneurysms associated with inflammatory conditions, such as pancreatitis or a rapidly enlarging aneurysm on serial imaging. For asymptomatic patients, the usually quoted conventional treatment threshold is 20 mm. During pregnancy, there is an increased incidence of rupture of visceral artery aneurysm, hence treatment is often recommended in women of childbearing age intending pregnancy.

If the aneurysm is <20 mm, then further follow-up imaging is often advised. The interval will depend on how close the aneurysm is to the treatment threshold.

Consent

In addition to the standard risks of angiography, you must mention major complications to the patient:

- Aneurysm rupture
- Non-target embolization, e.g. loss of the kidney, bowel infarction.

The consequences of these can be life-threatening and might require major surgery to salvage. There is not sufficient evidence to allow these risks to be quantified, particularly for false aneurysm. The risk of rupture in uncomplicated true aneurysm is probably <5%.

Equipment

Treatment of visceral artery aneurysms is often complicated by the need to preserve circulation. Some visceral aneurysms (e.g. splenic aneurysms) can have the parent artery occluded, this may result in splenic infarction if gastric collateral flow is lost. Other visceral aneurysms (e.g. SMA) will need preservation of the parent artery and either stent-grafting or packing of the aneurysm sac should be considered. If considering stent-grafting, it is vital to remember which branch vessels may be occluded.

The precise equipment depends on the therapeutic approach. However, as a guide:

- Consider using guide catheters/guide-sheaths as stability is vital, particularly for aneurysms close to the vessel origin.
- Many of these aneurysms will be occluded using microcatheters – use the best you can get your hands on.
- Coil embolization is the most frequently performed treatment; even if performing a conventional 'back and front door' embolization, consider using detachable coils as this offers much more control.
- Coil embolization by packing the sac is much more commonly performed by our neuroradiology friends; get their help for kit and technique. At a minimum, consider using framing coils and hydrogel coils.

- Stent-grafting is usually confined to proximal lesions. Delivering the stent graft is harder than it looks – remember to use a suitable guide catheter/sheath.

Tip: If in doubt about the coils, speak to your friendly interventional neuroradiologists; they have the *crème de la crème* of coil systems and can help you with deployment.

Procedure

Choose an access point which will afford a stable catheter position. The caudal angulation of the visceral arteries means it is worth considering access from the arm.

Conventional coil exclusion

Aneurysms can be excluded by closing the parent vessel across the aneurysm neck. This technique has the advantage that it is fairly straightforward from a technical perspective and uses familiar equipment. However, closing the parent vessel has consequences. Either you know that there is a collateral pathway that will take over the work and preserve the distal circulation or you are accepting the consequence of distal infarction. This technique is often used for gastroduodenal artery (GDA) aneurysms and sometimes used for branch visceral artery aneurysms.

Stent-grafting

Stent grafts are available for arteries from around 3 mm diameter upwards. If there is a sufficient length of artery without vital branches and the arteries are not too tortuous, then this is usually the easiest and safest option. The procedure is planned from pre-procedure CT imaging. Suitable reformats should demonstrate the anatomy and allow stent-graft sizing.

Stent-grafting: a step-by-step guide

- Follow the basic principles of catheterization and stent-grafting to access the target vessel, confirm the anatomy and establish the optimal angiographic view.
- Obtain a reference image and navigate beyond the aneurysm using selective catheters and wires, take care when doing this not to cause rupture by injudicious prodding.
- Exchange for a supportive guidewire.
- Introduce a guide catheter/long sheath into the target vessel as close to the aneurysm as possible.

Tip: In some cases it helps to pass the guide catheter beyond the aneurysm, as this simplifies introducing the stent graft.

- Pass a catheter into the vessel beyond the aneurysm and introduce a wire compatible with the stent platform.
- Repeat angiography to confirm anatomy and then position the stent graft.
- Repeat angiography before deploying stent graft to confirm position, using a reference image can help maintain position.
- Deploy the stent graft.

Endpoints
- Perform check angiography.
- If there is endoleak consider balloon modelling using a suitably sized angioplasty balloon. If necessary, deploy a further stent graft to manage a type I endoleak.

Tip: The visceral arteries are prone to spasm, so have a vasodilator on hand and consider prophylactic usage.

Stent-assisted coiling

Stents are placed in the parent artery/arteries across the aneurysm neck. The stent acts as a 'cage' that prevents coils herniating from the aneurysm into the lumen. Not all stents are suitable for this technique and our friends, the neuro-interventionalists, have special stents for this situation.

Stent-assisted coil deployment: a step-by-step guide

- The initial steps are the same as for stent-grafting. Once access has been secured, a stent is deployed across the aneurysm neck.

Alarm: This procedure is dependent on using an open cell structure stent to allow a microcatheter to pass into the sac. Specific stents are available. If you are uncertain, check whether the stent is suitable.

- A microcatheter is passed into the aneurysm through the stent struts; ideally the catheter should form a loop in the aneurysm sac for stability.
- Once a stable position is achieved start deploying coils. Begin with coils which correspond to the diameter of the aneurysm sac; these will be the longest and hardest to pack.
- If you have the luxury of a loop within the aneurysm sac, then the catheter can sometimes be backed off to create more space to pack coils.
- As the sac fills, it may be necessary to use smaller/shorter coils.

Endpoints
- When there is a dense coil nest in the sac or there is difficulty extruding further coils, wait a few minutes and then perform a check angiogram via the guiding sheath.
  - If there is no flow, it is time to stop.
  - If there is minimal flow and there was no difficulty introducing coils then add one or two more, wait and review again.
  - If there is a lot of flow, further embolization may be necessary. Either proceed as above or, if there was difficulty, consider using shorter, more flexible coils or finishing packing using Onyx.

Balloon-assisted embolization

This technique can be used with liquid agents, such as thrombin and Onyx. A microcatheter is placed in the aneurysm sac and an angioplasty balloon is placed across the aneurysm neck. The balloon is inflated to occlude the artery and prevent leak of the Onyx from the sac. As this causes distal ischaemia, the balloon may be deflated periodically during the procedure.

Alarm: The use of kissing balloons at a bifurcation can allow leaks of Onyx due to incomplete occlusion of the arteries. This may result in non-target embolization.

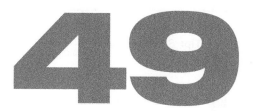

Treating haemorrhage

If you practice vascular intervention you will find yourself called to stop haemorrhage. This is one of the most challenging and rewarding aspects of practice and frequently life-saving. There are three ways you can help:

- **Inflow occlusion balloon:** this is the 'radiological tourniquet' and is used to buy time in severe haemorrhage by controlling bleeding until definitive treatment is provided.
- **Stent grafting:** this is used to treat bleeding from medium to large vessels in situations where preservation of flow is desirable.
- **Embolotherapy:** this is the most common treatment and is used when the target vessel can be sacrificed.

Bear in mind the principles of embolization (Ch. 35) and stent grafting (Ch. 33). This chapter will help you to select the appropriate treatment for patients with haemorrhage.

General principles

Speed is of the essence in the management of patients with haemorrhage, irrespective of origin. Interventional radiology sits alongside surgical and endoscopic management and is often favoured, as it is relatively non-invasive and offers less of a physiological challenge than surgery to elderly and infirm patients.

Clinical considerations

The vast majority of patients will present with traumatic haemorrhage and gastrointestinal bleeding. A small minority will have massive haemoptysis or bleeding in other contexts. Management is obviously context-dependent but there are some broadly applicable basic principles.

Patient safety

Patient safety is dependent on achieving a balance between the phases of resuscitation, diagnosis and treatment. Deciding when it is safe to move from one stage to another comes with experience and it pays to seek senior help as early as possible. There are some important considerations.

- **Blood pressure and pulse:** Is the patient already, or likely to, become haemodynamically unstable? If so then make sure that there is appropriate vascular access and plans for fluid and blood product resuscitation and that the place of care can offer an appropriate level of support and monitoring. In conditions where bleeding is intermittent, use the shock index as an indicator of whether the patient is actively bleeding.

Tip: Shock index $= \dfrac{\text{Heart rate (beats per min)}}{\text{Systolic BP (mmHg)}}$

Alarm: Elderly patients with a shock index >1 frequently become agitated and confused and you will need assistance looking after them.

A shock index of <1 suggests that the patient is not actively bleeding and hence the yield from investigation with contrast-enhanced multislice CT scanning (CECT) is reduced. There are caveats to this, e.g.:

- Patients taking a β-blocker may not mount a tachycardia
- Young patients may sustain their blood pressure through vasoconstriction, despite considerable blood loss
- In the 'metastable' patient, effective fluid resuscitation keeps up with the bleeding.

Patients with haemorrhage usually require high-dependency or intensive care. Remember that resuscitation can continue during imaging and should not lead to a delay in diagnosis, e.g. a central line can usually wait and, in any case, you may be the best person to place one.

Alarm: Don't be in such a rush that the patient comes to you without appropriate support, you won't be able to focus on your job and the patient may die.

- **Diagnosis:** this gets tricky and really depends on the clinical scenario, your role will usually be to divert the correct patients to early CECT. Remember to consider the shock index as an indication of whether there is ongoing bleeding.

Alarm: If the bleeding has stopped, CECT will be negative unless there is a structural abnormality.

Endoscopic imaging

Endoscopy is the usual first step for patients with haematemesis; this allows both diagnosis and in many cases treatment. Patients with bright red per rectum (PR) bleeding should have proctoscopy to exclude and manage haemorrhoidal bleeding. Colonoscopy is frequently futile as the blood will obscure the view. Patients with haemoptysis will normally have bronchoscopy to try to localize the bleeding to one lung and, if necessary, as a prelude to single-lung ventilation.

Radiological imaging

Almost everyone else needs a CECT, this has replaced diagnostic laparotomy, peritoneal lavage and the vast majority of diagnostic angiography. In general, you are looking to identify the site/s of active bleeding, abnormalities likely to be associated with repeat bleeding, e.g. false aneurysm, and other important pathologies which might change patient management, e.g. inoperable cancers.

Tip: Use structured reporting forms for trauma patients to make sure that you check everything.

Alarm: Do not let teams of clinicians harass you during image review. Once you have made an immediate review of the images, seek some privacy for a few minutes while you check your findings and perform reformats. The clinical team will find plenty to do with transfers and treatment.

- **Treatment:** Interventional radiological techniques (balloon occlusion, stent grafting and embolization) complement medical, endoscopic and surgical treatments. The attraction of interventional radiology is to provide expedient and definitive management with the benefit of reduced morbidity. A good example of this is sparing the patient a laparotomy and bowel resection for lower GI bleeding. In order to decide this, the imaging must be of sufficient quality to identify the target for treatment and to plan all aspects of the procedure. Reconstructions from CECT have revolutionized the decision-making process and, in the majority of cases, the information should be sufficient to decide the approach and the techniques you will use.

 Alarm: Avoid falling into the trap of 'if all you have is a hammer, everything looks like a nail' – make sure that the dialogue with a senior member of the clinical team considers all the options.

Specific clinical scenarios

Trauma

The importance of traumatic haemorrhage is that it tends to continue unabated. Early control of haemorrhage reduces morbidity, mortality and coagulopathy and transfusion requirement. The role of imaging and intervention in trauma is changing rapidly, whole-body CECT is revolutionizing diagnosis and the value of early embolization is increasingly recognized.

 Alarm: In order to be effective you need to be a part of the trauma team, which means being called and preparing for angiographic intervention whenever a patient with major trauma is imminent/being scanned. If not, both you and the patient are likely to be 'late'.

Reviewing and reporting the CECT

Emphasis is on saving life, so remember to use a template and provide an immediate report covering a 'primary survey' of the CECT looking for imminently life-threatening problems. The ABCD approach can be used:

- **Airway:** clear or obstructed, ETT position
- **Breathing:** flail chest, pneumothorax and lung injury
- **Circulation:** where and what is the site of haemorrhage
- **Disability:** brain and intracranial injuries plus obvious spinal injury.

 Alarm: Don't forget to notify the clinical team of the findings and document who you have informed.

Perform a radiological 'secondary survey' review of the CECT to look for other important injuries and pathologies and use a template for the report. Remember to look for the signs of arterial injury, which can be overlooked in the excitement of multiple fractures or solid organ injury. In the case of bleeding, consider whether it will be optimally treated by interventional techniques.

Arterial injury

Arteries can be injured by blunt and penetrating injury and there is a spectrum of CECT and angiographic findings depending on the mechanism and severity of the injury and whether it affects the full thickness of the vessel wall or just one of the component layers. Extravasation and dissection are often obvious. Conversely, false aneurysm and abrupt occlusion of an artery due to spasm or dissection may be difficult to spot unless you review reformatted images. These 'cut-offs' usually indicate a significant arterial injury (Fig. 49.1).

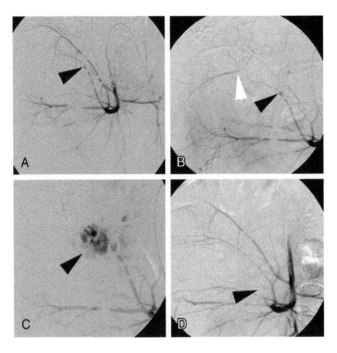

Fig. 49.1 ▪ Pelvic fracture post-internal fixation. (A) Cut-off in superior gluteal artery adjacent to metalwork (black arrowhead) and (B) reconstitution of distal artery via collateral flow (white arrowhead). (C) Extravasation following selective catheterization (black arrowhead). (D) Occlusion of the superior gluteal artery following coil embolization (black arrowhead).

 Tip: When an artery is injured remember to assess the territory it supplies for signs of ischaemia and consideration of endovascular or surgical revascularization.

Penetrating arterial injury is usually manifest by *contrast extravasation* or *false aneurysm*. Spasm or dissection may lead to 'cut-off' and haematoma may compress or displace the parent vessel. Remember to look for abnormality in the vessel wall, a significant adventitial and medial tear in the absence of intimal injury may leave an almost normal lumen. Sometimes, bleeding will have stopped.

Blunt arterial injury occurs through compression and stretching of the vessel. Minor injury causes *spasm*; more severe injuries cause tears in the intima, media or adventitia, leading to *intramural haematoma, dissection, occlusion* (Fig. 49.2), *transection* or *avulsion/rupture* of the artery.

 Alarm: Remember that a bone fragment may lacerate an artery following blunt trauma (Fig. 49.3).

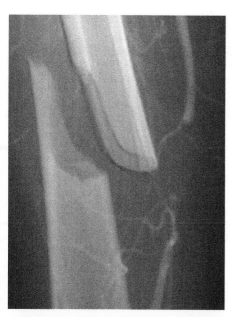

Fig. 49.2 ▥ Acute occlusion of the superficial femoral artery secondary to femoral fracture. At surgery, there was extensive dissection causing the obstruction; the patient made an uneventful recovery after a short jump graft was inserted.

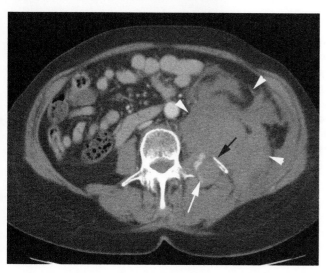

Fig. 49.3 ▥ Axial CECT demonstrating fractured right L3 transverse process (black arrow) with associated arterial extravasation from the lumbar artery (white arrow) with a large retroperitoneal haematoma (white arrowheads).

Indications for intervention

The aim of immediate intervention is damage limitation by rapid control of haemorrhage. Definitive reconstructive treatment is increasingly deferred and performed after an interval when the condition of the patient has been stabilized. In a patient with arterial bleeding from a pelvic fracture, embolization should precede surgical fixation. Patient selection is not an exact science and the decision should be based on your treatment being expedient and associated with reduced morbidity, e.g. avoiding or simplifying laparotomy or thoracotomy. If a bleeding source is identified, ask the following questions:

- *Does the amount of extravasation explain the patient's condition?* It is possible to overlook another more significant source of blood loss or alternative cause of hypotension, e.g. cardiac tamponade. Make sure that this is the only site of bleeding.

- *Is the bleeding vessel supplied from a single territory?* This has implications for treatment, as both the 'front and back doors' may need to be 'closed'.
- *What would be the consequences of occlusion of the vessel?* This must always be considered and is particularly important when dealing with end arteries. Do not think too long; at the end of the day it is better to be alive with a single kidney than a corpse with two.
- *Is embolization or surgery the appropriate intervention?* Embolization is appropriate if it is likely to lead to prompt cessation of bleeding without causing significant collateral damage. Discuss the situation with a senior surgical colleague.
- *Is it possible to use a stent graft?* This is important where preservation of flow is desirable or essential.

Tip: Don't forget that coronary artery stent grafts are available and suitable for use in small vessels (2–5 mm).

Suitable candidates for interventional radiological treatment are:

- Thoracic aortic injury
- A focal active bleeding source
- A significant arterial injury likely to re-bleed
- Any other injury likely to re-bleed.

Trauma intervention

Trauma patients should invariably have had a contrast-enhanced CT. Use the CECT reformats to plan the procedure and organize your thoughts for the surgical safety check. Consider:

- What is the most appropriate access?
- Are there any arterial variants in the territory that require treatment?
- What catheter shapes you may require?
- Whether a microcatheter is necessary?
- Whether you will need to perform any non-selective angiography, e.g. to localize a bleeding lumbar artery in a diseased aorta?
- Is the injury suitable for stent graft repair?
- The embolic agent?

Tip: Gelfoam can be particularly useful where there are multiple bleeding points in one vascular territory, e.g. liver trauma. Use coils or vascular plugs to embolize larger proximal arterial injuries as selectively as possible and spare as much normal tissue as you can.

Stent grafting in trauma

Consider stent grafting whenever preservation of flow is desirable in a patient with a vascular injury with extravasation or false aneurysm.

Aortic trauma

The thoracic aorta is injured either by direct compression and rupture (usually fatal) or because of shearing forces of the thoracic aorta distal to the left subclavian artery during rapid deceleration. Traumatic aortic injury (TAI) is a life-threatening condition and the vast majority of patients with complete transection of the aorta will die at the scene of the accident. Patients who survive to reach hospital will usually have a pseudoaneurysm secondary to an intact adventitia or contained haemorrhage in peri-adventitial tissue. This is an unstable injury and should be treated as though catastrophic haemorrhage is imminent. CECT should be performed on patients with a suitable mechanism of injury. Stent graft repair has become the first-choice treatment for TAI (Fig. 49.4).

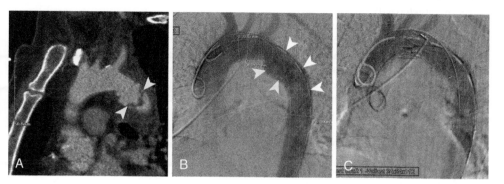

Fig. 49.4 ▨ Aortic trauma: the chest X-ray showed mediastinal widening. (A) CT reformat showing intimal/medial tear (yellow arrowheads) and adjacent haematoma. (B) Arch angiography with calibrated catheter (white arrowheads) shows false aneurysm (yellow arrowheads) distal to the left subclavian artery. (C) Following stent-graft repair.

Other vessels

The range of clinical scenarios is virtually endless and the scope of stent grafting is always increasing, such that it is reasonable to consider using a stent graft whenever flow preservation is paramount. It is probably the first choice for significant arterial injury in the thorax and abdomen and anywhere where surgical repair would be challenging. Each case should be discussed on its own merits as there are circumstances where surgery may be preferred for other reasons.

Embolization in trauma

Hepatic trauma: Embolization is increasingly used in major hepatic trauma and is indicated in the presence of false aneurysm or active extravasation.

Blunt hepatic trauma: Hepatic injury is often associated with other major injuries in the abdomen, thorax and pelvis. Haemorrhage is more commonly due to venous injury rather than arterial injury. Arterial bleeding is often focal and suitable for coil embolization. However, when there are extensive lacerations, the liver may be bleeding from multiple points, then Gelfoam is particularly useful. This type of injury pattern combined with embolization is associated with a risk of hepatic necrosis or biliary injury but these can be treated at a later date if required.

Penetrating hepatic trauma will either be due to stabbing by the public or by doctors. Percutaneous transhepatic cholangiography (PTC), biliary drainage and hepatic biopsy are all common sources of referral. The typical iatrogenic injury is a small pseudoaneurysm, which will require meticulous review of the CECT for detection. Hepatic arteries are not end arteries and there are multiple intrahepatic collaterals; if possible, start coil deployment distal to the lesion to prevent collateral 'back-door' filling.

Splenic trauma: Blunt injury is the commonest cause and embolization is indicated in the presence of false aneurysm or active extravasation; splenic laceration alone is not an indication for treatment. Unlike the liver, the spleen is an end organ, and vigorous embolization will lead to splenic infarction with the associated risks of hyposplenism. Hence, the aim is to preserve splenic function. Two distinct forms of splenic embolization should be considered:

- **Selective embolization:** this is the preferred option for any focal abnormality that can be readily catheterized.
- **Proximal embolization:** this is appropriate when there is diffuse injury, e.g. multiple bleeding sites that would take too long to embolize selectively. The splenic artery is occluded proximal to the short gastric arteries; the Amplatzer plug is good for this. The aim is to maintain collateral blood supply to the spleen via the short gastric and gastroepiploic arteries, while reducing perfusion pressure sufficiently to stop haemorrhage. This technique minimizes the risk of splenic infarction but does preclude further intervention if bleeding continues.

Pelvic trauma: Major pelvic trauma is often accompanied by significant arterial and venous injury. Bleeding from bone and veins stops when the fracture is stabilized with a pelvic wrap. Arterial bleeding does not respond to this and the patient requires CECT to look for pelvic arterial injury and other sources of haemorrhage.

Remember, even relatively minor pelvic fractures involving the pubic rami can cause major arterial haemorrhage (Fig. 49.5). If arterial bleeding is suspected, then embolization should take precedence over surgical fixation of the fracture.

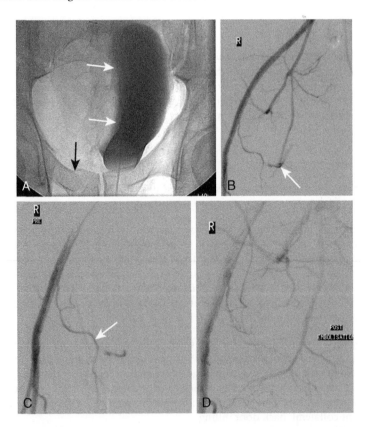

Fig. 49.5 ▨ Haemorrhage secondary to pubic ramus fracture. (A) Displacement of bladder by haematoma (white arrows), fracture (black arrow). (B) Initial angiogram suggesting extravasation (arrow) is from the IIA. (C) EIA angiogram showing bleeding from its corona mortis branch (arrow). (D) Post-embolization, the patient stabilized.

Tip: When performing angiography, the injured vessel almost inevitably lies over the fracture site.

Renal trauma: This is often iatrogenic following biopsy and can usually be embolized highly selectively. Make sure that there are two kidneys before embolization of a large amount of renal tissue. Renal arteries are end arteries, therefore there is no need to worry about collaterals, just infarction.

 Tip: Be pragmatic. If the patient is haemorrhaging and unstable, stop the bleeding and sacrifice the kidney; do not waste precious time trying to perform highly selective embolization (Fig. 49.6).

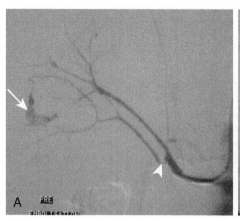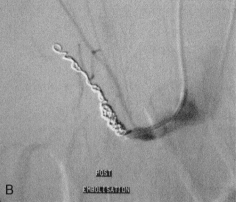

Fig. 49.6 ■ Post-biopsy haemorrhage. (A) Selective renal angiogram showing brisk extravasation (arrow) from a lower polar branch vessel with stenosis at its origin (arrowhead). The entire kidney is displaced upwards by the retroperitoneal haematoma. (B) Post-non-selective embolization.

Peripheral arterial injury

This is not uncommon in the context of penetrating injury, fractures and dislocations. Familiarity with the anatomy and understanding of the therapeutic options by you and the vascular surgeons makes endovascular treatments very popular. The increasing availability of stent grafts makes flow-preserving strategies more attractive but the management strategy depends on the needs of the patient.

Troubleshooting

The list could be endless but really distils down to you controlling the bleeding in a prompt fashion. If there is delay, then deploy a proximal occlusion balloon and discuss the situation with the clinical team and either agree that the patient's condition allows further time for catheterization and embolization or that they should have surgical repair.

Re-bleeding

Remember it is not rare for patients with trauma to re-bleed often when their blood pressure improves. This may be a result of one or more of the following possibilities:

- Bleeding which had stopped at the time of CECT when the patient was hypotensive. This is often a result of spasm in smaller muscular arteries, this will restart as perfusion pressure improves.

 Tip: When performing catheter angiography consider giving an antispasmodic drug in the presence of spasm or 'cut-off' to reveal the true condition of the artery and reveal the run-off.

- False aneurysm, this is particularly common if there is leakage of bile or pancreatic secretion
- Inadequate/incomplete initial embolization
- Coil migration: a coil which was appropriately sized for a constricted artery in a shocked patient may be too small when the patient is normally perfused and spasm has resolved.

If there is uncertainty regarding the cause or the site of recurrent bleeding, then repeat CECT is usually warranted.

Gastrointestinal bleeding

Gastrointestinal bleeding is a term which encompasses a wide range of clinical causes. Understanding the different presentations helps to localize the source of the bleeding and the likely vascular territory (Table 49.1). Improvements in diagnostic endoscopy, colonoscopy, capsule endoscopy and CECT have dramatically reduced the role of mesenteric angiography in the diagnosis of both acute gastrointestinal haemorrhage and occult gastrointestinal bleeding. In occult bleeding, diagnostic angiography should only be resorted to when all other forms of investigation have failed. Even with excellent technique, the study is likely to be negative! This is a case for expertise and it is worth considering referral to a specialist centre.

Table 49.1 Likely sources of gastrointestinal bleeding

Blood loss	Likely source	Target vessel
Red blood PR	Left colon	IMA (Fig. 45.18)
	Right colon	SMA (Fig. 45.19)
Altered blood PR	Small intestine	SMA/Coeliac axis
Haematemesis/malaena	Oesophagus, stomach or duodenum	Coeliac axis (Fig. 45.20)
		SMA (pancreaticoduodenal arcade)

PR, per rectum.

'Occult blood loss'

There are two forms of unexplained long-term blood loss:

- **Repeated acute episodes of bleeding** are often associated with a structural lesion, such as angiodysplasia. Smaller bleeds may only be recognized by the passage of blood or malaena and a drop in haemoglobin. Herald symptoms, typically abdominal pain, are usually associated with heavy bleeding, e.g. from a pseudoaneurysm. These cases should be treated as repeated episodes of acute bleeding and CECT should be performed during active bleeding.

- **Chronic insidious blood loss:** these patients are more likely to present with anaemia, and angiography has no role in their investigation.

Gastrointestinal bleeding: 'the usual suspects'

There are many causes of bleeding from the upper and lower GI tract. The following conditions are the most common causes:

Variceal bleeding: Usually in the context of portal hypertension and chronic liver disease. Most variceal bleeding is from the oesophagus and stomach but occasionally from other sites, e.g. haemorrhoids. Variceal haemorrhage is dealt with in the section on TIPS. Sinistral portal hypertension is a syndrome which occurs in the presence of splenic vein thrombosis and is not helped by TIPS.

Peptic and stress ulceration: Frequent and may be multifocal in patients in intensive care.

Oesophageal tears (Mallory–Weiss syndrome): associated with a characteristic history of vomiting.

Diverticular disease: A common cause of bleeding in middle-aged and elderly patients. Most cases settle with conservative management. Arterial bleeding characteristically fills the diverticulum before spilling into the colon (Fig. 49.7). Inflamed diverticula will give a patchy hyperaemic blush.

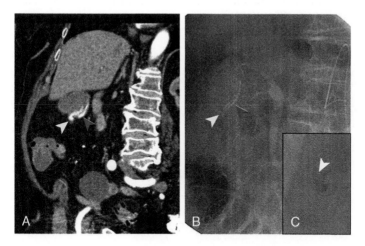

Fig. 49.7 ▦ Diverticular bleeding. (A) CT reformat and (B) non-subtracted angiogram showing typical appearance of blood filling the diverticulum (yellow arrowhead) before 'spilling' into the colon (red arrowhead). (C) Highly selective angiogram immediately prior to embolization, showing the supplying vessel (white arrowhead).

Angiodysplasia: Almost universally suspected in the elderly, but less frequently convincingly demonstrated. Angiodysplasia most often occurs in the caecum and ascending colon, though it can occur elsewhere, and is seen as a focal area of increased vascularity with dilated tiny arterioles with a prominent early draining vein (Fig. 49.8).

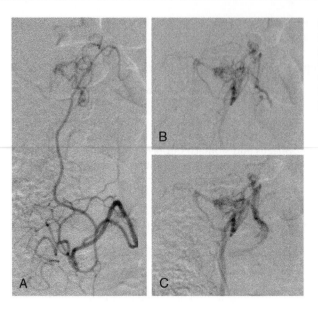

Fig. 49.8 ▦ Angiodysplasia in the ascending colon. (A) Early arterial phase shows a subtle blush. (B) Mid-arterial phase. Note the dilated arterioles and venous staining. (C) Late arterial phase shows prominent draining veins.

Meckel's diverticulum: Bleeding rarely occurs in the absence of ectopic gastric mucosa, hence the diagnosis is usually made on technetium isotope scanning. The feeding vitelline artery characteristically extends beyond the mesenteric border, has no side branches and ends in a corkscrew appearance (Fig. 49.9).

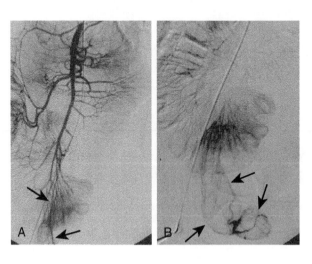

Fig. 49.9 ▦ Meckel's diverticulum. (A) The superior mesenteric artery run shows a vessel (arrows) extending beyond the mesentery; not all of the vessel is seen. (B) The subsequent run shows the typical blush (arrows) of a large Meckel's diverticulum; the vessel is the vitelline artery.

Tumour: A rare cause of acute GI bleeding. Angiographic signs of bowel tumours are often subtle. Examine the venous phase carefully – veins are larger and thinner-walled than arteries and are therefore involved earlier. Look for vascular displacement, encasement (constant narrowing – be careful not to misdiagnose spasm) and truncation (Fig. 49.10).

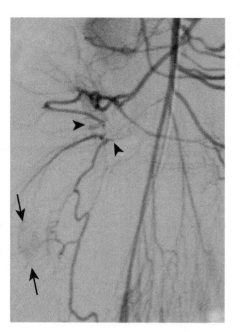

Fig. 49.10 ▓ Carcinoid tumour. There is a blush in the right iliac fossa (arrows). Invasion of the mesentery is demonstrated by occlusion of the ileocolic artery and distortion of the adjacent vessels (arrowheads).

Upper gastrointestinal bleeding

Bleeding from the oesophagus, stomach and duodenum usually presents with haematemesis. The patient is resuscitated and should have urgent upper gastrointestinal (GI) endoscopy, as this can be both diagnostic and therapeutic. The most important causes of bleeding are ulceration and varices. Embolization is reserved for cases of non-variceal bleeding which cannot be controlled endoscopically, particularly in high-risk lesions with a visible artery. Focal gastric (Fig. 49.13) and duodenal (Fig. 49.11) bleeding can usually be safely treated by coil embolization because of the extensive collateral supply in the foregut. It is essential to

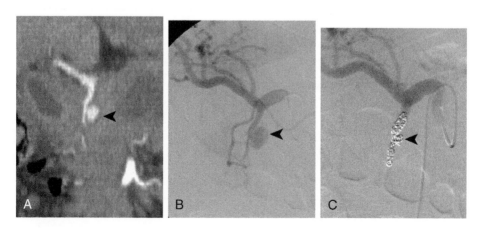

Fig. 49.11 ▓ Recurrent haemorrhage in a patient with pancreatitis. (A) Coronal CT reformat shows false aneurysm of the gastroduodenal artery (GDA) (arrowhead). (B) Selective hepatic artery angiogram showing near-identical appearance (arrowhead). (C) Completion angiography showing aneurysm exclusion. Note that the coils extend beyond the aneurysm to 'close the back door' and also prolapse into the false aneurysm through the arterial defect (arrowhead).

ensure that embolization does not simply occlude the inflow circulation leaving the 'back door' wide open. Re-bleeding may occur, which will be much harder to treat. The classic scenario is a posterior duodenal ulcer leading to gastroduodenal artery aneurysm. This will normally have supply from the gastroduodenal artery (front door) and pancreaticoduodenal arteries (back doors). Effective treatment requires placement of coils starting distal to the aneurysm and extending backwards to the inflow (Fig. 49.11). If you cannot directly catheterize the bleeding vessel, then consider blocking the parent artery proximal and distal to the bleeding branch.

 Tip: Always ask the endoscopist to place clips to mark the bleeding site. If you are lucky these will still be in the correct place when you perform the angiogram.

Lower gastrointestinal bleeding

The lower GI tract is everything distal to the duodenum. Patients with lower GI bleeding (LGIB) present with a rectal passage of fresh or altered blood (malaena); this often continues in between bleeds. Malaena implies bleeding from the small intestine or right colon. Fresh blood suggests bleeding from the left colon or rectum but heavy upper GI bleeding can present in this way, so patients will often have a preliminary upper GI endoscopy.

The pathway of investigation for LGIB is different and it is important to work to an agreed algorithm (Box 49.1). Colonoscopy is usually futile when faced with a torrent of blood/ malaena. Contrast extravasation into the bowel lumen on CECT is the critical sign of bleeding. We cannot go into the detail of the best CT technique other than to say do not give oral or rectal contrast and a triple phase scan should demonstrate any active bleeding.

Timing of CECT is everything; the patient must be scanned during an episode of active bleeding. This is where your friend 'the shock index' can help. If the shock index is >1 they are much more likely to be bleeding so do not delay getting them to CT for anything except basic resuscitation. If the patient is genuinely too unwell for investigation, they require

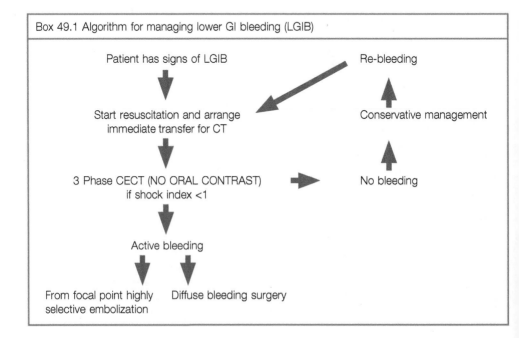

Box 49.1 Algorithm for managing lower GI bleeding (LGIB)

Patient has signs of LGIB → Start resuscitation and arrange immediate transfer for CT → 3 Phase CECT (NO ORAL CONTRAST) if shock index <1 → Active bleeding → From focal point highly selective embolization / Diffuse bleeding surgery

3 Phase CECT (NO ORAL CONTRAST) if shock index <1 → No bleeding → Conservative management → Re-bleeding → Start resuscitation and arrange immediate transfer for CT

immediate laparotomy and bowel resection with the associated morbidity and mortality. Conversely, investigating patients with a shock index <1 has a very low positive yield, as there are usually no other signs of the underlying cause. Therefore, if the shock index has normalized by the time the patient reaches you, it is best to send the patient back to the ward. The exception to this is postoperative bleeding, which is often associated with structural abnormalities such as false aneurysm.

Bleeding sites in the small and large bowel can both be embolized but should only be undertaken if it can be performed highly selectively (Fig. 49.12). The small bowel has a greater collateral supply via arterial arcades and therefore a greater risk of re-bleeding. In the colon, there are limited potential collateral arcades, this increases the risk of infarction – particularly near watershed areas.

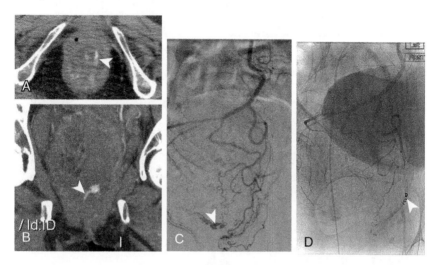

Fig. 49.12 ▥ Embolization for rectal bleeding. (A,B) Axial and coronal CT reformats showing contrast extravasation in the rectum (arrowhead). (C) Superior rectal artery angiogram showing extravasation (arrowhead). (D) following coil embolization (arrowhead) the patient stabilized with no ischaemic sequelae.

Mesenteric digital subtraction angiography and embolization

The techniques required for mesenteric digital subtraction angiography (DSA) are set out in Chapter 45. You must be capable of super-selective catheterization of the mesenteric arteries to reach the point of extravasation for embolization. Use the endoscopy or CECT findings to direct you to the correct vascular territory (Table 49.1).

Most common sources of bleeding:

- The **gastroduodenal artery** (GDA) lies posterior to the duodenum and is frequently the source of haemorrhage from a duodenal ulcer (Fig. 49.11). The GDA arises from the common hepatic artery and is most easily catheterized with a forward-facing catheter such as the Cobra II or RDC.
- The **left gastric artery** (LGA) is often the source of arterial bleeding from the stomach. It is a terminal branch of the coeliac axis and can be catheterized using a Sidewinder II. The catheter is initially advanced into the splenic artery and then slowly pulled back until the tip flicks up and engages the LGA. In reality, this vessel is seldom catheterized unless there is a very strong clinical suspicion of gastric bleeding (Fig. 49.13).
- Colonic bleeding most frequently arises from *ileocolic* and *right colic* branches of the superior mesenteric artery (SMA) (Fig. 49.14). Catheterizing these and other more distal

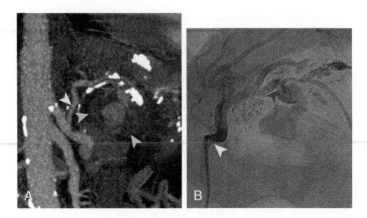

Fig. 49.13 ▓ (A) CT reformat and (B) DSA showing haemorrhage into the stomach (red arrowheads) from a pseudoaneurysm (turquoise arrowheads) of the left gastric artery (yellow arrowheads).

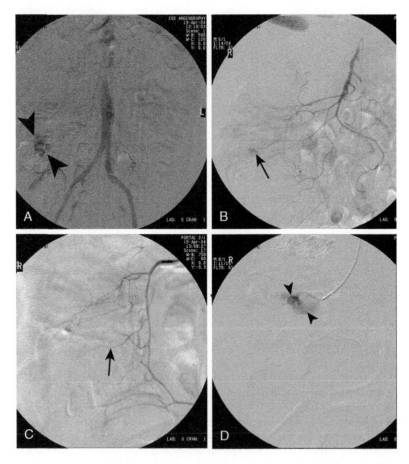

Fig. 49.14 ▓ Intermittent gastrointestinal bleeding. (A) Initial aortic run CO_2 angiogram showing extravasation in the caecum (arrowheads). (B) Selective SMA contrast angiogram: the extravasation is just visible (arrow). (C) Highly selective run from the right colic artery. The bleeding has stopped (arrow = target artery). (D) Extravasation (arrowheads) is seen again immediately prior to embolization.

branches of the visceral arteries usually requires a forward-facing catheter, e.g. Cobra. Hydrophilic catheters and microcatheters are often required.

As in any emergency investigation, studies for LGIB may be performed out of hours with relatively inexperienced staff. Using a systematic approach to acquire and interpret the images will greatly increase the chances of success.

What to look for: Gastrointestinal bleeding: A few conditions are responsible for the majority of cases and it is essential to know what to look for.

- **Active bleeding:** contrast extravasating into the bowel lumen
- **Spasm:** vessels which appear truncated
- **Early venous filling:** a sign of angiodysplasia
- **Abnormal vessels:** false aneurysm, chaotic tumour circulation, collaterals, encasement, etc.

 Tip: CO_2 may demonstrate the site of extravasation from a flush aortogram and will sometimes display bleeding that is not readily shown with conventional contrast (Fig. 49.14).

Interpretation

Examine the run frame-by-frame, looking carefully at the whole field. Take the time to re-mask each image. Review each phase of the angiogram, looking for the following abnormalities:

1. Arterial phase
   a. Active bleeding: extravasation appears as an irregularly shaped contrast stain that persists beyond the arterial phase of the angiogram (Fig. 49.15). If you are not performing embolization, decide if the bleeding is from a named vessel. This aids the surgeon by localizing the site of bleeding.
   b. Structural vascular abnormalities: look for false aneurysm, arterial encasement, displacement or occlusion.
   c. Early venous return: the appearance of a vein in the arterial phase is abnormal and may indicate angiodysplasia.

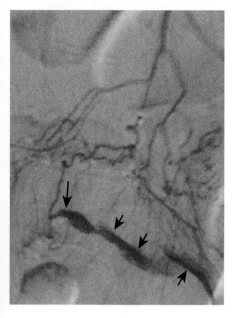

Fig. 49.15 Bleeding from the inferior mesenteric artery; contrast is extravasating (arrows) into the sigmoid colon.

Alarm: The ileocolic vein often opacifies before other mesenteric veins in normal subjects.

2. Capillary phase
   a. An area of increased capillary stain may indicate angiodysplasia or inflammatory or neoplastic involvement; look for supporting evidence. *Beware*, in the normal intestine, the capillary phase may appear patchy, particularly in the large bowel.
   b. Remember, areas of overlapping bowel can simulate increased vascularity – be particularly careful in the sigmoid colon. If there is a genuine lesion, the abnormality will be seen on every view.
3. Venous phase
   a. Look carefully for evidence of venous invasion, occlusion or hypertrophied collateral veins, as these may be the first angiographic evidence of a tumour.
   b. Normal veins have a similar branching pattern to the arterial tree; tumour venous circulation is often chaotic and tortuous.

If a bleeding site is identified

- Discuss the findings with the surgeon (ideally they are watching from the control room). You are deciding whether to embolize or operate.
  - Consider embolization if the bleeding vessel can be catheterized highly selectively (Fig. 49.14).
  - Consider surgery if you can only perform non-selective embolization. Remember, the surgical alternative is likely to be a quite extensive bowel resection, e.g. hemicolectomy.
- If the site will be difficult for the surgeon to identify in theatre, consider marking the abnormal area with a guidewire or coils, or by leaving a microcatheter in situ for injection of methylene blue or saline.

Troubleshooting

The commonest causes for failing to spot an identifiable lesion are due to poor imaging:

- Failure to get good subtracted images owing to peristalsis and respiratory artefact
- Missing out part of the intestine
- Failing to image through to the venous phase
- Lack of understanding of the relevant pathologies.

Variceal haemorrhage: transjugular intrahepatic portosystemic shunt and other techniques

Transjugular intrahepatic portosystemic shunt (TIPS)

The TIPS procedure involves forming a tract between the hepatic vein and the portal vein, thus shunting blood away from liver sinusoids and reducing portal venous pressure.

Indications for treatment

The principal indications for TIPS are variceal haemorrhage not controlled by endoscopic therapy, refractory ascites and Budd–Chiari syndrome. Trial evidence supports that in terms of re-bleeding, TIPS offers a considerable advantage over endoscopic therapy. TIPS is a complex procedure that requires careful clinical assessment, follow-up and re-intervention in a significant number of patients.

Consent issues

Patients who will undergo elective TIPS should be seen in the outpatient clinic. There is a 1–2% immediate procedure-related mortality and a risk of new or worsening hepatic encephalopathy.

Alarm: Patients with poor synthetic liver function (Child–Pugh scores >12) are at greatest risk of encephalopathy.

Anatomy for TIPS

Conventional TIPS tracts are formed between a hepatic vein and either the left or right branch of the portal vein. Although any of the hepatic veins can be used, it is easiest and safest to pass from the right hepatic vein (RHV) into the right portal vein (RPV) (Fig. 49.16). The central RHV bears a reasonably consistent position posterior and superior to the RPV. Bile ducts and hepatic artery branches frequently lie between the RHV and the RPV and are often opacified during the procedure. The middle hepatic vein may lie anterior to the RPV and therefore punctures may need to be angled posteriorly. Anterior punctures from the middle hepatic vein risk capsular perforation. It can be difficult to differentiate the RHV from the middle hepatic vein in the anteroposterior projection but this is easily done from a lateral projection.

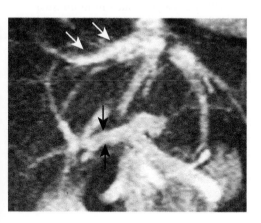

Fig. 49.16 MRI showing the relationship of the hepatic veins to the portal bifurcation. The right hepatic vein (white arrows), which lies posterior and superior to the right portal vein (black arrows), is the optimal approach.

Guidance for TIPS procedure

The principal difficulty with the procedure is targeting the portal vein puncture. It is common for patients to have had magnetic resonance (MR) or computed tomography (CT). Use these to assess patency and relative positions of the portal and hepatic veins. During the procedure, the portal vein can be imaged by wedged hepatic venography. CO_2 can be used to fill the portal vein retrogradely (Fig. 49.17). Ultrasound allows real-time targeting, but relying on a colleague to direct the puncture with ultrasound will strain all but the best relationships.

Equipment

- Basic angiography set
- Guidewires: 3-mm J, curved hydrophilic wire (regular and stiff), Amplatz wire (regular and short tip)
- Cobra catheter, angioplasty balloons 8-, 10- and 12-mm by 4-cm
- 5F sheath
- TIPS set – the contents vary between manufacturers; the Cook set includes:
  - 40-cm 10F sheath with end marker
  - 51-cm curved guide-catheter with metal stiffener
  - 60-cm long sheathed needle
- TIPS stent grafts 8-, 10- and 12-mm in a variety of lengths (it is impossible to be certain of the length until you have accessed the portal vein)
- Vascular pressure transducers to measure portosystemic pressure gradient. This is a time for simultaneous measurements
- Ultrasound for right IJV puncture.

Procedure

TIPS is a complex procedure, which can take anything from 30 min to 4 h to complete. Dilating the TIPS tract is very painful so it pays to have anaesthetic support for strong analgesia and deep sedation or general anaesthesia. Anaesthetic assistance is mandatory in variceal bleeders who are often agitated and may become confused with sedation.

Approach

Ultrasound-guided internal jugular vein (IJV) puncture; there is some evidence that puncturing the left IJV gives a more stable position. TIPS can be performed from unusual access approaches but this is a much more complicated procedure beyond the scope of this book.

TIPS: key steps

Catheterization

Pass the curved hydrophilic wire and Cobra catheter into the IVC, taking particular care steering through the right atrium. The RHV is the target vein. Rotate the catheter so that its tip points towards the patient's right, and slowly withdraw it until the tip engages the vein. Advance the hydrophilic wire and Cobra catheter into the vein. Exchange the hydrophilic wire for an Amplatz wire and carefully advance the TIPS sheath with metal stiffener into the proximal RHV. Next insert a 4F catheter over the Amplatz wire; putting the TIPS sheath and stiffener in at this stage means that the portal vein will be in exactly the place imaged on the wedged venogram.

Runs

To perform a wedged hepatic venogram, advance a 4F catheter into a distal and peripheral tributary of the hepatic vein (Fig. 49.17). If the catheter is wedged, there will usually be a satisfying sucking sound when the wire is removed. A gentle injection of contrast or CO_2 will demonstrate enhancement of the hepatic parenchyma and may even show the portal vein. If the catheter is not wedged, try a different position; if it is wedged, perform a run centred over the portal bifurcation (about 4 cm lateral to the spine, on the right!), including from the bottom of the right atrium down. This will show the relative positions of the portal vein confluence and the hepatic vein origin. If wedged venography fails, consider arterioportography with simultaneous hepatic venography.

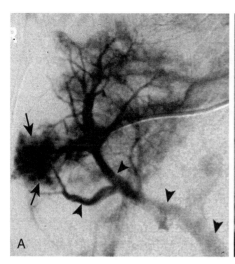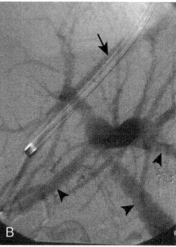

Fig. 49.17 ■ Wedged hepatic venography. (A) Conventional contrast is forced into the sinusoids causing a dense parenchymal blush (arrows) and then flows retrogradely into the portal vein (arrowheads). The portal bifurcation is clearly seen. (B) CO_2 wedged venogram showing the portal vein (arrowheads). Contrast can be seen adjacent to the sheath in the hepatic vein (arrow).

Puncturing the portal vein

This is easy to describe but is one of those practical procedures that takes quite a lot of experience to really get the hang of. Remove the guidewire; remember that the RPV lies anterior to the RHV; and turn the guide-catheter so that the metal arrow points anteriorly and slightly to the right. Slowly pull the guide-catheter back until its tip is 2–3 cm into the RHV. Now advance the sheathed needle through the guide-catheter; aim to hit the RPV 1–3 cm from the portal bifurcation. Resistance is felt as the needle passes into the liver parenchyma; cirrhotic liver is particularly tough. Do not go beyond the projected portal vein position. It is common to feel increased resistance as the portal tract is reached and a 'give' as the portal vein is entered. Withdraw the needle and attach a 5-mL syringe containing 2 mL of contrast to the catheter. Slowly pull the catheter back, aspirating as you go. Stop as soon as it bubbles or you aspirate blood; perform a short contrast run. There are three possibilities:

• Contrast flows towards the right atrium – you are still in the hepatic vein.
• Contrast flows towards the periphery of the liver – you are either in the portal vein or the hepatic artery. Portal vein branches are larger and are often visible to the periphery of the liver.
• Contrast flows towards the portal bifurcation if there is reversed flow in the portal vein. If it does not clear – you are in the bile duct.

If you are in the portal vein, congratulations! If not, continue pulling back until the catheter is in the guide-catheter. Put the needle back, redirect the guide-catheter and try again. Remember a degree of tenacity may be required and be prepared to try, try and try again, until the portal vein is entered.

Catheterizing the portal vein

Once the vein has been punctured, introduce a hydrophilic wire well down into the main portal vein. Advance the catheter from the sheathed needle until it is in up to its hub. If there is any lingering doubt regarding whether you really are in the portal vein, check now with an injection of contrast. At this stage, there are two options: some will advance the entire guide-catheter and sheath through into the portal vein; this seemingly brutal assault is the defining moment of the procedure; more often, the safest route is to exchange the hydrophilic wire for an Amplatz wire and initially insert a calibrated pigtail catheter to measure the tract length and measure the portosystemic pressure gradient between the pigtail in the portal vein and the sheath in the proximal hepatic vein/right atrium.

Forming the TIPS tract

Once you are in the portal vein, make sure that you do not lose access! Keep the tip of the Amplatz wire under control; it will readily perforate the liver or the mesentery. If the patient is awake, now is the time for some heavy sedation and analgesia, as dilating the tract is very painful. Dilate the tract with an 8-mm angioplasty balloon. The balloon will usually waist at the wall of the hepatic vein and the portal vein.

Stenting the TIPS tract

The tract must be stented if it is to stay open. Most operators now use a stent graft (e.g. Gore Viatorr). Obtain a venogram by simultaneously injecting into the portal and hepatic veins (Fig. 49.18A) and measure the length of stent needed; either use a calibrated catheter (Fig. 49.18) or the measurement software on your angiography unit. Do not leave stent protruding into the right atrium or dangling down the main portal vein as these can interfere if the patient subsequently requires a liver transplant!

There is excellent evidence to suggest improved TIPS patency with PTFE-covered stent grafts. The Viatorr (Gore) has been designed specifically for TIPS and comprises a bare stent that extends into the portal vein and a PTFE-covered portion intended to cover the intrahepatic tract and hepatic vein. The length of the covered part of the stent graft is the distance from the portal vein end of the TIPS tract to the end of the hepatic vein, the diameter is that of the desired shunt. The tract is dilated according to the pressure gradient. As neo-intimal hyperplasia does not narrow the stent graft, there is a

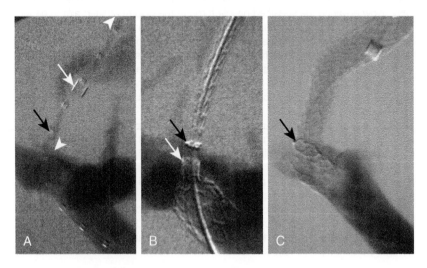

Fig. 49.18 ■ Using a Viatorr stent graft. (A) Portal and hepatic venogram using a calibrated catheter (black arrow); the end of the TIPS sheath is in the hepatic vein (white arrow). White arrowheads indicate the end of the hepatic vein and the portal end of the TIPS tract. (B) The sheath is placed in the portal vein, the stent is positioned so that the marker indicating the transition between the bare stent and covered stent is at the distal end of the TIPS tract (black arrow); the sheath (white arrow) is then pulled back to deploy the bare stent. (C) Completion venogram showing correctly positioned stent graft (arrow).

tendency to use smaller grafts. Most operators would use a 10-mm stent graft for bleeding and an 8–10-mm stent graft for ascites.

Placing the stent

Reinsert the Amplatz wire and dilate the tract to allow the TIPs sheath to be advanced into the main portal vein. The Viatorr stent graft is deployed by retracting the sheath with the distal stent in the main portal vein. The bare metal stent section will expand and while watching the radio-opaque ring at the distal extent of the stent graft, the expanded distal stent is pulled back until it sits against the portal vein. Next, look at the position of the proximal graft marker – it should be at the top of the hepatic vein. Make sure you have retracted the TIPS sheath and pull the rip-cord to deploy the stent. Dilate the tract to 8 mm and then measure the portosystemic gradient. If the gradient is <12 mmHg, dilate the tract to 10 mm and ensure the gradient is below 8 mmHg.

If the gradient is <12 mmHg, perform a completion venogram. A satisfactory venogram shows almost all portal vein flow passing through the stent into the hepatic vein (Fig. 49.18C).

Troubleshooting

Unable to catheterize the hepatic vein: This is either due to an obstruction or unfavourable angulation. Review the previous imaging to ensure vein patency and perform a venogram to look for obstruction (Fig. 49.19). If there is a hepatic vein web, consider angioplasty rather than TIPS. If there is modest cranial angulation, consider shaping the introducer accordingly.

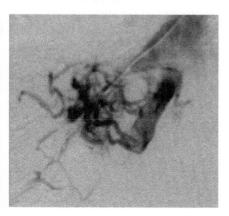

Fig. 49.19 Budd–Chiari syndrome. The hepatic veins could not be catheterized. Injection into the stump of the right hepatic vein reveals the network of spidery veins typical of Budd–Chiari syndrome.

Unable to hit the portal vein: Only practice helps here. Check that you are in the RHV and not the middle hepatic vein (MHV). Try puncturing from different points along the RHV and different degrees of torque on the metal stiffener. Consider bending the sheathed needle to alter the approach.

Hit an intrahepatic bile duct: This is of little consequence in its own right. The cholangiogram will help indicate the position of the portal bifurcation. The main importance is that TIPS tracts contaminated by bile have an increased incidence of pseudointimal hyperplasia and thrombosis.

Hit the hepatic artery: This is less common than biliary puncture but more likely to cause problems. If intrahepatic, you are likely not to be in too much trouble – simply carefully observe the patient during the remainder of the procedure. If extrahepatic, the potential to bleed is higher. Wait a few minutes and perform an angiogram. If necessary, embolize to stop the bleeding.

Hit peripheral portal vein: You are unlikely to succeed unless the tract has a favourable course. If you are not too far peripheral and too angulated, proceed as normal. If not, start again.

Hit the main portal vein: This is a dangerous thing to do, as there is a risk of massive bleeding if the vein tears, e.g. during angioplasty/stenting. Consider leaving a guidewire in situ to mark the position of the vein while you try again.

Unable to advance the TIPS catheter/sheath into the portal vein: Not uncommon in cirrhotic livers. Exchange the sheathed needle catheter for an 80–100-cm 4F catheter and advance the 4F catheter into the portal vein, then exchange for the Amplatz wire. If it is still impossible, then carefully remove the curved guide-catheter, keeping the Amplatz wire in situ and dilate the tract with a 4-mm angioplasty balloon. If this fails, exchange for a supportive 0.018-inch wire (e.g. platinum plus) and use a low-profile angioplasty balloon to dilate the tract.

The portal vein tears: This is a life-threatening emergency. Call for help and resuscitate the patient. The best advice is to stent or stent-graft the tract immediately. The drop in portal pressure will usually stop the bleeding. If this fails, gain control by placing an occlusion balloon in the portal vein, and breathe deeply. Surgery is the only solution.

Residual pressure gradient post TIPS: If a >12 mmHg gradient persists following stenting and angioplasty, perform a venogram and measure pressures to identify the point of obstruction. Use further stents and repeat angioplasty as necessary. If a gradient persists, a second 'parallel' TIPS may, rarely, be necessary.

The patient is still bleeding: Embolize the dominant varices through the TIPS tract. There is no need to embolize varices routinely. Glue can be very effective when there are large varices but make sure to perform a venogram to look for other portosystemic collaterals and take care not to glue the TIPS tract or cause pulmonary embolism.

Tip: If using glue consider placing an occlusion balloon in the varix to help direct flow.

Encephalopathy: Severe encephalopathy is usually associated with a large shunt and a very low portosystemic pressure gradient. Mild encephalopathy can be managed medically but more severe encephalopathy will require further intervention. There are two options: either reduction of the diameter of the TIPS tract or occlusion. There are a variety of different ways to reduce the flow through the TIPS shunt. The simplest method of controllably decreasing the TIPS shunt is by using a reducing stent graft. This is simply a stent graft with a waist. To achieve this, tightly tie a Prolene suture around the centre of an angioplasty balloon sized to match the diameter of the TIPS. The suture will cause a constriction when the balloon is inflated. Mount a balloon-expandable stent graft on the balloon and then deploy this in the TIPS tract. Measure the pressure gradient and progressively dilate the waist until a suitable pressure gradient is obtained, usually 8–12 mmHg.

TIPS follow-up

Make sure that the patient is followed-up with Duplex ultrasound to confirm shunt patency and exclude stenosis. Stent grafts have revolutionized patency rates; bare stents have only 50%

primary patency at 1 year, however 85–90% of stent grafts will remain patent. At any sign of trouble, perform a venogram and measure pressures. If the gradient is >12 mmHg, then intervention is indicated. Stenoses tend to occur in the hepatic vein proximal to the stent graft. These are normally treated by stenting. Repeat angioplasty and stenting is not usually anywhere near as painful as forming the primary tract, therefore, these procedures can usually be performed as a day-case via a jugular puncture.

Alternative strategies for managing variceal bleeding

There are limited therapeutic alternatives if TIPS has either not controlled the bleeding or is not technically possible or suitable. A modified TIPS technique with direct inferior vena cava (IVC) to portal vein puncture has been described; this is higher risk, as it is usually an extrahepatic puncture. Some patients may be considered for liver transplant, which may be curative. The following treatments can be used to stabilize a patient:

Obliterating the varices via an alternative approach

The options include:

- Via a portosystemic anastomosis: there is often a large shunt into the left renal vein. This can be accessed from a femoral vein puncture
- Direct ultrasound-guided transhepatic portal vein puncture
- Direct ultrasound-guided transplenic puncture: this is reserved for patients with occlusion of the main portal vein.

Once secure access has been established in the portal system, perform venography to establish the anatomy. It is usually necessary to use an occlusion balloon to direct flow into the varices. The varices can be treated by sclerotherapy or glue injection. Take care in the presence of anastomoses with the systemic circulation, as it could lead to serious consequences if filled with glue or sclerosant. While this may stop bleeding, it does not reduce the portal vein pressure and hence new varices are likely to form, possibly in less typical locations.

Partial splenic embolization

This is usually reserved for patients with splenic vein occlusion who have splenomegaly, massive varices and may have hypersplenism. The aim is to reduce the spleen in size, consequently reducing portal flow and hence the pressure.

Bronchial and pulmonary artery bleeding

Massive haemoptysis is much more commonly due to bleeding from the bronchial artery than from the pulmonary artery or from leaking thoracic aortic aneurysm. Remember that the problem with massive haemoptysis is drowning and not exsanguination, hence CECT and embolization may be undertaken after the patient has stopped bleeding. Do not expect to see bleeding on the CT – that really is rarely visualized in massive haemoptysis. Look for hypertrophied bronchial arteries (Fig. 49.20) and also for non-bronchial systemic supply, e.g. from subclavian, lateral thoracic and inferior phrenic arteries. A Rasmussen aneurysm is a pulmonary artery aneurysm in the context of inflammatory pulmonary disease. Classically this occurs in a tuberculous cavity. Therefore, there is usually also bronchial artery hyperplasia, hence it can be difficult to determine the source of the bleeding. Bleeding from a Rasmussen aneurysm is less common, hence bronchial embolization would normally be the primary intervention unless the aneurysm is large.

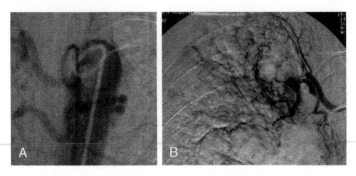

Fig. 49.20 ■ Bronchial angiography. (A) Flush aortogram showing origins of a right bronchial artery and a combined trunk. (B) Selective catheterization of the right upper bronchial artery prior to embolization.

Bronchial artery embolization

Bronchial angiography is almost exclusively performed as part of treatment for massive haemoptysis. It is invaluable to have good-quality CECT angiography as the bronchial circulation is complex tiger country. A little knowledge will help you and the patient survive.

Consent

It is essential to discuss the potential risk of non-target spinal artery occlusion leading to paraplegia (accurate risk is difficult to quantify but is <1 in 100) or very rarely, myocardial infarction secondary to coronary artery collateral flow.

Indicate that there is a tendency for patients to require further episodes of embolization as the cause is typically a chronic inflammatory process. Treatment becomes more challenging with each episode as all of the simple routes tend to thrombose.

Procedure

The target should be the section of the lung thought most likely to be the source of the haemorrhage on the basis of bronchoscopy or CT. This can be very difficult to ascertain as blood will be spread through the bronchial tree by aspiration.

Equipment and approach are as for bronchial angiography (see Ch. 45). Even if you can catheterize the bronchial artery with a standard catheter, use a microcatheter to gain more distal access and for embolization.

Embolization agent: This is a case for distal embolization using polyvinyl alcohol (PVA). Typically PVA 300–500 micron size will be used but this may be varied depending on the presence of shunting. Do not be tempted to use proximal coil embolization, this will not be effective and will simply prevent you from gaining access in future.

Alarm: Before embolizing, review the imaging, looking specifically for anastomoses with the spinal artery or coronary arteries.

Start embolizing from a distal position beyond any crucial branches and bring the catheter progressively more proximally as flow slows. Take care to flush through the loaded catheter before performing check angiography. Continue embolization until there is complete pruning of the bronchial artery circulation, unless further embolization is considered likely to lead to significant non-target embolization.

Troubleshooting

- The commonest problem is failure to catheterize a bronchial artery, in which case seek help and try different catheter shapes and alternative approaches.
- The bronchial arteries are thrombosed following previous embolization. This is when things get really complicated. Review the CECT looking for collaterals. If you cannot see them, then try angiography from the subclavian arteries and its branches which supply the chest wall starting with selective internal mammary artery angiography. You may also need to catheterize the intercostal arteries.

Pulmonary artery embolization

This is most commonly performed in the context of pulmonary arteriovenous malformation and very occasionally for a Rasmussen aneurysm. The latter is treated by selective coil embolization.

Postpartum haemorrhage

Postpartum haemorrhage (PPH) is a life-threatening emergency you may be asked to assist with:

- **Prevention of haemorrhage:** in patients with abnormal placental location (placenta praevia) or abnormal placental implantation (placenta accreta/percreta). The aim is to be able to provide immediate control of the arterial inflow during a caesarean section. There is wide variation in how this is done. Probably the commonest technique is to place (uninflated) balloons in the common iliac arteries usually using a cross-over technique to allow rapid catheterization after initial balloon occlusion. More rarely, some will catheterize the internal iliac anterior division; this can be challenging when there is a baby in the way of the screening (not forgetting the radiation exposure)! Do not be tempted to try to catheterize the uterine artery, as this can lead to spasm and reduce fetal blood flow. Place a Steri-Strip on the balloon shaft to mark the position. Accompany the patient to the obstetric theatre and be prepared to inflate the balloons when asked or, at the first sign of trouble. Once the baby is safely delivered, a trial of balloon deflation is agreed with the obstetric team. If there is no further bleeding then it is time to stop. If there is PPH, then the options are to try to control surgically or to offer angiography and embolization.

 Tip: Take a spare occlusion balloon just in case.

- **Management of a patient with severe PPH:** If you are called to the obstetric theatre take an aortic occlusion balloon. If there is severe bleeding and hypotension an aortic occlusion balloon offers the most rapid method of stopping haemorrhage. Unless you have excellent mobile DSA, the patient should then be transferred to the angiography theatre. Gain access from the contralateral femoral artery and perform angiography; you may need to deflate the balloon for a few seconds to allow flow. Haemorrhage will normally come from the uterine arteries or if there is a cervical or vaginal laceration, from the vaginal branches of the internal iliac artery. If possible, embolize selectively, however, if no focal source is identified, then embolize both uterine arteries with Gelfoam (see Ch. 23).

Troubleshooting

The bleeding does not stop following balloon inflation: Either the balloon is not properly inflated or it is in the wrong place.

Balloon has moved:

- Check the position of the Steri-Strip on the balloon shaft and if necessary deflate the balloon and advance to the correct position and re-inflate.
- If you have fluoroscopy, screen to check the position and apposition to the aortic wall just above the bifurcation.

Balloon appears to be in the correct position:

- In the absence of fluoroscopy, fill the balloon a little more.
- Still bleeding? Aspirate the balloon, if you get blood then it has ruptured and needs to be replaced (you did bring a spare?).
- If bleeding continues, then it is possible that the source is the ovarian arteries, in which case the balloon will need to be positioned above the renal arteries. This will markedly increase the risks of renal and bowel ischaemia.

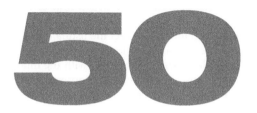

Treating haemodialysis access

Referrals for management of vascular access problems are among the most common requests for vascular intervention in centres where haemodialysis is performed.

 Tip: Embrace the dialysis patients; they will be one of the most important training grounds for vascular access, catheter and wire manipulation, angiography, angioplasty/ stenting and thrombolysis!

For patients on haemodialysis, their fistula, graft or dialysis catheter is a lifeline. Unfortunately, problems are common and anyone working on a site with a dialysis unit will frequently see patients with problematic access. Stenoses lead to inadequate dialysis, prolonged bleeding, arm oedema and thrombosis. Large shunts may cause steal phenomena. The key to these procedures is to understand the anatomy and the physical examination.

Permanent dialysis access

Arteriovenous fistulae: Patients with chronic kidney disease should have a fistula formed several months before they require dialysis, this allows the fistula to 'mature'. The commonest fistula is the radio-cephalic (Brescia–Cimino) fistula fashioned at the wrist of the non-dominant arm (Fig. 50.1). If this fails, it may be revised or a more proximal fistula formed, usually between the brachial artery and the cephalic or basilic vein. Sometimes the basilic vein is 'transposed' onto the brachial artery to increase the options. Once the non-dominant arm sites are exhausted, the dominant arm is used; if this fails, a fistula may be formed at the groin.

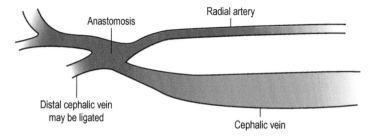

Fig. 50.1 ■ Brescia–Cimino fistula (distal radial artery to cephalic vein).

Haemodialysis grafts: These are an alternative to fistula formation and have the advantages of being ready to use immediately and allowing higher flow rates. The price for this is the frequency with which they develop stenoses and thrombose. Grafts often have a loop configuration. Typical sites are between the brachial artery and the cephalic or basilic vein or between the femoral artery and vein.

Fistula examination: Feel the fistula for the 'thrill' at the anastomosis and in the draining vein. The vein adjacent to the anastomosis usually has a spongy feel. If the fistula is underfilled, there is a problem with the inflow. A tense, distended vein indicates venous outflow obstruction. Venous stenoses are often palpable as 'defects' in the draining vein associated with a change in the degree of venous filling and thrill.

Tip: Hone your examination skills by trying to establish the problem and then confirming with ultrasound.

Dialysis access imaging

Imaging may be required to assess suitability for access formation and then to evaluate a maturing fistula. The majority of imaging comes about because of problems with the access.

Imaging is required whenever there is a problem relating to dialysis or the examination of the fistula. Typical problems are:

- Pre-dialysis: reduced thrill, aneurysm development, difficulty needling, arm swelling
- During dialysis: poor flow rates, recycling
- Post-dialysis: prolonged bleeding.

The same questions need to be answered for both fistulae and grafts, namely, the state of the inflow, the condition of any anastomoses and the condition of the draining veins from the periphery to the central veins. Ultrasound is invariably the first-choice investigation and is ideally suited for the evaluation of anastomoses, as access sites are superficial. Ultrasound cannot demonstrate the central venous anatomy or the origins of the subclavian arteries. If there is a fistula in situ, then a DSA study of the fistula (fistulogram) will also image the central veins. Magnetic resonance angiography (MRA) or computed tomography angiography (CTA) are alternatives for central venous imaging.

Alarm: CT is generally preferred to contrast-enhanced MRA due to the risk of nephrogenic systemic sclerosis.

Digital subtraction angiography technique

Equipment

- Basic angiography set with a micro-puncture set
- Ultrasound to guide puncture

Procedure

Positioning: You will need an arm-board to support the patient's arm slightly out from their side. Start with the patient's arm palm up. To cover from the chest to the wrist you will probably need to rotate the angiography table. Multiple oblique views are often necessary to sort out the anatomy.

Tip: To obtain oblique views, consider turning the patient's arm rather than rotating the C-arm.

Access: Retrograde arterial puncture of the ipsilateral brachial artery or the inflow limb of the loop graft is the ideal method. Performing the study via a 3F arterial puncture optimizes visualization of the inflow and allows complete assessment. The alternative, which seldom produces satisfactory images, is to place a needle in the draining veins of the fistula and use a supra-systolic tourniquet to achieve retrograde flow through the arterial anastomosis.

 Alarm: Remember that the patient will be heparinized during dialysis so do not perform the study straight afterwards.

Catheterization: Selective catheterization is only required for intervention.

Runs: The principle is the same as in bypass graft angiography and shows the anastomosis in profile. Because of the high flow rates through fistulae, a high frame rate (4–6 frames per second [FPS]) may be needed to study the anastomosis and the peripheral draining veins. As flow slows in the more central veins, the flow rate is decreased to 1–2 FPS. For arm haemodialysis access sites, the venous return should be studied as far as the right atrium. Central venous stenoses are particularly common in patients who have had multiple central lines.

Interpretation

- Significant stenoses are those causing >50% diameter narrowing.
- There are often occluded venous segments with collaterals and retrograde flow. This may only be appreciated when the runs are reviewed frame by frame at the console.
- Filling of collateral veins around the central veins is always abnormal. If you cannot see a lesion, try another view.

Troubleshooting

Unable to puncture the fistula: Use ultrasound to target the puncture.

The arteries distal to the fistula do not fill: This is usually secondary to a steal phenomenon through the fistula. Apply a tourniquet to occlude the venous drainage. The arteries will normally now fill.

Angioplasty and stenting

There is controversy about whether to intervene on asymptomatic dialysis access stenoses but symptomatic stenoses must be treated to improve dialysis, relieve swelling and prevent thrombosis. The commonest sites for stenoses are at the venous anastomosis and dialysis puncture sites. Before treating any stenosis or occlusion, make sure that everyone is aware of the objectives of the procedure, i.e. to preserve the function of the dialysis access site. Restenosis is frequent and repeat intervention is often necessary. Explain to the patient that treatment is a temporizing measure and not a miracle cure.

Access: Choose the approach according to the location of the lesion and the condition of the adjacent vessels. Think about where to position the ultrasound, trolley, C-arm, etc. It is often useful to stand towards the patient's head and sometimes helps to work from the contralateral side across the patient's chest when working on the basilic vein.

Fistulae: For direct arteriovenous fistulae, the dominant draining vein is usually catheterized; this is almost always the vein that is used during dialysis. Punctures can be retrograde (i.e. towards the hand) to treat an arterial anastomotic problem or antegrade (i.e. away from the hand) to treat venous stenoses. An alternative is to identify a suitable branch or tributary vein and use this for access. This has the advantage of avoiding the need for a sheath in the principal vein. It is sometimes necessary to approach Brescia–Cimino fistulae via an antegrade brachial artery puncture.

Haemodialysis grafts: There is nearly always a problem at the venous anastomosis. The graft is usually directly punctured at a point that allows space to manoeuvre under the C-arm with respect to the lesion.

Tip: The apex of some loop grafts is reinforced to prevent kinking. Check with the surgeon, or puncture away from the apex.

Angioplasty is performed in the conventional fashion (Fig. 50.2). The patient may require dialysis immediately after treatment, in this case the sheath can be exchanged for a dialysis catheter, which is left in situ; discuss the best arrangement with the dialysis unit.

Stenting is reserved for those cases in which angioplasty alone is unsuccessful. Only stent if it will achieve good outflow; if not, the patient is better off with surgery. Take care when stenting the central veins, as stent compression is common between the clavicle and the first rib. Try not to stent across other vessels that may be needed for central access in the future, especially the jugular veins. Make sure that the patient and clinician are aware of the position of the stent so that it is not inadvertently punctured. Long-term stent patency, particularly in peripheral veins, is poor. There is evidence that stent grafts fair better for peripheral AV stenosis, particularly at the venous anastomosis – while patency overall is unchanged, the number of interventions required to maintain patency is reduced.

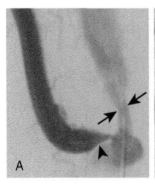
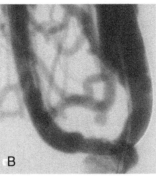

Fig. 50.2 ■ (A) Brescia–Cimino fistula with stenoses at the anastomosis (arrowhead) and in the draining vein (arrows). (B) Following angioplasty, excellent flow is restored.

A

B

Troubleshooting

Unable to puncture the draining vein: Use a tourniquet and ultrasound guidance; colour flow is invaluable for this.

Unable to dilate a stenosis: It may be necessary to consider using a high-pressure balloon or cutting balloon to overcome fibrotic strictures (Fig. 50.3). Make sure that you have suitable angioplasty balloons before starting. Never use a stent when you cannot eliminate the waist on the angioplasty balloon – you are simply lining a stenosis with metal!

Rupture: Rupture is more common during venous intervention than during arterial angioplasty. It is probably more common when using cutting balloons (Fig. 50.4). Extravasation is managed in a similar fashion to arterial injury; remember that occlusion is often an acceptable outcome if the fistula was not functioning adequately.

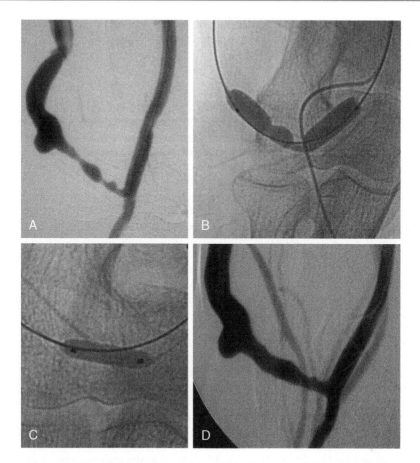

Fig. 50.3 ▨ Brachiocephalic fistula stricture. (A) Complex stricture in the cephalic vein. (B) Persistent waisting in a conventional angioplasty balloon. (C) Elimination of the waist with a cutting balloon. (D) Completion angiogram.

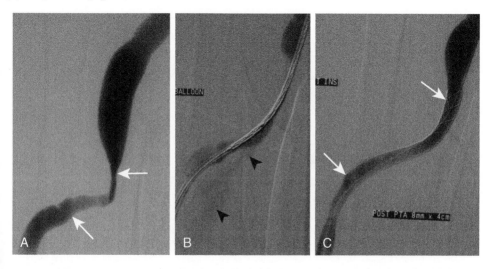

Fig. 50.4 ▨ Extravasation post-cutting balloon. (A) Pre-angioplasty flow-limiting basilic vein stenosis (arrows). (B) Brisk extravasation following cutting balloon angioplasty (arrowheads). (C) Completion angiogram following deployment of a covered stent.

Spasm: Spasm is common in the radial artery and in veins. Use vasodilators prophylactically and to treat spasm. Consider gentle dilation of areas of resistant spasm.

Thrombosis

Unfortunately, thrombosis is often the first sign of a problem. Radiological treatment options are thrombolysis and mechanical thrombectomy; the alternative is surgical embolectomy. Remember that there is almost always an underlying stenosis that must be treated when flow is restored. Ideally, treatment should be performed before the patient requires temporary venous access for dialysis as this preserves central veins. Typical thrombosis starts at or just distal to the arterial anastomosis; the artery nearly always remains patent.

Remember the contraindications for thrombolysis (see Ch. 47). CVA during thrombolysis is probably less common in a young dialysis patient than in an elderly patient with peripheral vascular disease. If the patient has a central line, check that there were no complications during placement, e.g. arterial puncture which might compromise thrombolysis. In reality, most units do not commonly use thrombolysis for fistulae; it is time-consuming even with modified techniques. Mechanical thrombectomy with rheolytic devices may be used though achieving complete removal of clot burden can be an issue. Surgical thrombectomy permits rapid clot removal, however it is essential that imaging is undertaken to reveal the underlying lesion and permit treatment.

Atrioventricular fistulae: Assess the extent of the thrombus with ultrasound. Puncture the main draining vein central to the thrombus and aiming towards the anastomosis. Perform gentle venography to confirm the anatomy. Position a 4F straight multi-sidehole catheter into the thrombus with its tip as close to the anastomosis as possible. Give a bolus dose of the thrombolytic agent (e.g. 5 mg rt-PA) and then start an infusion (see Ch. 47). Perform periodic check angiography to evaluate progress. When flow is re-established, perform check venography and treat any underlying stenoses.

Haemodialysis grafts: The thrombus is usually confined to the graft but may extend beyond it if there is a stenosis in the draining vein (Fig. 50.5). Occluded grafts can be treated by thrombolysis or thrombectomy using a crossed catheter technique (Fig. 50.6).

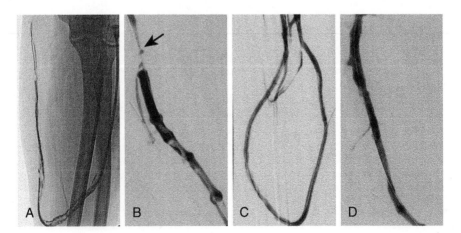

Fig. 50.5 ■ (A) Thrombosed forearm loop graft. (B) Stenosis in the draining vein (arrow). (C) Following mechanical thrombectomy, the graft is clear. (D) The cephalic vein is widely patent following angioplasty.

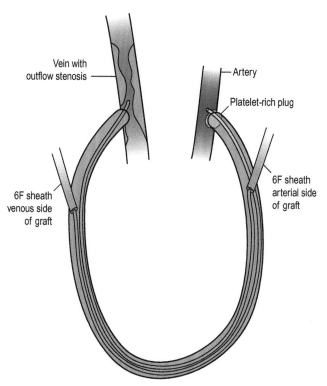

Fig. 50.6 Crossed catheter technique for loop graft thrombolysis.

1. Punctures are made into the arterial and venous limbs and catheters manipulated round the graft. Puncture of the graft is usually straightforward but if it is difficult to palpate, use ultrasound.
2. Using a hydrophilic guidewire and a Cobra catheter, negotiate into the draining vein beyond the venous anastomosis and perform a venogram to demonstrate the venous anatomy. If there is no direct venous drainage, stop now as the graft needs to be surgically revised. Ensure there is adequate central venous drainage, if the central veins are occluded or thrombosed the fistula will not run for long.
3. Either perform thrombolysis, usually with boluses of rt-PA, or thrombectomy using a mechanical thrombectomy device. Aim to treat the venous outflow first, then deal with the arterial limb. It is not essential to clear all the thrombus at this stage but just enough to allow flow to occur.
4. There is usually a platelet-rich plug of thrombus at the arterial end of the graft, which is resistant to thrombolysis. Use a hydrophilic guidewire to manipulate into the native artery and pass a small balloon catheter above the arterial anastomosis. Gently inflate it and pull it back into the graft (an over-the-wire Fogarty embolectomy catheter is ideal, although conventional angioplasty balloons will work). The platelet plug disimpacts and flow is restored.
5. Now is the time to tidy up the residual thrombus; often simple balloon angioplasty will macerate it.
6. Remember to look for the underlying lesion and treat it with angioplasty or stenting.

Troubleshooting

Uncertain anatomy: Try hard to establish the type of fistula or graft before starting. Look for operation notes and speak to the surgical team in charge. Ultrasound will often clarify the anatomy. If not, adopt a 'suck it and see' approach.

Extravasation occurs during thrombolysis: This is almost inevitable when treating dialysis access grafts that have had frequent punctures. Warn the patient about this in advance. It is usually possible to complete treatment unless there is marked extravasation.

Intra-procedural thrombosis: Particularly with thrombectomy, it can be difficult to stop re-thrombosis during the procedure. The key is avoiding delay between steps 4 and 5 above; it is essential to get flow through the fistula. Minor amounts of residual thrombus are easily resolved after flow has been established.

Treating venous disease

Percutaneous placement of inferior vena cava (IVC) filters and treatment of superior vena cava obstruction (SVCO) (Ch. 44) are the cornerstones of venous intervention. Venous angioplasty, stenting and thrombolysis are sometimes performed but remain controversial techniques, except in the management of haemodialysis access (Ch. 50). The principles of negotiating and treating venous stenoses and occlusions are exactly the same as in the arterial system. This chapter covers some established indications for venous intervention and details aspects of intervention specific to the venous system.

IVC filters

IVC filters are placed to prevent pulmonary embolism from sources in the lower limbs, pelvis and IVC. Contemporary devices are readily placed percutaneously via the right internal jugular vein (IJV) or femoral veins. Several permanent and retrievable filters are commercially available. Most retrievable filters can be left permanently in place.

Indications for IVC filtration

There is little evidence to support the use of IVC filters, and patients should be considered on a case-by-case basis (Table 51.1). Thrombosis rates vary between devices; overall, about 10%

Table 51.1 Indications for caval filtration and recommended filter type

Indication	Filter type
Unequivocal	
Recurrent PE despite adequate anticoagulation	P
Patients with PE and severely limited cardiorespiratory reserve	P
PE with contraindication to anticoagulation	P
Relative	
Free-floating iliofemoral/IVC thrombus with a high risk of embolization	P/R
Spinal cord injury with paraplegia	P
Severe trauma	P/R
Prophylactic – before surgery on patients at high risk of DVT or PE, e.g. before hip surgery in the presence of ipsilateral femoral DVT	R

P, permanent; R, retrievable.

of permanent IVC filters will thrombose within 5 years. Therefore, permanent filters should be avoided whenever possible in those patients with a long life-expectancy.

Introducer sheaths for IVC filters start at 7F; insertion of large catheters into the femoral vein is itself a cause of deep vein thrombosis (DVT), hence the jugular approach has a distinct advantage!

Equipment

- Ultrasound for right IJV puncture
- Basic angiography set
- Cobra catheter
- Three-mm J guidewire
- An appropriate IVC filter set (see below).

IVC filters are supplied with delivery systems designed for use from either the jugular or the femoral approach. These systems are not interchangeable, so make sure that you have the correct device! Check also that you have an appropriately sized device for the IVC.

Procedure

Access: The right IJV is the 'universal gateway' and can be used for access even in the presence of iliofemoral DVT. Make sure that there is a contemporary ultrasound to document the site and extent of thrombus. Placing a catheter through a thrombosed vein is likely to result in iatrogenic pulmonary embolism (PE)!

Catheterization: From the jugular route, use a Cobra catheter and 3-mm J-guidewire to carefully negotiate through the right atrium to the IVC.

Assessment is required for three reasons:

- To demonstrate the patency of the IVC, assess its size and any angulation
- To confirm conventional anatomy, i.e. single IVC
- To document the position of the renal veins.

Tip: In practice most patients will have had a contrast-enhanced computed tomography (CECT), which demonstrates the anatomy and IVC size, leaving you only needing to establish the position of the renal veins.

If digital subtraction angiography (DSA) is required it is usually sufficient to perform a simple IVC injection through a pigtail catheter placed just above the confluence of the iliac veins. An initial gentle hand injection will ensure that there is no thrombus adjacent to the catheter; perform a more vigorous injection to demonstrate the entire IVC. The position of the renal veins is usually apparent because of streaming of unopacified blood (Fig. 51.1). If the renal veins cannot be identified, use a Cobra catheter to engage them and perform selective hand injections to demonstrate their position.

Tip: Use the patient's spine as a reference for the position of the renal veins.

Once the position of the renal veins has been established, do not move the table or the image intensifier.

Alarm: If you did not measure it on the CT scan, do not forget to measure the diameter of the infra-renal IVC. Most IVC filters can only be used within a specified range of IVC diameters; if the filter is too small, the first place it will lodge is the tricuspid valve!

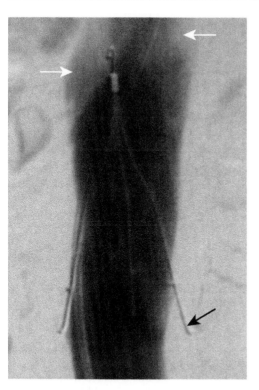

Fig. 51.1 ▪ IVC venogram performed prior to removal of IVC filter. Note the streaming effect of unopacified blood from the renal veins (white arrows). It is not uncommon to see a filter leg protruding through the IVC wall (black arrow); this does not preclude removal but should encourage you to be alert to possible difficulty.

Positioning the filter: There are two sites to place an IVC filter, and the position is determined from the cavogram.

- **Infrarenal:** this is the optimal site; if the filter causes IVC thrombosis, the renal veins will be spared. Conical filters should be placed with the filter apex at the level of the renal veins; the high flow promotes dissolution of thrombus trapped or formed within the filter.
- **Suprarenal:** in the presence of infrarenal thrombus, a filter can be sited between the renal and hepatic veins. In this position, filter thrombosis can lead to renal vein thrombosis and renal infarction.

Deploying the filter: Each type of filter is deployed differently and there may even be differences for a single type of filter, depending on whether the jugular or femoral route is used. Read the instructions carefully before use; if you do not understand them, seek help! It is traditional, but unnecessary, to perform a completion venogram to demonstrate the position of the filter; a single-shot image will suffice. If you must do this, consider injecting through the sheath and take great care if you pass a pigtail catheter or J-wire through the filter as they might become entangled!

Alarm: If there is no contraindication, the patient should be anticoagulated while the filter is in situ, to minimize the chance of filter thrombosis.

Filter removal: There is no absolute consensus on the length of time a filter can be left in place before removal is attempted. Longer dwell times are associated with greater complications and the filter should be removed as soon as it is no longer clinically required. Always perform a cavogram (Fig. 51.2) to see if there is any residual thrombus either in the

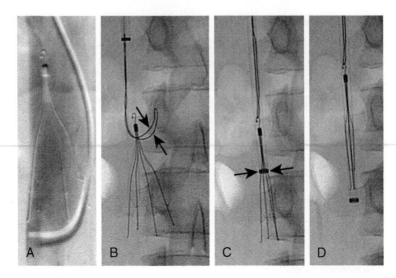

Fig. 51.2 ■ Removal of a Gunther tulip IVC filter. (A) Initial IVC angiogram demonstrates that the filter is free of thrombus. (B) The snare (arrows) is passed over the filter and the apex of the hook is snared. (C) The filter closes as the sheath (arrows) is advanced over it. (D) When the filter is fully inside the sheath, they are removed together.

filter or which would threaten significant PE. If there is <1 cm³ of thrombus in the filter, it can be removed. Most removable filters have a hook at their apex, this is snared from the jugular vein. The snare must be placed at the top of the hook; the snare is held in place and the sheath advanced over it to close the filter (Fig. 51.2). There is almost always thrombus/tissue on the filter struts (Fig. 51.3).

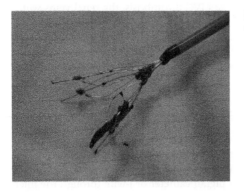

Fig. 51.3 ■ Thrombus on filter struts despite normal venogram.

 Alarm: If there is difficulty STOP! DO NOT USE FORCE. Accept that it may not be possible to remove the filter. It is better to leave a permanent filter than cause an IVC laceration.

If filter retrieval is difficult it is often worth stopping and obtaining a CT of the abdomen.

Complications

Significant procedure-related complications are rare and include:

Access site thrombosis: Femoral vein thrombosis was particularly common with early devices but is only seen in 2–3% of patients with smaller contemporary devices.

IVC perforation: Filter struts may perforate the caval wall (Fig. 51.1); this is rarely clinically significant but may make the filter irretrievable. Caval strut perforation is common and is best assessed on CT.

Incorrect deployment: There are four forms of incorrect deployment:

- Malposition in relation to the renal veins
- Incorrect filter sizing. At worst, this will result in fatal embolization of the filter. More commonly, it results in tilting or incorrect opening
- Conical filters can be tilted; this may reduce filter effectiveness
- The filter may open incorrectly so that the struts are not evenly distributed or appear not to reach the IVC wall. This may impair filter function. If you have any doubt, perform a limited CT to clarify the situation (Fig. 51.4).

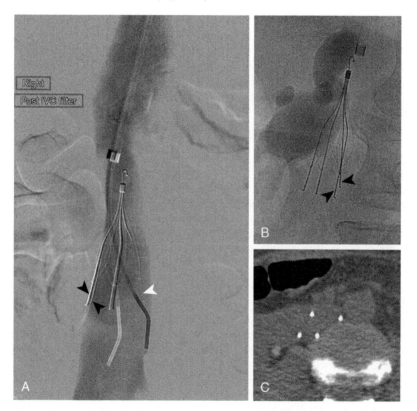

Fig. 51.4 ▪ Images of IVC filter. (A) The initial frontal projection shows two struts that appear to lie close together (black arrowheads) and a further strut (white arrowhead) that does not seem to reach the vein wall. (B) In the oblique projection, the filter struts appear crossed (black arrowheads). (C) The patient was sent for a CT scan, which shows the IVC is flattened, accounting for the proximity of the struts. The legs are all in apposition with the wall.

If you have placed a permanent filter, you are stuck, whereas a removable filter can be repositioned. If there is severe misalignment, a second filter may have to be placed above the first.

Tip: Try to deploy the filter in a straight portion of the IVC; it is more likely to be effective and much easier to remove.

Late complications

IVC thrombosis: This is seen in at least 10% of patients with Greenfield and bird's nest filters. Caval thrombosis is serious if suprarenal. Thrombosis of the infrarenal IVC is usually compensated by the development of ascending lumbar collaterals. Remember that surgical ligation of the IVC used to be the treatment for recurrent PE until recently!

Structural failure of the filter: This has led to several filter designs being withdrawn from the market and is another reason to remove filters whenever possible.

The long-term structural integrity and patency of the newer designs of IVC filters remain to be established.

Iliac vein obstruction

This often presents with iliofemoral deep vein thrombosis and massive leg oedema. The left side is more often affected due to compression by the overlying right common iliac artery (CIA) (May–Thurner syndrome). Treatment is by thrombolysis followed by placement of a large stent.

Venous lines

Venous lines comprise everything from peripheral cannulae to implantable ports. The access should be matched to the patient's needs and usually depends on the duration of required access and the nature of the intervention, e.g. dialysis versus chemotherapy (Table 51.2). Most peripheral access is inserted by ward staff and interventional radiologists tend to get involved in more complex access, such as lines and ports and to manage failed access and complications.

Line insertion

For the purpose of this chapter, line insertion can be thought of as lines placed over a wire in the conventional fashion and lines intended for long-term access, which are placed in conjunction with a subcutaneous tunnel. To place a conventional line, follow the principles of ultrasound-guided vascular access.

Tunnelled lines: It is essential you understand what type of line you are dealing with, as this affects the sequence of tunnelling and line positioning. There are multiple types of line: straight versus preformed curve (some dialysis catheters); single versus multiple lumen; low-flow versus high-flow designs. All tunnelled lines have a cuff on the shaft. This is positioned in the tunnel 2–3 cm from the skin exit site. Tissue ingrowth provides anchorage and a barrier to infection.

Tunnelled lines come in two main variants:

- **Lines that are cut to length**, e.g. a Hickman line. With this type of line, tunnelling is performed before being cut to length and inserted into the vein.
- **Lines that are fixed length**, e.g. some dialysis catheters and Groshong lines.

If the hub is an integral part of the catheter tunnelling is performed as above before insertion into the vein. If the hub is attached once the line is positioned tunnelling comes second and is performed away from the point of venous access towards the skin exit site.

Equipment

- A suitable line (Table 51.2). Most proprietary devices come complete with the basic equipment necessary for placement. It is helpful to have some catheters and wires in reserve for difficult cases
- Forceps for blunt dissection
- Guidewires: angled hydrophilic, Amplatz super-stiff
- Catheters: Cobra II
- Ultrasound machine: this is essential; a linear 5-MHz or 7-MHz probe with a biopsy guide is ideal
- Heparin solution to 'lock' the catheter.

Table 51.2 Options for venous access

Type	Indications	Cautions
Peripheral cannula	Short-term (days) access for infusion/antibiotics	Not suitable for some infusions as irritant to peripheral veins
PICC line	Medium-term (weeks/months) access for infusion/TPN, etc.	Not suitable for high flow, e.g. haemodialysis
Central line	Short-term (days) access – rapid infusion and pressures	Infection risk with longer-term access
Tunnelled line	Medium-term access (many months) infusion/sampling	May not offer high flow
Dialysis line	Medium-term access (many months)	
Implantable port	Long-term access particularly good if infrequent access required. Low infection rate	May not be suitable for high flow or when very frequent access is required

Choosing the correct line length: The line tip should reach the distal SVC and the cuff should lie within the subcutaneous tunnel approximately 2 cm from the skin exit site. Clearly, this distance will vary with patient size and point of venous access. As a general rule, you will need a longer line if you are accessing from the left jugular or if you have a tall patient.

Most lines are supplied in a variety of lengths, unfortunately, manufacturers may use a variety of methods to describe their device, e.g. total length from hub to tip (not very helpful) or length from cuff to tip (more useful). Curved catheters may also indicate the length from the curve to tip.

A few lines, e.g. Hickman catheters, come in a single size; these are cut to length after tunnelling.

Procedure

There are three stages to the insertion of all tunnelled lines:

- Venous access – this is always the first stage
- Tunnelling
- Line positioning.

Venous access: The right IJV is the first choice route for central venous catheterization. The jugular vein seems less prone to thrombosis than other routes. Access may be dictated by the presence of local disease, radiotherapy or stenosis/occlusion of the target vein (Ch. 28).

 Tip: Always use ultrasound to assess the target vein and guide the venous puncture.

A 1-cm transverse skin incision is necessary to allow side-by-side placement of the line and the tunnelling device. Use forceps to perform subcutaneous blunt dissection to create a space caudal to the incision. This will ease introduction of the catheter and allow it to form a curve before entering the subcutaneous tunnel.

Get the patient to hum to distend the vein, puncture and then advance the guidewire into the right atrium/IVC under fluoroscopic guidance.

 Alarm: Before you do anything else make sure you have established whether the chosen line is placed in the vein before or after it is pulled through the tunnel and perform these in the correct order!

Tunnelling: This dictates whether you tunnel towards or away from the skin incision!

The line exit site is usually on the anterior chest wall; you can check the line length again before committing.

 Tip: Think about the exit site, as a carelessly positioned line will cause discomfort by rubbing on clothing.

If your line is inserted prior to tunnelling: Place the tip in the optimum position and then lay the line on the skin. Mark an exit point roughly 3 cm beyond the cuff. The tunnel is then made from the venous access site to the exit site using the sharp tunneller provided.

If the line is tunnelled prior to insertion into the vein: Lie it on the patient skin and fluoroscope, position the tip over the SVC/RA junction then bend the line to lie over the proposed course of the tunnel. Mark the skin roughly 3 cm beyond the cuff.

The aim is to tunnel in the subcutaneous plane; this is painless for you and the patient. Introduce the tunneller and apply gentle forward pressure while rocking it from side-to-side. Tunnelling over the clavicle from an internal jugular entry can be difficult, particularly in a thin patient; if using a metal tunneller, bending the shaft makes it considerably easier.

 Alarm: If you are tunnelling back from the skin exit site to the point of venous access, go slowly and take care not to make a carotid jugular kebab!

Once the tunnel has been fashioned, the line is attached ready to be pulled through. Many tunnellers have a sleeve which is pulled over the line end to prevent detachment during passage through the subcutaneous tunnel. Remember the cuff should lie within the tunnel 2–3 cm from the skin exit point.

If you tunnelled towards the venous access site, the catheter is pulled through the tunnel until the cuff reaches the skin. Hold the catheter 2–3 cm further back and then pull the catheter until your fingers stop at the skin, the cuff will now lie 2–3 cm into the tunnel.

Alarm: If the cuff is further in than this, line removal will be difficult and can require significant dissection!

If the line does detach, either try again or pass a long sheathed needle through the tract, exchange the needle for a stiff guidewire and:

- **Either** – pass a suitably sized peel-away sheath (e.g. 16F) through the track. Once the sheath is in position this guarantees success and you will wonder what the fuss was all about
- **Or** – dilate the tract with serial dilators or an angioplasty balloon. Save this for cases where you do not have a peel-away sheath of the appropriate size.

Line insertion: The line is always introduced through a peel-away sheath (see Ch. 14).

 Alarm: Prevent air embolism: Once the sheath is in position, tell the patient to hum and take out the dilator and guidewire. Put your thumb over the end of the peel-away sheath and allow the patient to breathe normally. Repeat this process when you introduce the line.

Ask the patient to hum, advance the catheter well into the peel-away sheath. Stop humming.

Line positioning: The tip should be advanced just into the right atrium. The line invariably ends in the SVC when the patient is erect and takes a full inspiration for the chest X-ray. The sheath is then peeled away keeping your index finger on the catheter to hold it in position. Give a gentle pull on the catheter at the skin exit and the curve should pop under the skin leaving the cuff 2 cm in the tunnel.

For lines which are cut to length: The line is placed on the skin to mimic the curve of the guidewire and is then cut to the appropriate length to leave the tip in the right atrium.

Final assembly: Close the venous access site with a Steri-Strip. If your boss insists on a suture, try not to puncture the line as you insert it! Using a suture set with toothed forceps to hold the skin edge up will minimize the risk of a sharp-stick injury to you and the line.

Lines that are tunnelled towards the exit site need to have Luer lock fittings attached after tunnelling. The mechanism of attachment varies from system to system and is clearly described in the instructions. Test that blood can be aspirated and flush the line thoroughly. The line needs to be anchored externally for the first week until there is tissue ingrowth into the cuff. There is usually a proprietary device provided for this, if not, use a suture. Cover both sites with a clear occlusive dressing to minimize the risk of infection.

Dialysis lines

Successful dialysis depends on removing blood from one site (arterial line) and returning it to a separate site (venous line), typically more centrally in the venous circulation. If the lines are too close together or the venous line is proximal to the arterial line, dialysis will not be effective as the blood will simply recirculate. The separation is ensured in two ways:

- **Use of two separate lines,** e.g. Tesio lines. This requires two separate venous punctures and tunnels. The venous line is longer than the arterial line. Two lines are fine when there is good venous access but increases the problem when there is limited access.
- **Use of a dual-lumen line,** e.g. Ash Split catheter. These involve a single puncture and tunnel. The line is typically large, e.g. 14.5F.

All dialysis catheters are intended to have high flow rates. This can only be achieved if the line is not kinked. The dual-lumen lines are more prone to kinking and some come pre-curved with reinforcement intended to prevent this.

Troubleshooting

Arterial puncture: Take the needle/dilator out and get the ultrasound machine while you obtain haemostasis!

Doubt about position: Use fluoroscopy at the first sign of trouble. Put in a 4F dilator and inject contrast to confirm the anatomy.

Unable to advance the sheath: Put in a 4F dilator to secure vascular access.
- Use the hydrophilic wire and Cobra catheter to access the IVC.
- Exchange for an Amplatz wire and use this to introduce the sheath.

Unable to introduce the line through the sheath: This can be tricky, especially working from the left jugular; the sheath is thin-walled and tends to kink at bends.
- Try to pull the sheath back while maintaining forward pressure on the catheter. Do not split the sheath yet.

  If this fails:

1. Replace the dilator and use a hydrophilic guidewire to try to negotiate the kink. Then re-insert the sheath fully and this may straighten the sheath sufficiently to use.

   If this fails:

2. Insert the catheter as far as it will go and peel away the sheath. Remember to apply forward pressure to keep the catheter in position. The catheter can usually be advanced over a wire once it is within the vein.

Unable to aspirate blood from the line: Check the line position on fluoroscopy; check for kinking at the venous puncture site.
- Sit the patient up and try other postural manoeuvres to alter line position.
- If all else fails, inject contrast through the line to delineate the problem.

Kinking: This occurs most commonly deep to the puncture site at the point the line enters the vein. It can be difficult to rectify; try:
- Passing a stiff hydrophilic guidewire through the line to open out the bend (this seldom works in isolation)
- If using a dual lumen catheter, try gently rotating the shaft of the catheter during fluoroscopy
- Blunt dissection around the line to increase the space
- Exchanging for another catheter over a stiff hydrophilic wire
- Swapping for a pre-curved line.

 Tip: Try to prevent kinking. Use a more lateral puncture into the vein and make a two-stage tunnel come out 2–3 cm lateral to the puncture site and then tunnel across to the puncture site.

Awkward venous access

Last-ditch venous access can literally be a lifeline for some patients; this is particularly true of haemodialysis patients. By the time a patient has had multiple tunnelled lines, all of the central veins may be stenosed or occluded. At this stage, the renal team usually resorts to temporary femoral access, but this is uncomfortable and frequently results in infection. It is essential to re-establish long-term central venous access. There are descriptions of using the hepatic veins and the IVC but this is rarely necessary. The vast majority of patients can have access established via collateral veins using the same techniques to cross stenoses and occlusions that are described in the section on angioplasty and stenting. Remember that the aim is to establish venous access not venous patency: if necessary, dilate stenoses or occlusions to allow introduction of the line. Only place a stent if there is symptomatic venous obstruction.

The first stage in the procedure is to perform an ultrasound scan of the neck veins. If an internal jugular vein is patent, this is the optimal approach. There are always plenty of tortuous veins which cross the midline of the neck; these are seldom useful. Look for the patent anterior and external jugular veins or veins that lie more laterally in the neck.

Puncture the chosen vein under ultrasound guidance and insert a 4F dilator to perform venography. If there is a direct route to the central veins, then go for it. Dilate underlying stenoses as necessary in order to introduce the catheters. More often there is no direct route, but with knowledge of the likely course of the vein it is often possible to find a way through. Perseverance is the key – if the vein you have punctured is not 'the one', the venogram will often suggest an alternative (Fig. 51.5).

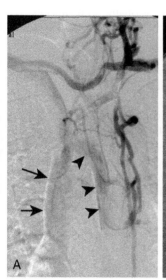
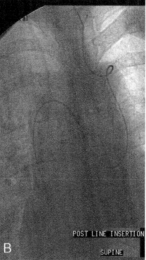

Fig. 51.5 ■ Awkward access. (A) Injection into a vein in the left side of the neck shows collaterals communicating with the azygous vein (arrowheads) and into the SVC (arrows). (B) The Groshong line follows this tortuous path.

Nigh-on impossible access – keys to success

- Good ultrasound
- Plenty of time and determination
- Use low-profile wires and balloons to cross tight strictures and occlusions
- Once you have access into a central vein, do not lose it! Get a supportive wire (e.g. an Amplatz wire) in place, preferably through to the IVC
- If dual catheters are required, e.g. for haemodialysis, resist the temptation to use the same puncture site for two wires. This only results in a venous tear and excessive bleeding. Instead, use ultrasound or fluoroscopy to perform a second puncture into the same vein about 1 cm from the first puncture. Better still, use a dual-lumen line!
- Use a long peel-away sheath – the sheath supplied with the catheter will not be long enough to support the catheter all the way through to the SVC/right atrium

- Leave a stiff hydrophilic wire through the sheath to minimize kinking when the dilator is removed
- Use a snare to grasp the catheter and pull it through very tortuous veins if the peel-away sheath kinks.

Maintenance of tunnelled central lines

All long-term central venous access is prone to four problems: infection, venous thrombosis, fibrin sheath and mechanical failure.

Infection limited to the exit site can be successfully treated with antibiotic treatment; however, for tunnel infections and infected lines, removal is usually required. Do not be tempted to place a new line until the patient has been clear of infection for several days or you will be removing that line as well. If access is needed in the interim, then use in-and-out catheters.

Line-related venous thrombosis is usually associated with symptomatic limb oedema, in which case the line is removed and the patient treated as for a DVT. If the thrombosis is asymptomatic, then anticoagulation alone is adequate.

Mechanical failure usually results in line fractures; extravasation then causes pain during injection and sometimes leak of fluid from the skin entry site. Occasionally, a line fractures or a totally implanted device such as a vascular port separates from its hub, leading to migration of the line and necessitating retrieval (Ch. 36).

Fibrin sheath formation is a common occurrence. Fibrin deposits envelop the line to form a condom-like cover. This obstructs the line tips, prevents aspiration of blood and may lead to extravasation. In dialysis lines, it results in markedly reduced flow, which compromises dialysis.

When there is a problem with a line, the first step is to fluoroscope to check the entire line from the skin to its tip. If this does not establish the diagnosis, the next step is a linogram. This is simply an injection of contrast down the line under fluoroscopic control. Look for:

- Line kinking, fracture or migration usually into the pulmonary artery
- Extravasation. This most commonly occurs at points of flexion or compression
- Free flow of contrast from the line lumen via the end- and side-holes. Sometimes it is necessary to perform a run to establish what is happening. Due to cardiac motion, unsubtracted images may be clearer
- Reflux of contrast back around the line, often with a thin radiolucent 'membrane'; this indicates a fibrin sheath.

If there is a fibrin sheath, the first-line treatment is to flush the line vigorously. This may disrupt the sheath sufficiently to restore flow. The next step will usually be to try a low dose of thrombolysis; this is best given by infusion rather than as a bolus. The ward team can do this without your help. If this fails, then mechanically stripping the fibrin sheath with a GooseNeck snare or over-the-wire line exchange with fibrin sheath disruption is usually the answer. Warn the patient that even if this is successful the fibrin sheath is likely to recur and require further treatment.

How to strip

The lines often abut the wall of the SVC, which makes them difficult to snare. In this case, simply pass a guidewire through the line and into the IVC if it will go. If you are dealing with a Groshong line, only a hydrophilic wire will pass through it. It may take a little pushing to get it through the valve but do not be deterred – it will go. Pass a Gooseneck snare from the femoral vein to catch the wire and then advance it over the line. If there are two lines,

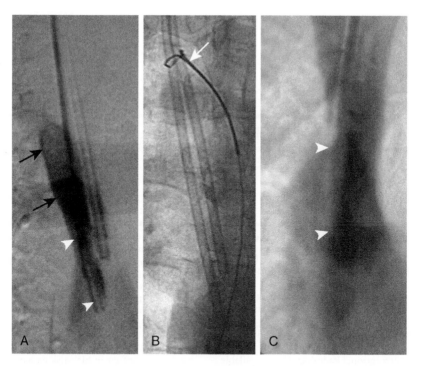

Fig. 51.6 ■ Stripping a poorly functioning Tesio line. (A) Injection through the venous line. The line tip is occluded (white arrowheads) and contrast outlines a fibrin sheath (arrows). (B) A GooseNeck snare (white arrow) has been placed around both lines. (C) Following stripping, the line fills to the tip (arrowheads) and contrast flows normally into the SVC. Normal function was restored.

e.g. dialysis catheters, both can be snared at once. Take the snare as far up the line as it will go. Tighten it so that it grips the line fairly firmly (Fig. 51.6).

Pull the snare back; if it is gripped tightly enough it will tug the line down when you pull. It is best to warn the patient that they will feel as though someone is pulling on the line, because they are. You are aiming to get enough grip to remove the sheath but leave the line in situ. Repeat this once or twice, then repeat the linogram. If flow is restored and the lines aspirate freely, then stop. If not, try again.

Sometimes when there are two lines that are stuck together, success is indicated by the line tips separating.

 Tip: Leave the wire through the catheter while stripping, as this allows the snare to be passed straight back up again. When performing the linogram, you need to remove the wire, so park the snare high up the line so that you do not have to catch it again.

Alternatively, perform an over-the-wire exchange of the line with fibrin sheath disruption. Insert a guidewire into the line and dissect out the tract to release the cuff. Remove the line and insert an angiographic sheath to the vein origin (it usually won't go round the steep turn). Insert an 8-mm angioplasty balloon over the wire and inflate it in the SVC – this disrupts the fibrin sheath. Remove and insert a new catheter over the wire.

Suggestions for further reading

Chapter 1

Patient information sheets

British Society of Interventional Radiology (BSIR). Available from: <www.bsir.org/patients/patient-information-leaflets>.

Cardiovascular and Interventional Radiology Society of Europe (CIRSE). Available from: <www.cirse.org>.

General information for patients; information on specific procedures.

Society of Interventional Radiology (SIR). Available from: <www.sirweb.org/>; <www.sirweb.org/medical-professionals>.

Screening tests

Payne, C. S. (1998). A primer on patient management problems in interventional radiology. *AJR. American Journal of Roentgenology, 170,* 1169–1176.

A useful overview of screening for and managing high-risk patients.

ASGE Standards of Practice Committee, et al. (2008). Position statement on routine laboratory testing before endoscopic procedures. *Gastrointestinal Endoscopy, 68*(5), 827–832.

Although this issue is about endoscopy, it is also pragmatic about levels of evidence and when a test might be useful.

High-risk patients

American Society of Anesthesiologists. (2014). ASA physical status classification system. Available from: <www.asahq.org/resources/clinical-information/asa-physical-status-classification-system>.

Explains how to assign ASA scores.

Contrast

Royal College of Radiologists. (2015). Standards for intravascular contrast administration to adult patients, 3rd edn. Available from: <www.rcr.ac.uk/publication/standards-intravascular-contrast-administration-adult-patients-third-edition>.

Explains how to manage patients at high risk from intravascular contrast agents.

The Renal Association, British Cardiovascular Intervention Society and Royal College of Radiologists. (2013). Prevention of contrast induced acute kidney injury (CI-AKI) in adult patients. Available from: <www.rcr.ac.uk/sites/default/files/publication/2013_RA_BCIS_RCR.pdf>.

Aspelin, P., Aubry, P., Fransson, S.-G., et al. (2003). Nephrotoxic effects in high-risk patients undergoing angiography. *The New England Journal of Medicine, 348,* 491–499.

Evidence supporting the use of iodixanol in high-risk patients.

Mueller, C., Buerkel, G., Buettner, H., et al. (2002). Prevention of contrast media-associated nephropathy: randomized comparison of 2 hydration regimens in 1620 patients undergoing coronary angioplasty. *Archives of Internal Medicine, 162*(3), 329–336.

Level 1 evidence on why to use normal saline.

Rihal, C., Textor, S., Grill, D., et al. (2002). Level 1 evidence the advantage of iodixanol (Visipaque) over non-ionic contrast media. Incidence and prognostic importance of acute renal failure after percutaneous coronary intervention. *Circulation, 105,* 2259–2264.

The true incidence of ARF and its significance in a real population; sobering reading!

Waksman, R., King, S. B., Douglas, J. S., et al. (1995). Predictors of groin complications after balloon and new device coronary intervention. *The American Journal of Cardiology, 75,* 886–889.

Big holes, big patients and deranged clotting. Platelets less than 200 and dual antiplatelet = false aneurysm.

Medical practice and consent

General Medical Council. (2013). Good medical practice. London: GMC Publications. Available from <www.gmc-uk.org/guidance/good_medical _practice.asp>.

Up-to-date and informative booklet outlining reasonable practice in the UK. Mandatory reading. There are also interactive case studies on the GMC website. Available from: www. gmc-uk.org/guidance/case_studies.asp.

General Medical Council. (2007). 0–18 years: guidance for all doctors. London: GMC Publications. Available from <www.gmc-uk.org/ guidance/ethical_guidance/children_guidance _index.asp>, download from: <www.gmc-uk.org/ static/documents/content/0-18_years_-_English _1015.pdf>.

Informative booklet outlining how to deal with children and those under 18 years of age (and their carers) in the UK. Mandatory reading.

General Medical Council. (2008). Consent: patients and doctors making decisions together. London: GMC Publications. Available from <www.gmc-uk.org/Consent___English_1015.pdf _48903482.pdf>.

Informative booklet describing all issues regarding consent in the UK. Mandatory reading but does not cover changes from 2015.

Department of Health. (2009). Reference guide to consent for examination or treatment, 2nd ed. Available from: <www.gov.uk/government/ uploads/system/uploads/attachment_data/ file/138296/dh_103653__1_.pdf>

Clear information regarding consent and capacity.

Sokol, D. K. (2015). Update on the UK law on consent. *BMJ (Clinical Research Ed.)*, 350, h1481.

BMA. (2005). Mental Capacity Act. Guidance for health professionals. Succinct explanations of the principles of patients' rights and ability to make informed decisions. Available from: <www.bma.org.uk/health_promotion_ethics/ consent_and_capacity/mencapact05.jsp>; download from: <www.bma.org.uk/images/ mentalcapacityact_tcm41-146891.pdf>.

Chapter 2

Royal College of Radiologists. (2013). Guidance for Fellows in implementing surgical safety checklists for radiological procedures. BFCR (13)1. Available from: <www.rcr.ac.uk/sites/ default/files/publication/BFCR%2813%291 _safety_checklist.pdf>.

Angle, J. F., Nemcek, A. A., Cohen, A. M., et al. (2008). Quality improvement guidelines for preventing wrong site, wrong procedure, and wrong person errors: application of the Joint Commission 'Universal Protocol for Preventing Wrong Site, Wrong Procedure, Wrong Person Surgery' to the practice of interventional radiology. *Journal of Vascular and Interventional Radiology*, 19, 1145–1151.

Joint Commission on Accreditation of Healthcare Organizations. (2005). Healthcare at the crossroads: strategies for improving the medical liability system and preventing patient injury. Available from: <www.jointcommission.org/ assets/1/18/Medical_Liability.pdf>.

Strategies to minimize preventable patient injuries – daft not to think about this really.

WHO. (2009). Surgical Safety Checklist. Available from: <www.npsa.nhs.uk/nrls/alerts-and -directives/alerts/safer-surgery-alert>.

Gawande, A. (2011). The Checklist Manifesto: how to get things right. Picador.

Yes, this is a whole book – but it is an easy and compelling read setting out the origins of checklists and the clear evidence for their benefits. A must for doubters.

Chapter 3

RCR. (2015). Standards for intravascular contrast agent administration to adult patients, 3rd edn. BRCR (15)1. Available from: <www.rcr.ac.uk/ publication/standards-intravascular-contrast -administration-adult-patients-third-edition>.

Gupta, R. K., & Bang, T. J. (2010). Prevention of contrast-induced nephropathy (CIN) in interventional radiology practice. *Seminars in Interventional Radiology*, 27(4), 348–359.

Ansell, G., et al. (1996). Complications of intravascular iodinated contrast media. In G. Ansell, M. A. Bettmann, & J. A. Kaufman (Eds.), Complications in diagnostic imaging and interventional radiology (3rd ed., pp. 245–300). Oxford: Blackwell Science.

An old but excellent summary with everything that you might ever wish to know about iodinated contrast and more besides.

Alternatives to iodinated contrast media

Caridi, J. G., & Hawkins, I. F. (1997). CO_2 digital subtraction angiography: Potential complications and their prevention. *Journal of Vascular and Interventional Radiology*, 8, 383–891.

How to work with CO_2. A useful starter.

Bettmann, M. (2004). Frequently asked questions: iodinated contrast agents. *Radiographics: A Review Publication of the Radiological Society of North America, Inc*, 24, S3–S10.

Kessel, D. O., Peters, K., Robertson, I., et al. (2002). Carbon dioxide guided vascular interventions: technique and pitfalls. *Cardiovascular and Interventional Radiology*, 25, 476–483.

Massicotte, A. (2008). Contrast medium-induced nephropathy: strategies for prevention. *Pharmacotherapy*, 28, 1140–1150.

Rao, Q. A., & Newhouse, J. H. (2006). Risk of nephropathy after intravenous administration of contrast material: a critical literature analysis. *Radiology*, 239, 392–397.

Chapter 4

American Society of Anesthesiologists Task Force on Sedation and Analgesia by Non-Anesthesiologists. (2002). Practice guidelines for sedation and analgesia by non-anesthesiologists. *Anesthesiology*, 96, 1004–1017.

Royal College of Radiologists and the Royal College of Anaesthetists. (1992). Sedation and anaesthesia in radiology: report of a joint working party. Available from: <www.rcr.ac.uk/publications.aspx?PageID=310&PublicationID=186>.

A good overview compiled jointly by anaesthetists and radiologists.

RCR. (2003). Safe sedation, analgesia and anaesthesia within the radiology department. BFCR(03)4. Available from: <www.rcr.ac.uk/sites/default/files/publication/Safe_Sedation.pdf>.

Shabanie, A. (2006). Conscious sedation for interventional procedures: a practical guide. *Techniques in Vascular and Interventional Radiology*, 9, 84–88.

Chapter 5

Keyoung, J. A., Levy, E. B., Roth, E. R., et al. (2001). Intraarterial lidocaine for pain control after uterine artery embolization for leiomyomata. *Journal of Vascular and Interventional Radiology*, 12, 1065–1073.

Lang, E. V., Berbaum, K. S., Pauker, S. G., et al. (2008). Beneficial effects of hypnosis and adverse effects of empathic attention during percutaneous tumor treatment: when being nice does not suffice. *Journal of Vascular and Interventional Radiology*, 19, 897–905.

Lee, S. H., Hahn, S. T., & Park, S. H. (2001). Intraarterial lidocaine administration for relief of pain resulting from transarterial chemoembolization of hepatocellular carcinoma: Its effectiveness and optimal timing of administration. *Cardiovascular and Interventional Radiology*, 24, 368–371.

Chapter 26

Matalon, T. A. S., & Silver, B. (1990). US guidance of interventional procedures. *Radiology*, 174, 43–47.

Essential ultrasound techniques; well-illustrated.

Yeuh, N., Halvorsen, R. A., Letourneau, J. G., et al. (1989). Gantry tilt technique for CT guided biopsy and drainage. *Journal of Computer Assisted Tomography*, 13, 182–184.

An invaluable technique for many lesions.

Index

Page numbers followed by 'f' indicate figures, 't' indicate tables, and 'b' indicate boxes.

A

W

X

Printed and bound by CPI Group (UK) Ltd, Croydon, CR0 4YY

03/10/2024

01040451-0006